Letting Go
Of Depression

Dr. Scott Graves, AP, MA

ISBN: 9798543186909

ACKNOWLEDGEMENTS

Mom and dad, without you I wouldn't be the man I am today and would not have had the privilege of being able to help others on the path of healing and freedom. You are the embodiment of love and selflessness as human beings and for that, I am eternally grateful.

My heartfelt gratitude goes out to Richard Gretsky for being kind, inquisitive, thoughtful, detailed and critical in the editing of this book. Thank you for your hard work and for the friendship shared along the way.

To all my patients, friends and family, I have learned so much about how to be a great physician and person because of your giving, love and patience. You inspire me and have taught me well how to help guide others to heal physically, emotionally and spiritually. I thank you with all my heart.

TABLE OF CONTENTS

PART 5: **Living in Surrender**

INTRODUCTION

In 2001, I went through an experience that sent me spiraling into a dark depression for 11 long, painful years. I felt so powerless to do anything about it. As time went on, ending my life seemed like the only realistic option to stop the emotional pain. After this experience, I searched and searched for answers to feel better. I didn't know where to look. I felt powerless against my feelings. I didn't know answers existed.

Feeling depressed is much like waking up in the morning and going into a nightmare, instead of coming out from one. You start to realize how badly you feel when the only thing you look forward to throughout the day is when you can shut off and go back to sleep. The alarm clock goes off and you feel the massive, heavy and terrifying sense of dread about facing the day. The nightmare is filled with so many awful experiences. It is like running in a dream to try to escape something only to look down and realize that you aren't moving at all. The effort becomes useless. Frustration builds. Despair sets in. You feel the stinging fear of constant failure because you have no idea what to do to feel better and to make the problem go away.

I desperately wanted things to be different. I tried to find relief, but slowly, day after day, every effort to find relief was met with an even greater sense of darkness, isolation and pain. I felt like no one understood me or what I was going through. Eventually, I began to somehow live with the pain. I pushed it down as far as I could because I knew that sharing it with others was only a heavy burden that no one seemed to know what to do anything about. I no longer wanted others to have to bear this burden for me. So I pretended. I pretended that life was ok. Other people asked how I was and I mustered up a pretend smile and said, "I'm good." But the pretending actually becomes tiring and I found myself utterly exhausted at the end of every day. What I carried around was so heavy and painful, that the weight of carrying it sucked all the life out of me.

Those around me who knew of my affliction didn't know how to help, even though they really wanted to. Eventually, I pushed people away in my life because I was hard to be around. People don't enjoy being around a lifeless, gloomy, and hopeless person - one who is trying so hard to just make it from one day to the next. Even my own father, who is an amazing human being, and who has his doctorate in counseling, said one day to me in helpless frustration, "I want to help you so badly, I just don't know how." When the most capable person you know doesn't have the answer, the hopelessness further solidifies. Where are you going to find answers at this point?

At first, I tried conventional treatments including talk therapy and medications for hypothyroidism and depression/anxiety. While drugs can be necessary and do work for some people, ultimately they do not address the root causes of depression. Many people also see benefits from talk therapy, but the thousands of dollars that was spent on talk therapy personally didn't help me much. The drugs didn't make me feel much better either.

I was still a wreck and things only got progressively worse. I read scores of books and talked to anyone who would listen to me. But over time, nothing changed my emotions. Nothing altered how I felt. Eventually, numbness set in. Numbness is a feeling that covers over all of the other feelings you have. You just don't want to feel anything anymore, and a part of you just continues to die. Yet, despite all this pain, light broke through and hope began to trickle back in. Does any of this story resonate with you or the experience of your loved ones?

Here's the good news. The root causes of depression are known and treatments are available through natural means. Our medical model desperately needs to change. Depression is not a chemical imbalance that a pharmaceutical drug will solve if taken for the rest of life. Western medicine hasn't done well to address the true, root physical or emotional causes of depression. It does not offer much treatment outside of keeping one dependent upon a pharmaceutical drug for the rest of life. As a result, people all over are starting to try things that fall outside of this paradigm of medicine.

And it's working!

This book is about the answers that I found to deal powerfully with the depression I felt. My mission in sharing this with the world is so that you or those you love can heal powerfully too. My recovery began when I went through Chinese medical school and started learning about the incredible wonders of Chinese medicine. Practitioners of Chinese medicine have been perfecting this healing system for thousands of years. Chinese medicine is one of the most sophisticated, brilliant, deep, and incredible systems of medicine this world has ever known. It is a completely natural system of medicine and was the only system of medicine that existed in China for thousands of years, successfully treating any and every health problem during this time in history. It addresses every level of health in the body-physical, energetic, and emotional. People have been depressed across all cultures and times for thousands of years. The answers contained in this medicine were just as valid then as they are now. Additionally, in my quest to feel better and obtain answers, I learned about other powerful tools which I will share with you that are helping thousands of people to heal today.

If you struggle with depression, you are not alone and things can be done immediately to help you feel better in a short period of time. Dealing with the root physical causes of depression may make a significant difference for you and be all you need to heal. Medical science exists that points us not only in the direction of the true root causes, but what can be done to powerfully heal. But depression for many is not just a physical problem. We are not just a physical body. We are so much more than that. Chinese medicine has proven treatments for the other non-physical parts of us too.

For many, depression starts after going through a traumatic event. A traumatic event triggers a deep fear inside. The emotional scars left over from one or multiple events then begin to replay over and over again. This trauma is what perpetuated how depressed I felt every day. It is my firm belief that negative emotions are far more powerful causes of disease and health problems than anything in the physical world. Things such as diet, supplements, massage, chiropractic, acupuncture, exercise, and many other things are useful and necessary pathways that can help you to heal. These things have helped many people to heal from depression and I would encourage you to pursue these options, if you feel led to. My philosophy is that you should try anything to support healing that makes logical sense, is safe, and doesn't cost you a fortune.

While others have written brilliantly about how to heal from the physical aspects of depression, this book is largely about how negative emotions, held within from past experiences, can manifest in our physical body, creating an ongoing experience of depression and anxiety. It is also about how learning to release those feelings can alter our reality instantly and make one feel better right now. My experience, both as a physician and a patient, reflects this and, after having tried everything, I had to walk the tough road of entering straight into the deepest and darkest emotional parts of me. When I set the emotions free from those deep and dark places, I healed very quickly. This is a very different experience than simply talking about feelings.

Diving into our darkness is not the path that most people willingly choose. Many want the easiest path to healing. Taking a pill will never release our negative emotions from the past experiences we have had. Walking this path has been the most difficult thing I have ever done. I wish that it was as easy as taking a pill and instantly healing. While opening to these parts of oneself may be extremely painful, I am quick to remind people that on the other side of the surrender of our emotions is always love, joy, and inner peace. Inner peace and freedom can be yours with the courage to truly see yourself as you are and surrender what may be fueling the depression you experience.

Depression is not your identity; It is not who you are. Anger is not your identity. Hopelessness is not your identity. Fear is not who you are. Apathy and giving up are not who you are. Your physical body is not your identity either. You may not *feel* this right now, but the reality is that you are strong, resilient, brave, and courageous. You have a universe of love, joy, and peace inside of you waiting to be accessed and discovered. Love—not anger, fear, or hopelessness—defines who and what you are. I hope my journey of healing inspires you to heal and that you are able to experience the freedom that is already yours and is waiting to be uncovered from within. You can heal from depression and here is how.

PART 1:
THE PHYSICAL WORLD OF DEPRESSION

1 WHAT IS DEPRESSION?

"Here is the tragedy: when you are the victim of depression,
not only do you feel utterly helpless and abandoned by the
world, you also know that very few people can understand, or
even begin to believe that life can be this painful. There is
nothing I can think of that is quite as isolating as this." -
Giles Andreae

People desperately want relief from depression. People want to feel better now. Depression affects us all, directly or indirectly. According to the Journal of the American Medical Association, "Overall, 16.7 percent of 242 million U.S. adults reported filling one or more prescriptions for psychiatric drugs in 2013."[1] Of this 16.7%, 12% reported taking antidepressants. Therefore, almost 25 million people currently take antidepressants! More than eight out of ten of those take them long-term—84.3% having refilled at least three prescriptions in 2013 alone. These numbers don't seem to be decreasing. Additionally, 7 percent of all visits to a primary care doctor end with a prescription to an antidepressant drug.[2]

Depression is estimated to cost the U.S.A. about $210 billion a year in productivity loss and health care needs. Global revenue for antidepressants is anticipated to grow to nearly $17 billion by 2020. Depression has become a very serious problem, affecting many people. And these are only the documented cases of those taking an antidepressant. Many millions more have never been diagnosed, but may also be suffering from the effects of depression. Chances are, perhaps without being aware, you know someone who is depressed.

In the hopes that a pill can help to deal with the suffering one carries around on the inside, most desperately look to modern medicine for some coveted relief. What doctors and pharmaceutical companies have led us to believe is that depression is a "chemical imbalance." We have been told this imbalance requires a drug to manage and manipulate these special chemicals in your brain so that you feel better. The only problem here is that this model isn't working and a pill is not fixing how depressed people continue to feel.

If depression wasn't enough, many other symptoms coexist with depression, which are commonly found in many of the people that come in for help with depression. When people, who are depressed, come into my clinic they normally have some combination of these other symptoms as well: fatigue, insomnia, anxiety, difficulty making decisions, dry mouth/skin, getting easily angered, poor memory, headaches, dizziness, weight gain, constipation, loose stools, acid reflux, and heartburn. I see variations of these symptoms in almost nine out of every ten people in the clinic. In many cases, we are not dealing with someone just feeling depressed as their only symptom, but with a whole combination of many of the above symptoms.

Upon seeing these symptoms in the clinic, the most common drugs that are prescribed for people with such symptoms are antidepressant and thyroid medications. Yet, often it is seen that in spite of taking these drugs they still don't feel well. This is why they find themselves going outside of Western medicine for answers. Over time, people are realizing that taking these drugs hasn't delivered in truly making them feel better. In fact, over longer periods of time, many people report that the symptoms get worse, and it takes higher doses of the same drugs to help people maintain.

People are starting to wake up to the fact that many doctors mainly use just one tool for what ails people – drugs. If those drugs don't work, some try other drugs. But ultimately patients seen in the clinic frequently comment on the severe limitations, short sightedness and dangers inherent in taking these drugs. People begin thinking out of the box saying to themselves: "There must be a better way than taking drugs to heal my body." Furthermore, secondary side effects accompany the taking of these drugs and oftentimes create even bigger problems. Symptoms are traded for other symptoms. Then, more drugs are prescribed to deal with those side effects. It is a vicious cycle and a better way exists. Has this been your experience so far? If so, you are not alone.

Many people bring "a drug to heal everything" mentality to their medical doctor in search of relief. They hope and believe that a pill is going to help relieve them of the many complicated and difficult-to-deal-with symptoms being experienced in the body and mind. As many people are learning, taking a pill for depression isn't working well. People show up in my clinic every week waking up to the fact that something else must be possible to help them feel better. Taking a drug for symptoms, most of the time, does not address the root cause of the problem and only serves to hide it. With more and more people waking up to the fact that these drugs aren't correcting the root problem of their depression, many questions begin to arise such as:

- How can I actually feel better without taking a drug for the rest of my life?
- Are there better, natural health solutions to depression and anxiety?
- Does science support a natural healing way even though medical doctors may not be aware of it?
- Are the current medical solutions (drugs) for my good or are they meant to keep me as a paying customer for the rest of my life?
- What if the root problem to depression isn't entirely physical?

- What did/does the ancient Chinese system of medicine say about the root cause of this problem and is it still valid today?
- Will Chinese medicine and acupuncture help me feel better?
- How can I release these horrible feelings/emotions that I carry around every day?

These are the questions I started to entertain that led me on a long and very arduous road to healing from depression both physically and emotionally. While depression medication has been life-saving for many and in many cases it may be necessary for a short season; ultimately it is not the answer. Depression, like all other health problems, must be looked at and treated holistically. We need to see the whole picture, including any and all factors that may contribute to how you are feeling. This book addresses all of these questions. You can heal without taking a drug for years or for the rest of your life. Natural solutions exist that have been proven to work. Depression is a multi-faceted issue that is experienced differently in different people. Chinese medicine has successfully treated this issue well for thousands of years and can continue if we turn back to the wisdom it holds for human health.

Beyond the physical body, emotional trauma must be adequately addressed as well. The first part of this book covers the physical aspects of depression. The latter half of the book covers the emotional side of depression. Both are equally valid, though one might gravitate towards one aspect over another. Regardless of the root cause of depression, at the heart of it is the overall desire to want to feel better. Our unhealthy symptoms don't feel good. Behind wanting to change, stop hurting, and to heal is a desire to simply feel better.

We all want to be able to feel alive, have purpose, and be relatively free from physical symptoms, negative emotions and the suffering that can dominate our lives. What better way to start improving health than to take a very introspective look at what might be sitting behind your health symptoms? We need to ask what physical and environmental factors, traumas and emotions have contributed to or caused us not to feel good. How good would we feel if we cleaned up the toxicity in our lives both environmentally and emotionally? How good would we feel if we learned to let our negative emotions go? The path to healing from depression is different for everyone, but my hope is that this book covers many of the factors which may be contributing to the depression you have or those you love have.

It cannot be understated how powerful the mind is and how letting go of negative emotions can be very physically healing. While I feel the mind is the most misunderstood and neglected part of healing in the world today, physical things also do play a very big role in helping us to heal. Before we discuss the powerful role emotions have in our healing, we will first talk about depression and how it is understood from a Western perspective and the issues that we are facing from within this paradigm. Let's take a look at how depression is defined, what Western medicine recognizes as the causes, and the common interventions used today. After that we will discuss how effective this model has been and what the true causes of depression are in the world today.

Defining Depression

People often come into the clinic and describe feeling depressed. What does this mean though? When you ask people specifically how they define feeling depressed the answers are wide and varied, but do contain similar themes. Here are some of the ways that it has been described by people:

- "Depression is like a black hole that is dark, cold, lonely, and seemingly inescapable."
- "It is isolating, like being on a deserted, cold island all alone. It pushes everyone that is in your life away because they don't seem to understand."
- "It is not wanting to wake up every morning because the only thing you feel is the crushing weight of hopelessness that awaits you each day."
- "Depression is a cloud of not being able to see anything ever changing or being able to see any other possibilities other than the limiting ones you experience every day."
- "Depression feels like a needle that is directly injected into your soul, sucking all the life out of you, like mustering all the energy you have just to do simple things throughout the day."
- "It has pushed away many of my loved ones and friends because of how intense the suffering is inside."
- "I just want to sleep all day long and never wake up. Sleeping seems to be the only thing I 'enjoy' because I get to shut off every day."
- "I just want the pain to go away; I don't want to live anymore."

Persistent depressive disorder is defined as having five of any of the following symptoms on a nearly daily basis for at least two years:

- Persistent sad, anxious, or "empty" mood
- Feelings of hopelessness or pessimism
- Feelings of guilt, worthlessness, or helplessness
- Loss of interest or pleasure in hobbies or activities
- Decreased energy, fatigue, or being "slowed down"
- Difficulty concentrating, remembering, or making decisions
- Difficulty sleeping, early-morning awakening, or oversleeping
- Appetite and/or weight changes
- Thoughts of death or suicide or suicide attempts

- Restlessness or irritability
- Aches or pains, headaches, cramps, or digestive problems without a clear physical cause and/or that do not ease even with treatment"[3]

What Does Western Medicine Recognize As The Cause Of Depression?

According to WebMD, "Depression is an extremely complex disease. No one knows exactly what causes it, but it can occur for a variety of reasons." Listed as contributing factors are abuse, certain medications, conflict, death or loss, genetics, major events, serious illness, and substance abuse. Most of these factors can be attributed to having emotional bases (abuse, death or loss, major events, conflict).[4] The Mayo Clinic also mentions: "It's not known exactly what causes depression," but lists more physical reasons such as biological differences, brain chemistry, hormones, and inherited traits.[5] According to the National Institute of Mental Health, "Research suggests that a combination of genetic, biological, environmental, and psychological factors play a role in depression."[6]

This last definition is probably the best broad definition found so far, encompassing all of the contributing factors that play a role in this health condition. Depression is a mixture of both biological (physical), environmental and emotional factors. While these are very broad sweeping categories, more precise factors in each of these categories are involved in the formation of depression. These sites fail to mention the precise primary factors that are responsible for depression, which we will be discussing very shortly.

What Are Current Western Medical Interventions For Depression?

Drugs are by far the most used substances to treat depression in the USA today. Below are some of the most common drugs that have been used to treat depression since the 1950's.

- Selective serotonin reuptake inhibitors (SSRIs) were launched in the mid to late 1980s, including well-known drugs such as Paxil, Zoloft, Celexa, and Lexapro. They essentially flood the brain with serotonin in an effort to make you feel better. I took these for a few months but never saw any noticeable effects and they made me feel "funny" or "off," which many have also reported.
- Serotonin and norepinephrine reuptake inhibitors (SNRIs) are a newer type of antidepressant. In addition to flooding the brain with serotonin, these drugs also flood the brain with norepinephrine. This neurotransmitter is involved in the fight or flight response and mobilizes the body for arousal,

alertness and vigilance.

- Tricyclic antidepressants (TCAs) were some of the first medications used to treat depression and work in a very similar fashion to SNRI's.
- Monoamine oxidase inhibitors (MAOIs) were also among some of the earliest drugs used for depression. These drugs have high interactions with other drugs and can cause serious side effects.
- Other mood stabilizing drugs exist such as antipsychotics, lithium, stimulants (Ritalin and others) and anti-anxiety (Buspar) that also have been used to treat depression depending upon varying factors for certain people.

Psychotherapy Or Talk Therapy For The Treatment of Depression

Psychotherapy, next to drugs, is another intervention that is highly suggested for those suffering from anxiety and depression. Many people feel so isolated and alone that simply talking with another person on a deep level in a safe and trusting environment can be very helpful. In general, I love psychotherapy and think it is something everyone should go through.

Some people have such deep states of depression that directly addressing the emotions that are causing their problems can feel threatening, especially if they have a mountain of trauma that needs attention. Therefore, a strong therapeutic relationship may need to be built very slowly over time to foster trust and confidence with the practitioner before helping someone to completely let go of their emotions. Another approach is to focus on physical healing first as a foundation. Then, in the future, once people physically feel better they may feel ready to tackle emotional issues.

Ultimately though, learning how to surrender and let go of negative emotions, in my estimation, is the most direct path that can help people to heal the fastest. In the book, _Letting Go: The Pathway of Surrender_, psychiatrist Dr. David Hawkins, MD, who ran one of the largest psychiatric practices in the world for more than 30 years noted this about the surrender of negative emotions, 'Therefore, as a person constantly surrenders, physical and psychosomatic disorders improve and frequently disappear altogether. There is a general reversal of pathologic processes in the body and a return to optimal function.'[7]

So many people on this planet feel isolated and keep many of their feelings bottled up inside. Psychotherapy is wonderful to help people express and talk about the things they have buried for years. Simply voicing feelings can be very therapeutic and is a much needed form of initial release. In addition to this, I have observed profound changes in people when they surrendered the emotions that have imprisoned them for so long.

So many incredible psychotherapists are actually moving in the direction of total surrender and emotional release. Movements in this direction have often been spurred on by focusing on greater understandings in mindfulness and non-duality.

Mindfulness is "the practice of maintaining a nonjudgmental state of heightened or complete awareness of one's thoughts, emotions, or experiences on a moment-to-moment basis."[8] Mindfulness helps to bring the unconscious conscious.

Mindfulness is an amazing way to bring awareness to one's deep and rich inner life. Having an awareness of one's emotions is the first step towards freedom. The second step is total freedom through the complete surrender of those emotions. The surrender of emotions was my pathway to healing. Everything changed once I learned how to release emotions. That whole process is outlined here and is why this book was written. If you have found psychotherapy useful for you, I highly urge you to continue it.

How Effective Are Pharmaceutical Drugs For Treating Depression?

Depression is not a chemical imbalance in the brain. It can be dangerous when we start tinkering around with select chemicals in the body and brain, especially when not one study exists to support the idea that depression is a chemical imbalance that will be fixed with medication.[9] The drugs for depression are not only failing to produce lasting relief, they are making people even sicker, while deepening their sense of hopelessness. One of the known side effects of antidepressant drugs such as Prozac (fluoxetine) is an increased risk of suicide. Other side effects of anti-depression drugs are loss of appetite, dry mouth, rash and abnormal dreams.[10] Another phenomenon of side effects is called "serotonin syndrome" including symptoms such as high body temperature, agitation, increased reflexes, tremor, sweating, dilated pupils, diarrhea, seizures and muscle breakdown.[11]

In 2007 the FDA required all antidepressants to carry a black box warning stating an increase risk of suicide for those younger than age 25.[12] It is not uncommon for people who are severely depressed to express a desire to commit suicide, yet we give them a drug that may potentiate this symptom? Is this responsible medicine? Is it worth it to try to fix depression only to expose oneself to the many side effects that people experience by taking this medication? Is this the best we have today in our technologically advanced world?

Evidence-based, drug-free treatment for depression exists and works very well, yet is not on the forefront of medicine due to pharmacological influence. One of the most astounding things that psychiatrist Dr. Kelly Brogan states is, "Antidepressants have repeatedly been shown in long-term scientific studies to worsen the course of mental illness." She goes on noting, "The dirtiest little secret of all is the fact that antidepressants are among the most difficult drugs to taper from, more so than alcohol and opiates."[13] We are hearing so much in the news about the opiate crisis, but what about the profound changes that occur detrimentally in the brain as a result of taking antidepressant medications for years. The damage and dependence on these drugs in our world is extensive. But, with the right healing protocol the damage can be reversed.

Pharmaceutical Brainwashing

We have been brainwashed by the pharmaceutical companies that a cure/fix to all health conditions will be found in a pill. A pill/drug will never be able to heal most chronic health conditions. Yet, as a society, we continue to buy into the brainwashing that a "magic bullet" pill will cure our diseases. For example, we are encouraged to "Run for the Cure" to raise money to develop drugs that supposedly, one day, will be the cure for cancer. Believing in drugs to save us is psychological manipulation of people's biggest hopes and fears. If we acknowledged the rather obvious causes of cancer (environmental and food toxicants), we would know that a drug will never be able to do what's necessary to deal with those causes. We are encouraged to take the "Ice Bucket Challenge", dunking ourselves in water to raise awareness for ALS (Lou Gehrig's Disease), all the while donating money to the pharmaceutical companies to create a magical, mythical pill that will one day cure people of this and other health conditions. I'm all for awareness, but I don't buy into the model that cancer, ALS or other chronic "incurable" conditions will be cured with a pill. This is especially the case when the etiology or origin of many such diseases is still unknown by Western medicine. It is just brainwashing, pure and simple.

Drugs will never be able to solve the majority of health issues that ail society today. As we continue to go against the flow of nature with the health of our bodies, the consequences will become even more devastating. Occurrences of the worst diseases continue to escalate and the only seeming solution from Western medicine is the hope for more drugs. We still use horrible toxins like radiation and chemotherapy to deal with cancer. The irony is that toxins are one of the primary causes of cancer. We are using toxins to deal with toxicity in the body. It is sad that the best we have in 60 years of cancer research is just more sophisticated forms of radiation and chemotherapy. Radiation and chemotherapy destroy an already weakened immune system. Instead of destroying the immune system, medicine should be focusing all its efforts on discovering what weakens the immune system and how we can make it stronger so that it can deal with cancerous cells on its own.

Cancer and many other chronic health conditions are preventable, if we implement healthy, life-giving habits <u>early</u> in life that correspond with nature and what Chinese medicine has said for millennia. Chinese medicine is a system of medicine that was developed by watching and following the healing rhythm of nature and uses a deeper understanding of the nature of the human body to create health with minimal to no side effects. Chinese medicine has worked beautifully for thousands of years and now more than ever we need its wisdom to help deal with the catastrophic health problems we see in the world today. When we work in harmony with nature, health tends to abound.

The biggest problem with thinking that a pill will be what cures us from depression or any other health problem is that it largely negates personal responsibility for one's lifestyle choices and surrounding environment. I see this everyday in the clinic with my patients and have also wrestled personally with this mentality many times over the years. It is as if we think we can do whatever we want, live ignorantly of the natural rhythm of our body and live within a toxic physical and emotional environment only to think that taking a pill one day will fix the years of damage we have allowed our bodies to endure because of the poor health choices we have made. This mentality spills over into the natural health world as well with people chasing the next super supplement that will fix all that ails us.

Supplements can be very useful in healing, but are meant to "supplement" a healthy lifestyle, not be the sole solution to everything. If we truly believe as a society that a pill will one day be the magic bullet for every health problem, we will continue to perpetuate a mentality that the pharmaceutical companies will save us. Let me prophesy about the future and tell you that this will never work. Believing in a magic pill is not taking responsibility for our bodies or environment. Disease and health problems have been skyrocketing for many decades. During this time the drug companies have created drugs for every conceivable symptom and disease but, as a society, we are not any healthier. We need to start asking difficult questions about why disease is skyrocketing and what the true causes are for the majority of our health problems.

When people show up in my office they are, to some degree or another, ready to take responsibility for the many factors that may be contributing to their not feeling well. We have to start taking a closer look at the many foods we consume and things we are exposed to that contribute to people feeling depressed. When we take a closer look, not only does current scientific research expose the true offenders, but the solutions are stunningly simple.

Depression Drugs versus Placebo

It has been documented that depression medication, in many cases, does not perform better than a placebo.[14] A placebo is a substance, such as sugar in pill form, which is used in drug trials and is given to people to contrast how it fairs in efficacy against the drug. The placebo effect shows how powerful consciousness and the simple power of belief in a pill are. We literally create healing with our intention, emotions and thoughts. Imagine if we believed we were going to heal combined with things from nature that actually contributed to health and caused no side effects. The drug companies are not interested in things such as using healthy food and herbs, which have been used to help people heal from depression for thousands of years. You cannot patent and make billions from food and herbs. Therefore, the same research, time and money are not spent on such things.

Let's be perfectly clear that drug companies are not interested in symptom free health. Symptom free health would mean they would go out of business. They are primarily interested in making money. They are not interested in finding cures. They are interested in you needing a drug for years or decades, constantly refilling prescriptions, getting vaccines every year and making a killing in profits. They will go to great lengths to provide education to doctors and generate commercials promoting things that are dangerous in the long run only to make money. In many cases, the means does not justify the end, especially when tried and true options exist that are safe, healthy, have been studied, have virtually no side effects and are relatively inexpensive. This is the heart and wisdom of Chinese medicine.

Tried and true foods, herbs and formulas have been used for millennia that work in harmony with the body to restore balance and health to the body. Why are we not dumping tons of money into studying and promoting this more? It is simply because herbs cannot be patented (owned) and don't generate the billions of dollars that drugs do. Moreover, insurance companies don't cover the cost of herbs. They only cover drugs. This is our modern reality.

Addiction And Withdraw From Antidepressant Drugs

One study concluded that withdrawal symptoms from SSRIs (Selective Serotonin Reuptake Inhibitors) were comparable to trying to quit sedatives and barbiturates.[15] Many of my patients report feeling horrible after deciding on their own to stop their antidepressant medication. Unless the true causes of the problem are addressed, they continue to feel awful. Many times they also report returning to their primary care doctor with the complaint that the medicine isn't working anymore and they need something else in order to feel better. It is not surprising that coming off of depression medication is potentially the same as withdrawing from sedatives, barbiturates and other illicit drugs.

You cannot alter chemicals in the brain for long periods of time without damaging and addicting consequences. Yet, in spite of the damaging effects, the human body has a remarkable ability to heal within a short period of time with the right interventions. When the true causes of depression are addressed, patients will often report feeling better within weeks. Dr. Roger Williams summarized it best when he stated, "The basic fault of these weapons (drugs), is that they have no known connection with the disease process itself...Drugs are wholly unlike nature's weapons...They tend to mask the difficulty, not eliminate it. They contaminate the internal environment (with side effects), create dependence on the part of the patient, and often complicate the physician's job by erasing valuable clues as to the real source of the trouble."[16]

"The part can never be well unless the whole is well." -Plato

Reductionism Versus Holism

Western medicine is mostly reductionistic in nature. This philosophy began with Rene Descartes, a French philosopher that lived in the 17th century. It takes the whole and reduces things down to individual components or parts. In trying to figure out health problems, the body as a whole is reduced to figuring out which chemical or small part is problematic. We see this mentality at work in blaming our genes for our health problems. Two main problems surface from this mentality. First, we are blaming genes for our health problems. This, just like taking drugs and thinking a pill will save us, doesn't allow for taking personal responsibility for the real factors behind our health problems. Second, the ones behind propagating this mentality are oftentimes the drug companies. We have been wrongly taught that our genes are where our problems can be found and corrected.

Buying into this mentality is seen in the hysteria of Angelina Jolie undergoing a "preventative" double mastectomy cutting off both her breasts in an attempt to make sure she doesn't develop breast cancer due to a gene mutation. This is on the same level as absurd as medical doctors promoting cigarettes as healthy 60 years ago. However, this solidifies the narrative for the current medical industry, which continues to get us to believe that our genes are defective.

Chinese medicine sees the whole picture – body, mind and spirit – and seeks to identify and correct anything in each of these realms which would be contributing to one's health problem. The environmental and lifestyle influences on our genes are a much greater factor in affecting our genes than the actual genes themselves. Epigenetics is the study of environmental factors that lead to poor gene expression. Epigenetics takes a hard look at all the factors involved in someone's life that influence gene expression. In Chinese medicine, a large emphasis is placed on what has been or is present in the environment that may be a possible cause of a health problem.

Reductionist medicine treats the body much like a machine. A machine is just made up of a bunch of parts. If one can understand all of the parts, down to the very smallest part, and learn to influence, change or fix said parts, we should be able to "fix" what is wrong or at least explain why the whole body functions a certain way. If we can figure out which part is not functioning correctly and fix that part, the whole can be understood and should start to work again. Western medicine has looked for answers in the smallest parts of the body including our genes, chemicals, enzymes, and specific cell components. It then creates a drug to influence that small part of the body. Reductionism is like looking at a tree in the forest, whereas holistic medicine keeps the smallest components in mind but also looks at the entire forest as well.

Chinese medicine doesn't invalidate reductionism over holism. Looking at the smallest parts we have has given us incredible access to information and understanding into things that we didn't know 100 years ago. This information has been very helpful and insightful. Reductionism isn't bad and holism good, they are just separate models of understanding dis-ease in the body. We can hold a view that incorporates both into the picture, combining the best components of each view. The problem occurs when medicine is practiced only in a reductionistic way, which is largely the case today. This is evident in taking a drug for every symptom we seem to have. This can be very short sighted because symptoms start to look all like nails and the only tool to work with a nail is a hammer (drugs). This is changing in the medical world, but has a long way to go.

Epigenetics – The True Influence Of Health Issues

Dr. Bruce Lipton, Ph.D in his book, _The Wisdom of Your Cells_, states outright that our genes do not control our health.[17] Instead he talks about epigenetics or the environmental influences that turn on and off the expression of our genes. If you place cells (genes) in a healthy environment, they continue to be healthy. If you place cells (genes) in an environment lacking nutrients, full of toxins or induced stress, they will begin to express sickness or dis-ease. Genes themselves affecting less than 5% of the expression of health in our lives are not the largest contributing factor to sickness that we have been taught to believe.

Think of the human body as one large cell. It is critical to take a close look at the human body and the tremendous impact all factors in our environment play in determining our health. The environment that humans are in today is far more toxic than ever in our history. When combined with other environmental toxins and stress, what emerges is an understanding that the health we have today is a direct result of the many environmental factors we are exposed to. We must consider all of these influences. When we do, we realize that each one of us must be responsible for factors we allow to affect our health. It is in taking responsibility for the totality of our environment that we can reclaim our power to do something about it. The reversal and natural healing of cancer, heart disease, diabetes and depression will arise when we are taught to take full responsibility for our health from birth and live in a preventative environment, rather than waiting to take responsibility when we are diseased and toxic after a lifetime of environmental abuse.

Let's use an example about epigenetics in reference to heart disease. Heart disease is the number one killer of people in the USA today, accounting for over 610,000 deaths each year.[18] People commonly claim that since heart disease runs in the family, it must be a genetic problem. This is the farthest thing from the truth. If we look more closely, we see that horrible dietary practices, decades of toxic environmental exposure and the emotional stress inherent in that particular family are the actual factors behind the expression of heart disease. Heart disease is not a genetic problem and can be prevented and reversed in most cases.

T. Colin Campbell, Ph.D, Professor Emeritus of Nutritional Biochemistry at Cornell University, authored a book called _The China Study_, which analyzed the link between diet (environmental influences) and diseases such as cancer, heart disease and diabetes in China.[19] The conclusion was that environmental influence and certain consumed animal products altered genes in such as way that expressed disease. When these factors were addressed and animal products were removed from the diet, these diseases reduced significantly and reversed.[20] Dr. Caldwell Esselstyn, medical doctor and heart surgeon, wrote a book entitled *Prevent and Reverse Heart Disease*, which also states that natural solutions exist to this horrible health problem.[21] The environmental factors that contribute to the number one killer in the USA are the same factors that contribute to depression. You will not see this information given to aspiring medical doctors in school, nor will it be advocated for by pharmaceutical companies. This road to healing takes drugs off the table, which is not profitable and would be a threat to the current system of health.

Observations From Shadowing An Internist

In January 2018, I spent time following a medical doctor (internist) on his rounds. This experience gave me a wonderful view into the common state of reductionistic Western medicine as it is being practiced today across the USA. It was very eye-opening to see this experience firsthand. Here is what I observed after spending time in this environment:

1. The average appointment with the doctor was around 10-12 minutes.
2. No causes to health problems were discussed at all.
3. What I observed was symptom management through more drugs, nothing more.
4. No concrete lifestyle or dietary changes were recommended.
5. The doctor didn't appear to know concrete causes behind most of the issues presented as it applied to each person. Or if he did, no plan was put in place to deal with it outside of using drugs.
6. Patients honestly didn't know about many of the things that contributed to their health problems.
7. No incentive is given to patients to change their health either from the healthcare provider or insurance company.
8. A pill was commonly prescribed for every major symptom expressed.
9. Some patients were on between 5-15 different medications. Some of the medications taken were solely to deal with the side effects of other medications.
10. When I was given permission to offer advice, most of the people were not interested in hearing more, but simply wanted a pill to make their symptoms go away.

The only "medicine" I observed in this experience was very reductionistic. For every symptom that was named by each patient a new drug was suggested. In almost every case, this was the only thing that was recommended. The only other thing that was mentioned, in cases where it was required, was surgery. This was a very enlightening but sad experience for me. The doctor I followed is a wonderful, caring human being and is extremely intelligent. He was just following the model that he learned in school. This model is heavily influenced by drug companies. Pharmaceutical drugs are largely directed at influencing very small parts of the body in an attempt to effect a change that corrects a symptom. However, in my view, this really is not true medicine. Medicine is supposed to be an attempt at the full natural healing and prevention of disease. Most drugs do not cure or prevent disease.

It is impossible to try to get to the root of someone's health issues only by spending 10 minutes with them. While each patient was in the exam room, the doctor was looking at the computer and typing almost the entire time. This is because of the necessity to have the medical record updated with each visit as required by the insurance companies and for liability purposes, both of which cut into actual patient care. These things are not the fault of the doctor. How can you really be present with someone for a few minutes? How can you get to the root cause of a health issue? How can you keep people accountable for their life and choices? How can you inspire, educate or encourage someone to take a healing course of action by spending just minutes with them? These visits were mechanistic, short, encouraged the use of more drugs, and never got to the root of the issues. This is healthcare in the USA today. I hear the same experience from patients all day long. I have 50 minute sessions with people during a visit and oftentimes wish I could spend longer with them.

Treating people with drugs is mostly just sick care and managing symptoms. If the majority of the people stopped taking their medications, the symptoms would come roaring back, which is the primary indicator that the root cause is not being addressed. This is especially the case in the treatment of depression. The best treatment is not taking medication to stop a symptom; it is dealing with the underlying causes so that drugs don't need to be taken on a long term basis. Even in cases where "life saving" medication is needed another way to heal almost always exists.

This is certainly the case even with diseases such as diabetes. Arguably, the foremost expert in curing people from diabetes is Dr. Gabriel Cousens, MD. His book, _There is a Cure For Diabetes_, is full of scientific references along with his proven program to help people heal completely from diabetes. A good percentage of type 1 and most type 2 diabetics can be medication free within just 30 days with the right natural intervention.[22] For some type 1 diabetes, it is possible for the body to start producing insulin again if the factors are addressed which are destroying the beta cells in the pancreas. Yet, most doctors are unaware of this information or some may just find it easier to hand out drugs, rather than helping people heal naturally or keeping people accountable for their poor choices. This would require physicians to take a stand, educate themselves and orient their medical practices around a completely different model of health.

On a side note, this same medical doctor approached me not long after I spent time with him. He kept hearing over and over again from his patients about how cannabis oil (CBD) was powerfully helping his patients sleep better, feel less pain[23], experience less anxiety and depression[24,25], have diminished seizures and feel overall better. He couldn't ignore the overwhelming anecdotal evidence that many of his patients and his own family were experiencing by using CBD oil. I have also seen and heard this anecdotally from many of my own patients. CBD oil is just one product from one plant. In Chinese medicine, hundreds of plants are used that have stood the test of time and work just as well to help deal powerfully with any symptom that the body may exhibit. CBD oil can help, but in my experience, even more foundational things must be addressed for people to truly heal in the long run and not just become dependent upon something else like CBD oil.

Doctors should be doing whatever it takes to find the true causes of each problem and work to correct them through natural or organic means first. I'm not opposed to using life saving medication or any other medication in the short run, as long as the ultimate goal is to heal through natural means whenever possible, so that drugs don't have to be taken long term. This is truly doing no harm. In Chinese medicine, I have observed that when the right physical, electrical and emotional causes are identified and addressed, people can heal naturally. At the very least, symptoms decrease and few to no side effects occur. This is how medicine should be. True medicine is not taking a pill for the rest of your life when the possibility exists to correct a cause through natural means.

I hear people ask me constantly in public, "What supplement should I take for _______ problem?" True, vibrant health will NEVER be reduced to what one will find in a pill, even if the supplement was the best whole food supplement money can buy. I have people that come into the clinic all the time that take mountains of supplements, but still have many symptoms. If the supplement or drug fixes things, the symptoms should go away. But oftentimes they do not. People's hearts and intentions are good in trying to find relief for their symptoms, but some have replaced drugs with supplements because the mentality is the same. Our society has been conditioned by the drug companies to believe that a pill should solve our health problem, even if that pill is all natural.

Recently, I was with a different medical doctor, who has been in practice in Florida for the past 15 years and gets to the root of her patients' issues through what is called functional medicine. Functional medicine is the modern Western medicine equivalent of naturopathic medicine and even to a certain degree Chinese medicine. Functional medicine purports to determine why illness is occurring and to correct the problem at the root physical level through the most natural means possible. To be clear, functional medicine is a significant departure from conventional Western medicine and truly does try to get to the root causes of issues. Many of my acupuncture colleagues, including myself, have embraced this and incorporated it into their Chinese medical practices. Functional medicine has its limitations, but is far better than conventional medicine at addressing the root causes issues. When functional medicine is combined with the ancient wisdom of Chinese medicine, the possibility for healing is even greater.

As I spoke to this very passionate, informed and well spoken medical doctor, she said that in her third day out of medical school 15 years ago, she had this stunning realization that she was just going to be a "legalized drug dealer." These are powerful words coming from a medical doctor and there is much truth to this statement. She looked out into her future and realized how this was not what she signed up for and wouldn't make the difference she wanted to make in the world of medicine. We see the painful reality of this when it was documented by the CDC in 2016 that 63,632 deaths occurred due to drug overdose, many of them from properly prescribed medications.[26] Moreover, adverse drug reactions cost us $136 billion dollars annually.[27] She has a thriving practice with testimonials from many of her patients that have reclaimed their health and life from the plight of poor health through natural means. Functional medicine works, as does Chinese and Naturopathic medicine, and people are utilizing these branches of medicine to heal now more than ever.

In summary, the substantial limitations of Western medicine have become clear when looking beyond acute medical care. If you break your arm, no better medicine exists than Western medicine. If you need surgery, Western medicine is the best game in town. However, when it comes to prevention, understanding food and diet to help heal, identifying root causes, and using treatments that actually treat root causes to chronic health issues, Western medicine is not the best option on the planet. It is a system awash with programming from the drug companies that drugs are the savior we all will continue to need. Drugs don't heal most chronic health conditions. They have extensive and damaging side effects and are meant to be continued for years or decades, ensuring profits and retaining good customers for many years to come. We need to start taking responsibility for our health, one person at a time and be the change we wish to see in the world and in our healthcare system.

2 FIRST CAUSE OF DEPRESSION: TOXINS

"By cleansing your body on a regular basis and eliminating as many toxins as possible from your environment, your body can begin to heal itself, prevent disease, and become stronger and more resilient than you ever dreamed possible!" -Dr. Edward Group III, MD

"All truth passes through three stages. First, it is ridiculed. Second, it is violently opposed. Third, it is accepted as self-evident." -Arthur Schopenhauer

This quote speaks volumes about the world of medicine today. Many times, I have heard those in the Western medical world both ridicule and violently oppose the truths of Chinese medicine. Yet, history is not on the side of those that ridicule or oppose it. Nowadays, it seems that people are ridiculed or opposed if they question Western medicine, its practices or the scientific method. Chinese medicine is viewed skeptically today. However, it will become self-evident that Chinese medicine and its principles of living in harmony with nature will be the answer to our health both now and in the future. Those who question the official Western medical narrative, often get maligned, ridiculed or opposed from within and outside the system. Questioning the symptom management and drug model of medicine often results in being labeled a quack and, at times, being subject to ridicule.

Sadly though, when it comes to understanding the origin or etiology of many of the chronic health problems we have today, all that is known is as follows: "exact etiology unknown." So many people have shown up in my clinic over the years with a similar story where doctors don't know what is causing their health issues. They come looking for answers out of desperation. They don't know what else to do, but have a tremendous drive to heal.

This response is one that is commonly given when people are faced with a new diagnosis of chronic disease. Doctors will say, "We aren't completely sure what the cause is, but genetics and some other dietary and lifestyle factors MAY be a factor." I hear this all the time from my patients when they retell their stories to me. Genetics are blamed, which implies that not much can be done because we are just victims to the genes that we received from our ancestors.

Yet, I believe that we can state with certainty what the exact causes are of most chronic health problems today in the world, both on a macro and micro level. The truth of what is behind most chronic health problems has been ridiculed in our world today, even violently opposed. However, I am confident that one day in the near future, the truths of what are causing the chronic health issues today will become self-evident. As mentioned earlier, epigenetics leads us in the direction of our environment as the cause behind most health problems in the world today. It is not our genetics.

First, let's start on the macro level and talk about which broad environmental factors are behind chronic disease and depression. Three environmental factors stand at the root of almost every chronic health problem in the world today. Those three factors are toxins, nutritional deficiencies and stress. Understandably, these are very broad factors, and the mind instantly wants to know which specific toxins, nutritional deficiencies and sources of stress are the largest contributors. However, it behooves us to talk in broad strokes first about these things because, while specific things may apply to specific conditions, we must see the big picture first.

Before we expound on each of these topics, it is critical to understand on an even more simple level how these three factors create depression and ill health. When toxins, nutritional deficiencies and stress are present, they all contribute to creating a state of inflammation in the body. Depression has been aptly called by some as simply inflammation of the brain. Toxins, nutritional deficiencies and stress literally heat up the body and lead to the creation of inflammation in the organs, glands, muscles, tissues and skin. As a result of the rise of this state of inflammation that grows out of control in the body, opportunistic pathogens can then grow uninhibited.

Leading research is pointing in the direction of depression as being caused by chronic inflammation in the body. The sources of inflammation in the body must be dealt with and nourished properly. A study in the journal, *Neuropsychopharmacology,* indicated this connection between inflammation and depression, stating "Psychosocial stress, diet, obesity, a leaky gut and an imbalance between regulatory and pro-inflammatory T cells also contribute to inflammation and may serve as a focus for preventative strategies relevant to both the development of depression and its recurrence."[28] Australian researchers also concluded that "A range of factors appear to increase the risk for the development of depression and seem to be associated with systemic inflammation; these include psychological stressors, poor diet, physical inactivity, obesity, smoking, altered gut [function], [allergies], dental [cavities], sleep and vitamin D deficiency."[29]

Here is the progression towards depression and chronic health problems:

Toxins, Nutritional Deficiencies and Stress → Growth of Pathogens (Viruses, Bacteria) → Widespread Inflammation → Chronic Health Problems and Disease

This is the very simple progression of how depression and other health problems get started in our world today. When the immune system is not being supplied with the right nutrients that literally can cool the body down and quell the fires of inflammation, pathogens rise up to plague the body.[30] Behind most of the chronic health problems we see in the world today, you will find a viral or bacterial factor, or both. So the progression is straightforward. Toxins, nutritional deficiencies and stress destroy the immune system and lead to widespread inflammation in the body. When this inflammation occurs and goes unchecked, viruses and bacteria take note of this opportunity, begin to grow uninhibited by an already compromised and weakened immune system, which leads to long term chronic health problems and disease.[31]

Long term chronic inflammation in the body is being fueled by either a virus or bacteria.[32] When you have any kind of condition with an "-itis" on the end of it, you can be sure a viral or bacterial component is present and at work in sustaining the inflammation. Pathogens are opportunistic. Much like a lion will try to pick on the baby antelope or the smallest antelope of the group, pathogens seek out weak or injured parts of the body to set up camp and proliferate. This is especially the case when injuries occur. Parts of the body that have been weakened or injured over time are places that are ripe, fertile grounds for pathogens. Injuries aren't limited to physical injuries though. Organs and other parts of the body can be injured, especially by non-physical things such as emotional traumas. Any kind of injury must be considered when a part of the body is not functioning optimally. In fact, inflammation of any kind that is chronic should be a warning to us that systemic inflammation is occurring on some level.

Overuse (as in the case of athletes), underuse, misuse, exposure to metals and toxins over time, eating toxic inflammatory producing foods and emotional traumas cause and create inflammation leading to chronic inflammation sustained by pathogens. In order to heal, the offending metals and chemicals must be removed. The body and immune system must be strengthened with proper food and supplements. Emotional traumas need to be released from the mind and body. Once this occurs, people can heal from disease and health problems of all kinds including depression and anxiety. That is it. It really is quite simple. Health is simple; it is disease that is complicated. If people could learn what constitutes good health early in life, the risk of getting chronic disease would be significantly diminished.

Having said this, let's explore in further detail, some of the physical toxins and nutritional deficiencies that can create inflammation in the body and support a state of depression in the body.

Environmental Toxins

On some level, we all are familiar with the idea that toxins are a significant factor behind chronic disease. Yet, on a more personal level and as a society, we fail to see very common toxins that we are exposed to on a daily basis as the cause behind the many health problems we have. It is almost as if we are waiting for the media or the medical world to make an astonishing discovery in order to start taking responsibility for something in our world that is contributing to disease before we do something about it. Most of the toxins that we are exposed to are mild compared to some of the things that we have learned in the past that directly cause disease. As mild as they may be in toxicity, when they are combined with the hundreds of other chemicals and metals we are exposed to on a daily basis, the results in our current, societal health are catastrophic. Let's examine a few examples from history.

In 1977 the USA banned the use of lead paint, along with toys, car gasoline, and furniture containing lead. Apparently, children were ingesting paint chips that had fallen off of the wall and were getting very sick. So lead was labeled a public health hazard and was banned from certain products. Lead is an environmental toxin that causes nervous system damage, stunts growth, damages the kidneys and delays development.[33] It does much more than this, but these are a few of the many symptoms elicited in the average person. While we have banned paint, toys and other things with lead, it has not disappeared from our world today.

In 2007, the Campaign for Safe Cosmetics found lead in 61% of lipstick brands out of 33 studied.[34] I cringe when I see women using lipstick in the world today, knowing that there is an almost 2/3 chance that it contains lead. Lead contributes to damaging the hormonal system as well. We see women today with all kinds of hormonal issues, ranging from painful periods, infertility, and menopausal symptoms of hot flashes and night sweats. Lead may be a contributing factor to this in conjunction with other toxins. Lead is just one of the toxins found in lipstick.

While lead was removed from gasoline that we put into our cars, it was not removed from airplane fuel. Lead is in 70% of airplane fuel, so living under flight paths or near airports can be very harmful due to the lead that gets dumped into the air. Airports are common in big cities where the majority of the population congregates. This means that a good percentage of the population is still getting a steady dose of lead, in small amounts on a daily basis, through the air that we breathe and the things that we touch that have residue that has fallen from the sky.[35]

Pesticides and DDT

What are some other examples of things from our environment that glaringly contribute to chronic disease? Not long ago, we saw medical doctors advertising for cigarette companies, advocating how amazing smoking was. Very quickly we learned that this leads directly to lung cancer and other chronic health problems. This hasn't just been isolated to the smoking of cigarettes. We seem to blindly believe in anything that medical doctors and Western medicine push on us these days and determine to be "safe." Often times, we are not questioning if something is detrimental to our long term health or if a much better option exists outside of what we are being given and told.[36]

In 1972, the insecticide DDT was banned due to it being linked to cancer and the threat it was having on wildlife, especially birds.[37] If this insecticide was banned, should we not start looking at all insecticides as harmful and damaging?! These chemicals target and destroy the nervous system of insects. We absorb these chemicals too, but since we are much larger than insects, the reactions are not as pronounced and the damage is not done as quickly. They damage our nervous systems just as severely, but more slowly over long periods of time.

Asbestos

Not long ago, asbestos was commonly used in building materials as an insulator and for its resistance to fire. It was soon discovered that inhalation of asbestos fibers lead directly to lung cancer, mesothelioma, and other health concerns. Even as recent as 2018, 22 women won a lawsuit for 4.9 billion dollars from Johnson & Johnson claiming they got ovarian cancer from baby powder containing asbestos.[38] What we breathe in and put on our bodies in the form of powder can have a tremendous impact on our health. We need to question everything that we put on our body, breathe in and consume.

Chemicals Galore

In the world today, we have more than 84,000 chemicals on the market. Many of us are exposed to hundreds of these chemicals every day.[39] Yet, virtually none of them have been studied for safety or are deemed as safe up to acceptable levels. As time goes on, people are suing the manufacturers of chemicals (toxins) that are overtly contributing to chronic health problems. I would argue that many, if not most of the toxins that people are exposed to have direct consequences to health over years and decades of constant exposure. They may be "safe" and not have much of an effect in the span of weeks, but after months and years of exposure, the consequences to our health are anything but "safe." Just as it may take 20 or even 30 years for lung cancer to develop in the life of a chronic smoker, exposure to other common toxic chemicals on a daily basis, may lead to other forms of cancer. I'm convinced that exposure to hundreds of chemicals in our personal care products every single day for years or decades has already led us to chronic diseases and health problems.

These chemicals are contributing to the rise of cancer in the world.[40] Firefighters, for example, are 14% more likely to develop cancer than those in the general population, due to exposure to fire retardant chemicals that are commonly used in their profession.[41] Tampons and sanitary pads are actually considered "medical devices" and as a result, the ingredients that are used in them do not have to be disclosed on the packaging. Each sanitary napkin contains the equivalent of four plastic bags. Plastic comes from petroleum and contains BPA, BPS, Phthalates, and synthetic fragrances. These are all toxic. Chlorine, genetically modified cotton and other disinfectants are found in sanitary pads. These toxins are absorbed into the skin and surrounding tissues to which they are exposed. This creates an environment ripe for bacterial growth and symptoms that affect the reproductive area for women.[42] Organic, unfragranced, chemical free products exist that will not create environments of disease in women's reproductive areas.

Chemicals In Umbilical Fluid

Our exposure to chemicals doesn't just begin after we are born. Toxins being ingested, inhaled, and touched are finding their way to fetuses via the mother. The unborn are starting life out these days having to deal with a chemical cocktail that in time could prove to be devastating. Dr. Sanjay Gupta, neurosurgeon and CNN's chief medical correspondent notes that 200+ chemicals are found in umbilical cord blood of babies before they are born, potentially leading to asthma, autism, developmental disorders, childhood obesity and other unknown health issues.[43] Newborns have underdeveloped immune systems and may struggle with detoxifying these substances from their system. Never before in our history has this been something that the human body has had to deal with. Mothers carry these toxins in their bodies and pass them along to their children.

Armed with this knowledge, mothers should be guided, instructed and encouraged with the information necessary to provide them with what they need to detoxify and make their bodies as suitable as possible for pregnancy. It is no wonder that infertility rates have skyrocketed in recent years, with many women left wondering why they are having such a hard time getting pregnant. A toxic body is not suitable to support life. Instead of trying to isolate which chemicals are causing problems, we should start with the assumption that they are all creating some kind of adverse health effects and should immediately take a much deeper look at removing these toxins completely from our lives.

If we want to move in the direction of health, we must take conscious, responsible and swift actions to reduce the amount of heavy metals and chemicals we expose ourselves to. Most people don't even consider what chemicals and metals they are exposed to. Our personal care products and cosmetics are loaded with disease causing toxins. Over time, these chemicals build up, damage the liver, contribute to widespread inflammation and confuse and destroy our hormonal (chemical) system. "The average woman in the U.S. uses about 12 personal care and cosmetic products daily (168 chemicals on average). The average man uses about 6."[44] This means that the average woman is exposed to hundreds of chemicals before she even goes to work in the morning!

The risk of using hundreds of chemicals on a daily basis sets most people up for the perfect storm of disease and health problems, especially when combined with stress and nutritional deficiencies. You cannot use toxic chemicals with products that you put on your body every day and expect to be healthy over time. After years or decades of exposure, your body will begin to suffer. Chemicals alter enzymes, and decrease their function causing reproductive, nervous system and possible carcinogenic effects.[45] Enzymes accelerate chemical reactions and are necessary in almost every metabolic process in the body. When these chemicals are exposed to the skin, they are absorbed and quickly find their way into our blood. Your entire blood supply filters through your liver every four minutes.

Depression is an expression mostly of poor health affecting the liver as seen through the lens of Chinese medicine. It is the liver's job to filter the blood and detoxify the body. After exposure to hundreds of chemicals on a daily basis that goes on for years, the liver gets tired and burns out, leading to disease and chronic health problems.

Sodium Lauryl Sulfate

Let's make this personal. One of the most common ingredients in hand soap, shower soap and shampoo is sodium lauryl sulfate (SLS). It is commonly used because it is inexpensive and is a good foaming agent. The Journal of the American College of Toxicology has deemed it an irritant, causing skin reactions.[46] Yet, it has been deemed "safe" for consumer use.[47] How can something be considered safe when it is a known irritant, causing skin reactions such as dermatitis? The powers that be determine levels that are accepted as safe to a certain level for humans. Yet, in general, the immune system doesn't just launch attacks upon things that assimilate well with the body. This is not the only chemical present in soap and shampoo. Not only is this chemical known to be an irritant, but when combined with other chemicals, it is a toxic chemical cocktail. Many people aren't aware that organic, safe alternatives exist that come from 100% natural ingredients, including oils (like from coconut) and essential oils.

Changing your soap or shampoo to an organic/natural product is just one step that you can make to reduce the toxic load of chemicals and poisons that you are exposed to every day. This can go a long way in reducing inflammation in the body. But we need to go even further. Organic and natural products exist that can replace most of the toxic personal care products we use today.

Take any of your personal care products and look at the ingredients. Most of them are hard to pronounce. They are toxic man-made synthetic ingredients that contribute to disease, inflammation and long term chronic health problems. Let's take a look at one of the best selling shampoos in the USA, Pantene Pro V Nature Fusion, and see what kinds of ingredients are in this product:

1. Sodium Laureth Sulfate
2. Cocamidopropyl Betaine – In 2004 this substance was named "allergen

of the year" and has been implicated in skin reactions.[48]
3. Sodium Chloride – Common table salt.
4. Sodium Xylenesulfonate – surfactant, could elicit skin reactions.
5. Cocamide MEA – surfactant, foam builder and emulsifier. Contamination concerns are connected with the product together with Nitrosamines, which are carcinogenic (cancer causing).[49]
6. Sodium Citrate
7. Citric Acid – flavoring, preservative, emulsifier, corrosive, irritant, allergen, may cause genetic defects, carcinogenic, danger to fertility, organ toxic, very ecotoxic.[50]
8. Fragrance – irritant, allergen, ecotoxic.[51]
9. Dimethiconol
10. Cassia Hydroxypropyltrimonium Chloride
11. Sodium Benzoate – organ toxic, irritant.
12. Disodium EDTA – irritant, organ toxic, allergen, ecotoxic.[52]
13. Benzyl Salicylate – allergen, ecotoxic.[53]
14. Butylphenyl Methylpropional – Harmful if swallowed, skin irritant, allergen, fertility damaging, ecotoxic to aquatic life.[54]
15. Panthenol
16. Panthenyl Ethyl Ether
17. Hexyl Cinnamal
18. Hydroxyisohexyl 3-Cyclohexene Carboxaldehyde
19. Alpha-Isomethyl Ionone – corrosive, allergen, irritant, ecotoxic.[55]
20. Linalool
21. Persea Gratissima (Avocado) Oil
22. Bambusa Vulgaris Shoot Extract
23. Methylchloroisothiazolinone - preservative. Allergen, irritant, ecotoxic.[56]
24. Methylisothiazolinone – preservative. Allergen, neurotoxic, irritant, ecotoxic.[57]
25. Vitis Vinifera (Grape) Seed Extract
26. Cl 47005 - Yellow dye - linked to contact dermatitis
27. Cl 17200 - Red dye - linked to contact dermatitis
28. Cl 42090 - Blue dye - linked to contact dermatitis

Is there really a need to have 28 different chemicals in shampoo? As you can see above, many of the ingredients found in this product cause irritations, produce allergic responses, are toxic to the environment and are possibly carcinogenic. The levels of these chemicals in these products have been deemed "safe" for humans. They are anything but safe. If this wasn't bad enough, we use many other personal care products in the morning. Other products have chemicals in them that are just as harmful.

Here is a list of some of the most common personal care products that contain disease causing toxins: shampoo, shower soap, deodorant, mouthwash, toothpaste, nail polish, nail polish remover, makeup, lip balm, lip stick, hair products, hair dye, perfume, cologne, body spray, body lotion, shaving cream. Additionally, you are exposed to other toxicants in shower water, drinking water, laundry detergent, fabric softener, dry cleaning fluid, tampons, pads, household cleaning products, air fresheners, insecticides, lawn care chemicals, hydrocarbons, and plastics.

In many of these products, it is not just one carcinogenic chemical that is present, but many. They are combined together to create a toxic cocktail that you expose to your skin or breathe in day after day, year after year, without ever thinking about it. We have learned to blindly trust in the manufacturers of our personal care products without thinking if they are having slow, but catastrophic effects on our health. I find that when people are educated about this, a good majority of people will say this makes sense and will migrate over to using organic products.

Stop and ask yourself the following questions about your own awareness before reading these past few pages:

1. Have you ever considered that all the personal care products that you expose your body to may be one of the direct causes to your health problems, including anxiety and depression, but not limited to that?
2. Has anyone ever mentioned to you how these chemicals may be more of a problem than you have ever considered?
3. If you have heard something like this, have you dismissed it in your mind thinking that it couldn't possibly make that much of a difference?
4. When considering the toxicity of these products and switching to healthier products, did your emotional attachments arise in that moment to the products you already use and "Love!" Said in a different way, do you not want to give up certain products because you are attached to them?
5. Is smelling or looking good really more important to you than your health? Would you say the same thing if you were diagnosed with cancer? Would you have made better, more informed choices knowing the dangers that can arise from these chemicals?

It is worth repeating again and again that these personal care products and other toxic metals and chemicals are definitely responsible for the deplorable state of health that we see in the USA today. Before we move on, I wanted to address an attitude that I hear from time to time with regards to these things. People tend to think that as one person they couldn't possibly make a difference or that it really doesn't matter. Some people, when confronted with this information, may have the following response, "I'm going to die anyway, so what does it really matter?!" Here's the issue with this response. It is characteristic of irresponsibility for not only one's own body, but also for the world. At the end of the day, many of these toxic chemicals get flushed down the drain, only to poison our air, soil and precious water supply. The effects of these toxic chemicals are doing untold damage to our environment. When millions of people decide that this doesn't matter, it pollutes the world at large, in addition to their own bodies. We need to educate, take responsibility and think about future generations and the toxic world we are leaving them.

You can make a difference. Change in the world starts with the small changes that each individual makes. Take a detailed look at ALL of the common products that you put on your skin, breath in, and use that have toxic chemicals in them. The science may not exist that describes in great detail how toxic each chemical is, but that doesn't mean it's not toxic. Don't wait 30 years (like with cigarettes, asbestos, lead or DDT) to hear about how toxic your personal care products are. Err on the side of safety and invest in products that already exist that are safe, non-toxic, chemical free and organic. Decades of using such products can prove to be a decisive factor in your having health not only in the short term, but especially in the long run, not only for yourself but also for your children.[58]

"From the bitterness of disease man learns the sweetness of health." - Catalan Proverb

Toxins in Our Food

Perhaps the one area in our lives where we are exposed to the greatest quantity of toxins that contribute to poor health and disease is in the food we eat. Many people understand that what they are eating is not healthy, but when the toxins that are in the food are uncovered and exposed, it amplifies how important it is to make better dietary choices. Most people in the world know that they have to eat healthy, but few are doing what is truly healthy to ensure that cancer, heart disease, diabetes and depression are not in their future. Some of the most common things that people eat are actually very unhealthy. Additionally, not taking responsibility commonly masquerades as thinking that having a little piece of cake couldn't possibly make that big of a difference. The little things count much more than we think.

The problem is that people are not just making one poor dietary choice throughout the course of the day. People are making dozens of poor choices during the course of a day without even realizing it. Just as the hundreds of chemicals that we are exposed to via our skin that buildup, clog and pollute the body, all of the chemicals in our food do the same thing. We minimize the impact this is making in our lives, because we don't want to fully take responsibility for our health or change what we eat. We have the health we have because we have chosen our health in this way. Yet, we can take responsibility and make better choices. We can have vibrant, disease free health. Let's look at a couple of examples of common foods that we eat that are some of the primary toxic catalysts behind why we are depressed and have poor health.

Wheat – It's Bad for Everyone

Roundup (glyphosate) weed killer from Monsanto is the most common pesticide sprayed on food crops in the USA. In August of 2018, Dewayne Johnson was awarded a sum of $289 million dollars in damages against Monsanto, when Roundup glyphosate was linked to his development of non-Hodgkin's lymphoma (cancer).[59] This is the first time in history that someone has been awarded damages for a health condition linked to this herbicide. It is the most common herbicide used in the USA and is used in conjunction with "Roundup ready crops." Another name for these is genetically modified crops, which have been created specifically to survive when application of this herbicide is used to kill weeds but allows for the growing of such crops. So basically, this chemical kills and destroys everything around it, but leaves the genetically modified crops untouched. The most common genetically modified crops include wheat, corn, soy, canola, and beets (sugar).

In 2015, glyphosate was finally classified as most likely to be carcinogenic by the World Health Organization.[60] Glyphosate has been in use since 1974 and is also the most commonly used herbicide by other countries in the world. Americans consume heavy amounts of genetically modified wheat products that are loaded with this cancer causing chemical and have been doing so for much of the last 40 years. Wheat is a staple in almost every meal for some people. Some of the most common foods containing wheat are bread, pastries, pasta, English muffins, cereals, couscous, bagels, buns, crackers, chips, cakes, donuts, tortillas, beer and cookies.

This chemical has been used for over 40 years and we are just now waking up to the fact that it contributes widely to inflammation and disease. ANY chemical pesticide or herbicide that destroys smaller forms of life (weeds) is going to eventually destroy larger forms of life (humans). The rate of destruction is just a much longer period of time (years or decades). These chemicals are absorbed into the foods that we are consuming when they are sprayed directly onto these crops. No one should be eating wheat at all today, just like no one should be smoking. It doesn't matter if you think you have an allergy to wheat or not, it is a horrible toxic food for anyone to eat, even in small amounts. Glyphosate damages, pollutes and creates disease in the body. Some of the most common reactions to this food include coughing, sneezing, asthmatic reactions, itching, rashes, diarrhea, muscle spasms, headaches, fatigue, tingling, abdominal pain, vomiting, nausea, anxiety and feeling depressed.

Gluten is the protein that is found in wheat and is named so because it is a "sticky" protein, and is most commonly used in baked goods for being able to hold things together well. Gluten has been blamed and implicated in contributing to allergies and immune reactions of all kinds. The wheat that we use today is not the same wheat that has been used in cultures around the world for thousands of years. Genetic modification has changed all that and over 90% of the wheat in the USA today is genetically modified.[61] Gluten is hard for the body to break down and then contributes to rotting and inflammatory reactions in the digestive system and in the rest of the body.

It is not just those with celiac disease that suffer. Celiac disease is an autoimmune inflammatory disease that affects the small intestines. The small intestine gets inflamed due to a reaction from gluten. Everyone gets inflammation in the gut to some degree with the consumption of wheat. Gluten rotting in the gut leads to a rise in harmful bacteria and viruses and also the creation of gases, such as ammonia, that are very harmful to the body. The immune system is attacking this rise of pathogens in the small intestines, not the body itself. The immune system isn't confused; it is doing its job and trying to take care of a pathogen flourishing in this part of the body. This has led researchers to identify gluten in creating celiac disease and other digestive disturbances.[62] The genetic modification of the food and also the reaction the immune system has to glyphosate has proven to be catastrophic for humanity. This food should be avoided like the plague for every human being, whether you think you are allergic to it or not. When health continues to decline in the years to come, we will look back and see what a disaster wheat has been for humanity within the last century.[63]

We also have to make a distinction about what part of wheat is used most often in food products. Wheat is composed of three parts - bran, germ and endosperm. Bran is the hard outer layer. Germ is the reproductive part that germinates and is able to grow into a new plant. The endosperm is tissue that surrounds the germ and makes up the bulk majority of the grain (80%). The endosperm is the part that is removed from the bran and germ to make wheat flour. Most white wheat flour is made from the endosperm. What makes whole grain flour distinct from regular wheat flour is having the endosperm, bran and germ all together versus just having the endosperm. Oftentimes, the endosperm is bleached and made even whiter with a bleaching agent, which is a toxin chemical. These bleaching agents are permitted in the United States, but are outlawed in the European Union because it contributes to disease.[64] Wheat flour is often enriched with synthetic vitamins to "make up for" the loss of nutrients by not having the germ and bran present. Wheat flour that is bleached and "fortified" with synthetic nutrients obviously is not what the human body was designed for. The germ and bran are the parts of the grain that have most of the nutrients and these parts are absent from most wheat products on the U.S. market.

Whole books have been written about the dangers of modern day wheat products. Wheat has been genetically modified, so that it can be patented and owned. Only Roundup glyphosate can be used with this "franken-food" so that everything around it dies except the plant itself. In this process the gluten (protein) is changed and the plant absorbs this toxic chemical. This toxic chemical is consumed by most people in the USA today and over the decades has become a powerhouse of inflammation and cancer causing destruction. When wheat is harvested, it is bleached, and most of the nutrients (bran and germ) have been removed to make white wheat flour. Synthetic vitamins and nutrients have been added back into the flour because otherwise it is a lifeless, toxic, disease producing food. But the addition of the synthetic vitamins doesn't actually change how horrible this once nutritious food is. This is what our breads, bagels, muffins, donuts, cereals, cookies and cakes are made of. Modern wheat is a science experiment gone wrong and you, the consumer, are the one being experimented on. People have started demanding these products start being labeled, as they are in other countries, but until now, powerful lobbyists have prevailed. Genetically modified foods should be labeled so people have a choice in the matter of the food they consume.

Wheat Consumption and Depression

A strong correlation exists between the consumption of wheat (gluten) and depression. We know that wheat contributes to inflammation in the body and depression is simply another form of inflammation affecting the brain and other parts of the body.[65] I have seen incredible transformation with patients in the clinic when wheat is removed from the diet. Many of my colleagues have witnessed this too. Julia Ross, M.A. in her book *The Mood Cure* states, "Dozens of studies confirm that depression is a common symptom of gluten intolerance, one that usually disappears when wheat and the similar grains are withdrawn...gluten has been implicated in mental illness since at least 1979, tremendous improvement in the symptoms of patients with depression and manic-depression . . . who had been experimentally taken off gluten-containing foods."[66] Dr. Jeffrey Morrison, in his groundbreaking book *Cleanse Your Body, Clear Your Mind* shares how one of his patients had all symptoms of schizophrenia disappear after removing wheat/gluten containing products from his diet.[67] If you want to feel less depressed, it is imperative that you remove wheat from your diet completely.

As we mentioned, it is not just wheat itself that is a problem. Any food that has had commercial pesticides, insecticides and herbicides sprayed on them find their way into the food itself and when we consume these foods, these chemicals destroy our immune and nervous system, contributing to inflammation and disease. This is why it is imperative to advocate for and consume organic food. People grew crops for thousands of years just fine before the use of these chemicals entered our world. Genetically modified crops are not better for the world, do not solve a food shortage and do not yield higher crop volume.[6869] Monsanto has also been caught red handed in consumer fraud and other unbecoming business practices.[70] Many people have also touted Monsanto as being either the most or one of the most hated companies in the world.[71]

Here we have discussed how toxic wheat is, but other genetically modified foods are commonly consumed and people are mostly unaware of the damage they do. All of the other genetically modified foods should be avoided as well. Soy, corn, beets (where refined sugar comes from), and canola (commonly used to fry food) carry the same risks as wheat. The chemical companies have chosen these foods because they have been staples in the American diet for a long time. Why not target, patent, own and sell both the seed and herbicide to farmers? This ensures total domination of the food supply and the creation of disease in the general population.

The chemical companies exist to make money, control and own the planet's food. Once a food is patented, it can be owned. Once something is owned it can be controlled. The destruction of our food and health is due to greed, power, control and domination, not for the actual betterment of our world. Farmers are not better off with these foods; neither is the general public. Genetically modified crops do not offer higher yields and are poisoning our food supply.[72] Other chemical (pharmaceutical) companies give you more chemicals (drugs) to deal with the health problem pesticides and the horrible foods have created. Then, those drugs cause secondary side effects that require more chemicals/drugs to deal with the side effects. This is not working and will not work going into the future. Each of us must take our health back into our own hands.

When people are exposed to these chemicals every day, they rob and steal from the body and mind, until they no longer have any effective resources left. So frequently I hear such things from people as, "Nothing much in my life has changed and my diet remains virtually the same. My routine and health habits are as they have always been. But then one day, everything shifted and my health began a downward spiral." The same is heard often in the case of allergies as well. People mention that they have eaten the same things for decades and then from one moment to the next, the body "developed" an allergy to something, health shifted and oftentimes, very pronounced symptoms started cropping up. What is really going on in these cases? The body of the average human is so adaptive and forgiving, but without adequate levels of nutrients, over time, our resources get so depleted that the body cannot maintain things as they have always been. Then, one day, the resources are exhausted and all hell breaks loose in the body. The body reaches a breaking point.

Seeing it from another perspective, let's say you consume genetically modified conventional wheat every day, which is highly inflammatory for everyone. For most people, since it is biochemically in your system so frequently, the body gets used to the inflammation that such a food provokes. You may notice some symptoms, but choose to look the other way or do not know what to do about basic symptoms that may appear (gas, bloating, low energy after a meal, brain fog, headache, constipation, diarrhea, skin changes, etc).

When such a progression occurs, people are surprised that one day, out of the blue, they develop cancer. It is as if the cancer just came out of nowhere. You cannot eat gmo wheat, dairy, gmo refined sugar, gmo corn, gmo soy, fried food, eggs, pork and consume alcohol habitually for years and not expect something to happen. Those who live long lives despite consuming these things are the exception today, not the rule. Cancer doesn't just appear overnight; it takes years to develop. In the overwhelming majority of cases, many signs and symptoms were in place for decades before cancer was diagnosed. When I really press people for information about what they experienced in the decades before they "got" cancer, 9 times out of 10, I find many symptoms that have persisted for years. Even something as "small" as gas is a symptom that must be paid attention to. When you get gas for example, it is a symptom that something didn't break down well in the body. It is sitting in the gut fermenting and is creating toxic fumes. Other aches and pains, which people just attribute to "getting old" that have persisted for years before the development of a chronic disease, are a part of the canary in the coal mine. If you have persistent pain and inflammation in a certain part of your body for years, this is just one sign that you have reached a point where inflammation is already spreading in your body.

Refined Sugar (From Genetically Modified Beets)

Before the turn of last century, sugar was a commodity that was not easy to get your hands on. Therefore, sugar consumption was relatively low for much of the population. Refined sugar enters the body and creates inflammation. Sugar can even cause inflammation in the brain and endocrine glands which are responsible for giving you many of the chemicals that contribute to you feeling good. This inflammation can give rise to the start of disease and health problems in any part of the body. Processed sugar is very toxic to the body. A great book to read on this subject is *Suicide by Sugar: A Startling Look at Our #1 National Addiction* by Nancy Appleton, Ph.D.[73] In this book, she describes how sugar suppresses the immune system, artificially stimulates and elevates production of dopamine and serotonin (which is why it's so addictive), contributes to obesity, raises cholesterol and triglyceride levels, contributes to allergies, creates inflammation, and causes children to become hyperactive. The recent documentary entitled *Fed Up* is also a good tool to raise awareness about how damaging sugar is.

Refined sugar leaches precious minerals and nutrients from the body that are needed to help you feel better. It has been proven that sugar feeds cancer.[74] We see so much more cancer in the world than we did 100 years ago. The average American is said to eat more than 130 pounds of processed sugar per year (versus only 5 pounds in 1900). Added refined sugar makes up an astonishing 17% of the diet of an adult today.[75] It has been said that coronary heart disease is hereditary for many people, but research has concluded that sugar is a powerful promoter of this disease, much more than genetics ever will be.[76] Women may also be interested to know that increased consumption of refined sugar leads to aging and the appearance of more wrinkles on the face over time.[77]

Sweetened beverages, such as soft drinks and diet drinks, are associated with increased risk of depression.[78] Just consuming one can of soda per day equals 10% of one's recommended amount of calories, all in the form of refined sugar. Drinking soda is like pouring liquid inflammation straight into the body. Refined sugar feeds pathogens, such as viruses and bacteria, perpetuating inflammation leading to chronic disease. A study following 8,000 people for 22 years showed that men who consumed 67 grams or more of sugar per day were 23% more likely to develop depression than men who ate less than 40 grams per day.[79] Other studies conducted have led to the exact same conclusion – refined sugar consumption directly correlates with increased depression.[80] One symptom that is often experienced simultaneously with depression is feeling fatigued or drained. In this state it is easy to reach for sugar because it causes a rush of feel good chemicals in the body, giving one a boost of energy. However, the result is often a crash, making you feel worse than before you had the sugar in the first place. Research points in the direction of refined sugar consumption creating an overall feeling of draining the body, leading to low energy and lethargy.[81]

Sugar is in everything these days. It seems like it is almost impossible to avoid. Even brown sugars or "healthy" alternatives to sugar create inflammation in the body. The only safe sources of sweet things that I advocate for are raw, unfiltered organic honey, organic maple syrup, or stevia. These should only be consumed in very small amounts. Even though stevia (which are leaves from the stevia plant, dehydrated and ground into powder) has become more prominent and is natural (when it's organic), I have a good percentage of people clinically that do not test well for it. The liver's ability to process this may have something to do with it.

Many people, when they are going through emotional experiences, reach for sugar to make them feel better. Sugar creates the same feel-good euphoria as cocaine in the body because it influences the same chemicals in the brain. This is why many will reach for something sweet when they feel anxious, angry, afraid, guilty, etc. We must take note of the emotions we experience that drive us to the sugar and wanting to feel good and then spend time letting go of those emotions. Then you can feel good without needing something to artificially create this and cover up your negative emotions.

Another of the dangers of constantly consuming sugar is increasing your risk of hypoglycemia. When you consume sugar, your body will pump out insulin in order to use this hormone to facilitate pushing sugar into your body's cells for usage. The body may create too much insulin causing blood sugar levels to drop rapidly. This is known as functional hypoglycemia or the inability of the body to properly handle sugar. Cerebral dysfunction can happen in this state and in some cases people exhibit signs of psychosis, mental confusion, fatigue, nervousness, dramatic mood swings, headaches, depression and anxiety. By completely stopping consumption of refined sugar, many people have seen a dramatic decrease in symptoms.

High fructose corn syrup (HFCS) comes from genetically modified corn and has the same damaging effects as sugar. I have recently even seen marketing with certain products that advocate they don't have HFCS. But when looking at the ingredients, you see that the main sweetening ingredient is sugar. It is just more deception and hypocrisy from people wanting to sell their own products.

This is why it is critical to start looking at and questioning all of the ingredients that are found in the foods you regularly consume. As you do this and choose a healthier lifestyle, you will be making much of your own food, so that you can control what you eat. The healthier you become, the less you will be eating foods that are processed and come in boxes and bags. Even in most of the organic cereals, for example, you will find organic cane sugar. While organic cane sugar is a little healthier, it is still sugar that has been separated from its source.

I encourage people to reach for fruit when they have a craving for sugar. Fruit sugar is processed and seen by the body very differently than it sees refined sugar. Dried organic black mission figs are an amazing brain food, destroyer of bad bacteria in the gut and can instantly cool a sugar craving. Perhaps 50% of the time or more, it could be possible that your brain just needs a little sugar. The brain consumes a lot of glucose. If a craving doesn't go away after consuming fruit, then I would explore the possible emotional components to a craving.

Many people clinically mention sugar filling an emotional emptiness. They may say that life does not feel sweet (pleasurable) to them, only painful. The lack of sweetness can be the mask that parades around covering feelings of weakness, control, guilt, lack, and limitation. Sugar can also heavily mask a deep-seated craving for love and attention. These things can only be transformed by having an awareness of these feelings that drive the craving and then the dedication to surrender them. The bottom line here is that refined sugar is catastrophic for health, leads to chronic disease, including cancer and heart disease and also contributes to a rise in depression and anxiety. The answer is clear that refined sugar should be avoided at all costs. Moderation is not the answer.

Artificial Sweeteners

Artificial sweeteners are just that - artificial. They are not natural and are very destructive to the body. Splenda (sucralose), Equal, Sweet & Low, aspartame or any other artificial sweetener should be strictly avoided, especially if you are depressed, anxious or have a chronic disease. They are neurotoxic and poisonous to the brain. Many people have turned to these alternatives believing that they do not raise glycemic or blood sugar levels and do not affect the production and absorption of insulin. Yet, evidence is suggesting that this isn't the case and that blood sugar and insulin levels do rise upon consumption, particularly with those who are already obese or overweight.[82]

Artificial sweeteners are also bad for the health of your digestive system. In one study with male rats, it was shown that Splenda negatively impacts gut microbiome, decreasing the amount of healthy bacteria that normally contributes to good health.[83] Consumption of artificial sweeteners may also affect the reward system of the brain much like sugar. Although they are touted to be effective for weight loss, they may actually trigger cravings and a desire for more sweets leading to weight gain.[84]

Consumption of artificially sweetened beverages has been linked to an increase of type 2 diabetes, much the same as it is with consumption of beverages with refined sugar.[85] Diabetes is just another disease that is the product of widespread inflammation in the body. These artificial products are toxic and create inflammation in the body.

Cancer is another health problem driven by inflammation. One study showed a correlation between consumption of artificial sweeteners and increased risk of leukemia and lymphoma.[86] Artificial sweeteners have also been linked with other health conditions such as headaches[87] and seizures.[88] Adequate levels of neurotransmitters are critical for feeling well. In this study, antioxidants levels and neurotransmitters were severely reduced with rats' brains in just 40 days of exposure to aspartame.[89]

People were convinced a generation ago that fat was bad for us. So they removed fat from many products. The fat naturally found in foods is not necessarily bad. But fat was vilified, and they took fat out of everything and put sugar in everything. Then sugar was vilified, so they said that artificial sweetener was the way to go. The more our food is messed with and processed, the worse it becomes. Artificial sweeteners are very acidic, and the body will have to utilize alkaline minerals to neutralize the extreme acidity of these artificial sweeteners. People are already in short supply of the most abundant alkaline minerals: calcium, magnesium, sodium, and potassium.

When your body doesn't have enough of these, it will steal them ultimately from the bones (calcium), leaving us with a generation of people with porous bone issues (osteoporosis). In the short run, it may appear that these sweeteners aren't causing problems because symptoms don't appear right away. But over time, they will lead to grave health problems and need to be avoided completely because of their extreme toxicity.

Dairy Products

Dairy is one food that is often mentioned in Chinese medicine as causing a lot of problems, especially inflammation. Dairy (all products - conventional and organic) produces more dampness internally than perhaps any other food. Dampness is a pathogenic factor and term that is used in Chinese medicine. Dampness gums things up and slows things down in the body, causing dysfunction. People who are depressed feel down or "slowed" down. Dampness leads to phlegm buildup in the body because the longer something is stagnant the more potential it has to accumulate together. Phlegm buildup leads to things becoming hard and turning into what the Chinese called a nodule. Nodules can be cysts, fibroids or tumors. These are protective mechanisms for the body due to an imbalance that has occurred. People who are depressed typically are more stagnant in body, mind or both. Dairy, in all forms, is not good for anyone that wishes to be healthy. Dairy in its organic, raw, natural, non-altered form is the perfect food for calves, not humans.

One of the things that cause problems for many people in cow's milk is lactose.

Lactose, a naturally occurring sugar found in cow's milk, needs the enzyme lactase in order to be digested. After nursing, many people lose the ability to make lactase. In fact, over 75% of the population loses the ability to process this sugar after the age of four, especially if you are of Asian or African-American descent.[90] When one loses the ability to do this, one will begin to experience abdominal pain, bloating, flatulence, diarrhea and other gastrointestinal symptoms. These symptoms alone should be proof enough that when cow's milk is consumed, the body does not process it very well, which leads to more and more symptoms. Rotting and fermenting sugar and protein in the intestines leads to chronic inflammation. Strangely, many people don't think that the production of such symptoms like gas is abnormal.

For many though, not being able to process lactose is solved by buying a form of milk that doesn't have lactose or by consuming over the counter pills to break down lactose. However, as many have experienced, problems still continue with dairy consumption because it is not just lactose that is the problem. Not being able to process lactose is not an allergy. However, many people have very powerful allergic responses to dairy including hives, swelling, wheezing, congestion, diarrhea, nausea, headaches, joint swelling, abdominal pain, chronic fatigue and more. Reactions can be immediate or delayed, sometimes manifesting 24-72 hours later.[91] Delayed reactions make it more difficult to correlate symptoms with dairy.

One study confirms that consumption of cow's milk is directly correlated with acid reflux. If you drink milk and have acid reflux, it is advisable to stop immediately. Some of the most common medications in the world today are for acid reflux.[92] When people come into the clinic with acid reflux, one of the first things mentioned that should be cut out of the diet is all forms of dairy. In most cases marked improvement is seen within one week's time.

We don't consume the same dairy our ancestors did. Conventional dairy products today breed health problems because they are consuming the same disease causing foods that we are - genetically modified grains. Cows were meant to eat grass in a pasture that is pesticide free, not genetically modified grains. Cows today are so inhumanely treated that many of them grow up in a narrow bin and are rarely outside in the sun eating grass. They are just used for what we can get from them.

Cows today are injected with lots of growth hormones. Growth hormones ensure that calves grow faster so that they can be used for food as early as possible. Additionally, other hormones are given to cows so that they produce milk continuously throughout their lives. We would not expect a woman to nurse a child for 5 years straight, but cows are injected with hormones to ensure they continue to produce milk. We know that breast cancer is heavily influenced by too much estrogen, which is a hormone. Cow's milk contains extraordinary amounts of estrogen.[93] Cows are a commodity, and they need to be forced to grow so that a profit can be made off of them.

Humans are the only species that consume milk after infancy. Cow's milk was designed for cows, not humans. It was made to take a calf to a 700-1200 pound cow in a very short period (2 years). The protein in milk (casein and whey) is huge from a molecular perspective, much larger than humans can process at times. It is not a healthy protein option, even when it's organic. If you must have a protein powder, I suggest an organic plant-based protein powder. Clinically, when people are body building and it is suggested to stop using dairy based products, marked improvements in digestive symptoms have been noted anecdotally.

Cow's milk is legally allowed certain levels of blood, pus, and feces. One of the reasons for this is because of how commonly cows get mastitis, which is an infection of the udder. It is the most common reason for the premature slaughter of a cow and the second most frequent cause of death.[94] This occurs because many cows are milked continuously for much of their life. They become so inflamed (mastitis) that this pus and blood finds its way into the milk itself. Certain levels are allowable from a legal perspective. When you consume milk, you don't even realize you may be consuming blood, pus, and feces. It looks white and clean, but it is not.

Due to mastitis, the FDA has approved the use of over 80 different antibiotic drugs for factory farms. When the public is being told that they find no trace of antibiotics in the milk supply, it is because only 4 of the 80 are being tested.[95] Some people are highly allergic to antibiotics, which could be one of the main reasons why so many people are allergic to dairy these days. Furthermore, when cows are injected with so many antibiotics and then the bacteria become resistant to such drugs, that bacteria can find its way into the milk supply contributing to massive inflammation for the human digestive system.

We have been told that dairy is needed for us to get calcium and to have strong bones. Countries with the highest consumption of dairy have the highest incidences of bone fractures. Calcium itself, especially from dairy, does not necessarily make bones strong.[96] The calcium in cow's milk may not be well absorbed. Cows grow to be very powerful and strong animals, and what they eat naturally in order to get to this size is lots of grass, or plant food. The calcium found in green leafy vegetables is far better and more absorbable than the calcium found in dairy will ever be. So be sure to eat your kale, collard greens or any other green leafy vegetable.

Consumption of cow's milk has been directly linked with cancer. In one study, women who drank two or more glasses of milk per day showed a 44 percent increase in the risk of developing ovarian cancer.[97] The risk for men developing prostate cancer is also directly linked to the consumption of cow's milk.[98] The consumption of cow's milk has been linked to many other types of cancer and health conditions including joint pain, arthritis, heart disease, Crohn's disease, breast cancer, multiple sclerosis, Parkinson's disease, infertility, menstrual cramps, and many other conditions.

Lastly, cow's milk is homogenized and pasteurized. When the milkman brought people milk raw and fresh, in a very short period it would separate into water and cream/milk. The fat naturally separated from the water. People would simply shake the bottle to manually homogenize ("make the same") it. Homogenization alters the fat structure and makes it smaller so that this doesn't occur. Again, we are altering nature, and that is not good. Pasteurization heats the milk up to just below boiling to kill bacteria. However, people have consumed raw milk without problems for thousands of years. Not only does pasteurization kill bacteria, it pretty much kills everything else. Pasteurization kills all the enzymes in the milk and many of the vital phytonutrients.

Drinking milk straight from the cow (or goat or sheep) is the only way to consume milk, if at all. Even then, cow's milk was designed for baby calves and not humans. Dairy farms are also some of the most destructive, resource consuming foods on the planet. If we wish to help the earth be more sustainable for everyone, the decline of dairy consumption and beef is wise. Milk, cheese, cottage cheese, sour cream, kefir, and yogurt (yes, even this) should be avoided. If you have good eating practices and have strengthened your digestive system through other means, you will not need to supplement with probiotics. Trying to get probiotics through yogurt is pointless. Dairy feeds bacteria in the gut. It's like steroids for bacteria. Candida is a reaction to a growing bacterial problem in the gut. This is how antibiotics were discovered. Bacteria were left out in the air in a petri dish, and by the time Alexander Fleming returned to the lab, a fungus had completely consumed the bacteria. This mold or fungus became what we now know as the first antibiotic. Candida is not the problem in the body. Candida is simply a natural reaction the body is having to excess harmful bacteria. Target the bacteria, not the fungus. Probiotics and dairy (yogurt) is nothing more than a sneaky, deceptive marketing ploy to sell more milk and cause disease.

Milk does not do a body good. It is a horrible disease and inflammation spreading food. Chinese medicine is supportive of a healing role that grass fed beef can have in the diet, but most people consume far too much beef as it is. Additionally, most beef consumed today is not organic, which can further contribute to health problems. Try considering some of the organic nut milk options that exist today. Organic almond, coconut, and rice milk are good alternatives to regular animal's milk. It was tough to get used to at first, but then I just sucked it up and did it. Now I enjoy it! An even better option is to make these nut milks yourself at home. This will ensure freshness and lack of preservatives.

Polyunsaturated Vegetable Oils

The use of polyunsaturated vegetable oils is at the heart of so many health problems today, including depression. Foods that are fried, especially in polyunsaturated vegetable oils, (corn, safflower, soy, canola, sunflower) create a lot of internal heat/inflammation and are very unhealthy. This is especially true considering that these oils are made mostly from foods that are genetically modified (corn, soy, canola). We have been brainwashed to believe that polyunsaturated oils are the ones that are best for us. This isn't even remotely true.

Rancidity is the complete or incomplete oxidation or hydrolysis of fats when exposed to air (oxygen), light, heat and moisture, resulting in an unpleasant smell and taste. Polyunsaturated fatty acids (found in vegetable oils) have molecular bonds that break down easily when they react with oxygen, creating a free radical that turns normal fatty acids in your body into dangerous molecules that cause destruction in the body. Polyunsaturated fat found in vegetables is not harmful in and of itself, the way it is found in its natural, organic and unprocessed state, but becomes so if and when you eat too much of it, and/or especially when the oils degrade, which occurs during refining (exposure to oxygen), processing and heating (cooking).

All of the oils that are used in cooking in restaurants and homes are polyunsaturated oils such as corn, soy, sunflower, safflower or canola oil. Once these foods are processed for their oils, they immediately begin to go rancid. Unsaturated fats are not stable fats and are highly subject to oxidation creating rancidity. No one would eat rancid foods, but all of these oils go rancid very quickly after being exposed to oxygen. You would never know they are rancid though because when they are processed, they craftily remove the offending smell and taste.

When these oils are heated, they turn into trans fats. Over 30,000 deaths (some say as high as 100,000) per year can be directly attributed to the consumption of these oils (trans fats).[99] Even worse than direct correlation is that these fats have also been linked to coronary heart disease, which is the number one killer in the USA. Spanish researches, who analyzed the diet of 12,059 people over six years, found a 48% increase in major depression with those that consumed trans fats over those who did not.[100]

Every time you cook on the stove with these oils you consume this awful disease causing substance. Trans fats have been banned in food because of how destructive they are to our health. Every time you consume something fried at home or in a restaurant, you are essentially consuming trans fats. It takes great lengths of time for the body to get rid of these fats and they destroy the liver and gallbladder. In order to neutralize the free radicals and destruction these oils cause antioxidants are needed.

Antioxidants come from fresh organic fruits and vegetables. Today so many people eat fried food weekly and consume very little vegetables and fruits. This is another one of the reasons health has declined so fast in the USA in the last couple decades. No one should be consuming fried foods if you want to be healthy and depression free. Trans fats occur naturally in some animal products including butter, milk and cheese, which are dairy products and should be avoided.[101] The hydrogenation process, which produces trans fat, is responsible for the creation of products such as margarine and Crisco. They are almost chemically plastic and are awful. Partially hydrogenating a vegetable oil increases its shelf life and decreases the need for refrigeration. These oils are found in many baked goods. They have been linked to increased risk of heart disease, obesity, high blood pressure, cancer and type 2 diabetes.[102]

The story of the use of these oils is also just another example of greed, money, power, and control. Here is the short version of it. People used to cook with butter, lard and coconut oil until about 40-60 years ago. Saturated fat is stable and is not subject to the rancidity of unsaturated oils. Polyunsaturated oils were used commonly in oil-based paint. When they started using petroleum in paint instead of vegetable based oils, those who produced these oils realized they would lose much of their business. They decided to start very crafty marketing campaigns to deceive people into thinking that the "tropical" oils such as palm and coconut were bad along with butter and lard. The dominating idea birthed out of this is that saturated fat is bad for you and is the cause of heart disease, which is not true. So people stopped using these natural oils and sources of saturated fats and started consuming these polyunsaturated vegetable oils.

The best oils to use for cooking are saturated ones such as organic coconut oil and palm oil, which have been cold pressed and have not been exposed to light or heat. These are the ones that we should be consuming. Organic cold pressed olive oil is good if it is not heated and is best used on salads cold. If I cook on the stove, I always do it with coconut oil. Even though coconut oil is a stable fat, cooking with it does heat it up and destroys its nutrients. Being conservative is better when it comes to cooked food. Consuming a little raw cold pressed organic coconut oil per day helps to feed the brain and can have a powerful effect on clarity and brain fog. Coconut oil also gives the body a very powerful form of energy, medium chain fatty acids, which can give you a good pick-me-up during the day.

Today, I am convinced that the liver and gallbladder of most people are so gummed up with toxins that we need to be careful of how much fat we consume. If the liver cannot produce bile that it needs to, the gallbladder will not be able to help emulsify (breakdown) the fat that we do consume. This unprocessed fat is causing many people wide and varied health problems in the world today. We see this in blood work when triglycerides are elevated.

Raw fat naturally found in nature, especially in things such as nuts and seeds are very healthy for the body. We need fat for good health. Eating fat does not make you fat. Eating the wrong types of fat and too much fat will make you diseased and obese. Never consume processed vegetable oils, especially ones that are heated (either on the stove or used for frying). Consume fats in their natural forms. Coconuts, avocados, nuts and seeds are best consumed raw and uncooked. If you must cook or sauté vegetables, do so with moderate heat using organic coconut oil. Too much of any fat that is consumed today can cause the liver to work much harder. The liver is the main organ in Chinese medicine that contributes to depression. This is why it is necessary to only get fat that is absolutely necessary and avoid fats that are harmful to health.

Coffee

Non-organic coffee is regularly consumed by many people these days. Coffee shops abound all over major cities. Caffeine, found in coffee, is the most commonly consumed psychoactive substance (drug) on the planet. 90% of adults consume it regularly, with 2 cups per day being the average.[103] The looming question is whether coffee is good for or detrimental to health? Most people wake up and the first liquid that is consumed for the day is a fresh cup or two or three of coffee. Numerous studies exist that tout the benefits of coffee. One must be careful about who is conducting the studies because much like the pharmaceutical companies fund studies to support their drugs, those in the coffee industry use studies to promote and sell their product as well. A few good reasons exist why coffee should not be consumed, especially as it is related to depression.

First, coffee is sprayed with hefty amounts of pesticides, many of which are banned in the USA but are not in third world countries.[104] As we mentioned above, you cannot be exposed to these harsh chemicals and not expect them to be carcinogenic cancer causing agents. Secondly, coffee, from a Chinese perspective, focuses most of its action on the liver. The liver is the organ that is already overburdened, toxic, and malnourished. Coffee may, in some cases, put more pressure on this organ, promoting further stress. It creates heat and most people, from a Chinese perspective, already have conditions related to too much heat (inflammation) being present in the body. Thirdly, coffee today is not consumed black by many people. Many add sugar, fat or both to their coffee, which is not healthy at all. It is the liver's job to break down fat (with bile) and if you already have liver symptoms, adding more fat for the liver to process would be antithetical to healing. It would be like giving more work to someone who has already worked 60 hours per week. Fat is the most difficult thing for the body to break down digestively speaking. The added sugar, artificial sweeteners and creamer (fat) make this a horrible cocktail of toxins for people. Fourthly, coffee and the consumption of caffeine is known to be addictive and people may have significant withdrawal symptoms when stopping.[105]

Coffee, organically grown and consumed black in minimal amounts (1-2 cups per day), has been a wonderful beverage for people for hundreds of years. It is the heavy use of pesticides, added sugar, fat and overconsumption that causes problems for people in the world today, especially those with depression. If you do have coffee, it is suggested that it be consumed with a little raw organic honey or maple syrup only. Fat and sugar in coffee should not be combined together.

3 SECOND CAUSE OF DEPRESSION: NUTRITIONAL DEFICIENCIES

"Health is like money, we never have a true idea of its value until we lose it."
- Josh Billings

Recently, a friend of mine told me when her depression first developed. It was her first year of college and she moved out of state to go to a college about 500 miles away. She told me that she really didn't know why she got depressed but it definitely started that year. I began to ask her a few questions. My first thought was, "You ate in the cafeteria, correct?"

"Yes, I did, three times per day", she responded.

"What were some of the things you ate in the cafeteria on a daily basis for breakfast, lunch and dinner?"

She went on to tell me that she had eggs, bacon, cow's milk, cereal (Fruit Loops, Captain Crunch, Fruity Pebbles, and Raisin Bran), waffles (with corn syrup and butter or margarine), and some fruit. Many times for lunch and dinner it was pizza, French fries, macaroni and cheese, lots of soft drinks, more cow's milk, animal protein and other fried foods. Almost daily for lunch and dinner she ate a vanilla or chocolate sundae from the soft serve ice cream dispenser.

Very soon, it became very apparent to me why her body went into a downward spiral of depression and anxiety. Her brain was getting no real nutrients and began to starve and get super inflamed. For many in college, cafeteria eating sets a powerful foundation for poor health in college and the years beyond. All the foods she was consuming, with the exception of a few, promote depression and are horrible for health. Most of what cafeteria food offers is just basic unhealthy carbohydrates (as opposed to good carbohydrates), antibiotic and hormone infested animal protein and unhealthy fats (heated and separated from nature). If you put all of these things into your body for extended periods of time, the only factor that will determine when symptoms ensue will be relying on the foundation of one's genetics.

Unfortunately, this is a typical story for many people every day. College students, in the cafeteria, get to eat an unlimited amount of lifeless food. However, many children these days consume the same awful foods starting at a very early age. Pizza, fried foods, hot dogs, food loaded with cheese, microwave dinners, bagels, sugary cereals, cow's milk, donuts, muffins, pasta and so many other unhealthy foods are consumed resulting in low nutritional levels of vitamins, minerals and phytonutrients in the body. These foods are lifeless and destructive to health even in very minimal amounts. They counteract any kind of good things we may do for the body to build up our health reserves.

The second cause of depression, anxiety, and most of the other chronic health problems we have today is due to nutritional deficiencies. Due to the incredible increase in toxicity that the human body is faced with today, even more nutrients and resources are needed in order to counteract and deal with the toxins we are exposed to. We can liken nutritional deficiencies in the body to resources in an army. Just as an army needs a constant resupply of good quality materials and goods in order to keep the soldiers nourished, strong, healthy, ready for battle and functioning optimally, our body needs the same. Our body needs resources for rebuilding, cleaning, proper functioning, and for keeping the immune system strong and able to defend us against toxins and pathogens. If the body's immune system, for example, needs supplies and weapons to be able to "fight" against pathogens that seek to destroy and take over, the constant supply line of resources comes directly from what we eat. In the USA today, many people are giving their bodies the equivalent of BB guns to defend them through the diet, when bazookas, missiles and bombs are needed to do the job. A BB gun will not stop a tank, just as the resources many get through their diet these days will not stop the tanks of certain viruses and bacteria (and resulting disease) that seek to overtake us.

Many foods that are consumed by a good majority of people in the USA today have little nutrition beyond simple protein, fat and carbohydrates. We are the 12th most obese country on the planet, yet in spite of being so obese, people are literally starving to death for actual, good nutrients. Simple protein, carbohydrates and fats are not able to adequately give the human body what it needs to be healthy and remain disease free. I commonly stand in line at the supermarket waiting to check out and sometimes fail to find anything on the conveyor belt that does anything to prevent and reverse disease.

Health is simple; it is disease that is complicated. If we provide our bodies with the right nutrition and resources, stay away from toxins, avoid foods that create disease and inflammation and implement practices that are life-giving, health will abound for people. Three main deficiencies exist for people that are struggling with depression and other forms of ill health. The first is a deficiency of fruits and vegetables. The second is a deficiency of sunlight. The third is a deficiency of exercise.

"Don't eat anything your great-great grandmother wouldn't recognize as food. There are a great many food-like items in the supermarket your ancestors wouldn't recognize as food…stay away from these"
- Michael Pollan, New York Times Best Selling Author

Vegetables and Fruits – What Are Those?

The most protective, life giving, and nutrient dense foods in the world are organic vegetables and fruits. The 2015-2020 Dietary Guidelines for Americans outlined by the US Department of Health and Human Services recommends that adults consume 1.5-2 cups of fruit and 2-3 cups of vegetables per day.[106] Only 12.2% of adults meet the minimum for fruit consumption and only 9.3% of adults for vegetable consumption per day.[107] Among high school students, the numbers are worse with only 9% meeting the minimum for fruit and 2% for vegetable consumption. For most people in the USA, this boils down to consumption of less than 1 cup of fruit and 1 cup of vegetables per day.

At the end of the day, only 10% of adults meet the minimum requirements for vegetable and fruit consumption per day. How can we ever expect to be healthy if only 10% are just meeting the minimum? These amounts are minimums, but to be truly healthy, much greater amounts of vegetables and fruits are needed to protect and keep us disease free in the world today. Given this information, perhaps 5% or less of the population is consuming the very things that will keep disease away. Protein, complex carbohydrates and fats/oils will not save the health of humanity, vegetables and fruits will.

With the consumption of vegetables and fruits being so low for most people in the USA today, it is no wonder chronic disease has been rising exponentially for years and will only continue to get worse with time. You cannot eat less than 1 cup of vegetables and fruits per day and expect not to get cancer, heart disease, diabetes or depression.[108] Having abundant vital health starts with the dietary choices that you make every single day. These dietary choices are enabled by a powerful understanding of what gives life to the body, and not by emotional responses that drive people to eat only to feel good. When eating is driven by health, not pleasure (cravings and emotional responses), the body will respond with healing. Ironically, when you eat for health, your physical body will feel good and these more constant feelings of vitality will begin to drown out the temporary and short lasting "high" and good feelings of eating only for pleasure.

Per the recommendations above, it is recommended to have at least 2 servings each of fruits and vegetables per day for adults. However, this amount will never be able to reverse chronic disease in the USA today or heal those suffering from depression. It doesn't even come close to what is necessary. Physical depression is not such a difficult thing to heal from. My dietary advice for those who are depressed and anxious is basic. Stop consuming the foods that contribute to inflammation (ALL dairy, wheat, corn, soy, refined sugar, fried foods, eggs, pork and alcohol) and eat 6-8 servings of vegetables and 3-5 servings of fruits per day.

Consume moderate amounts of nuts, seeds, grass fed organic meats and clean carbohydrates. The vegetables and fruits need to be organic, free from pesticides and should be consumed raw or in the case of some vegetables lightly steamed or raw. If the vegetables and fruits are being boiled, baked or cooked they will lose much of their nutritional value and enzymes due to the application of heat. It really is this simple. This simple advice, started from early in childhood, would go a long way in keeping the majority of the population healthy. At a minimum, just consuming the necessary amounts of vegetables and fruits in spite of other unhealthy food will still make a big difference. No one likes to "diet", so just add these things into your diet daily and see if you don't experience big differences. As you begin to heal, you can then work on other aspects of your diet and continue making other adjustments to continue the healing process.

Consuming a <u>variety</u> of this many fruits and vegetables per day will provide your body with the minerals, vitamins, phytonutrients and other undiscovered disease protective substances it will need to be healthy.[109]

Recently a woman came to the clinic with extreme symptoms of depression, anxiety, insomnia, constipation, hot flashes, night sweats, skin rashes, headaches, nasal congestion and allergies. When I asked her how intense most of the symptoms were subjectively on a scale from 1 – 10, all were above a 7. I encouraged her to do a detoxification and dietary reset for 21 days just consuming only vegetables and fruits and nothing else. I gave her a very specific protocol for ensuring she got a variety of vegetables and fruits. She would be getting at least 9 cups of vegetables and 5 cups of fruits per day. She was advised to consume nothing else; no tea, coffee, alcohol, complex carbohydrates, fats/oils, nuts, seeds or animal protein. After the 21 day period, she reported that every symptom she had was reduced to a 1 or 2 out of 10 or less except for a skin rash, which still persisted. She lost 12 pounds and felt like a whole new person. This is what is possible for humanity, even just in 21 days! We can prevent and reverse depression and chronic disease through the consumption of whole foods, vegetables and fruits.[110]

While consuming nothing but vegetables and fruits for an extended period of time may not be right for everyone, raising our daily consumption of fruits and vegetables is. I have seen symptoms be reduced significantly or disappear when people do this. It never ceases to amaze me how food can be medicine and powerfully help people to heal.[111] Later in the book we will go over a plan that makes getting this amount of vegetables and fruits easy to accomplish.

Do Multivitamins Work To Prevent Nutritional Deficiency?

Many people in the USA today take multivitamins. According to the CDC, "The percentage of the U.S. population who used at least one multivitamin/multimineral product increased from 30% in 1988–1994 to 39% in 2003–2006, with use more common among women than men."[112] This number now is probably even higher than it was in 2006. It may be safe to say that up to 50% of the population in the USA might be taking multivitamins at this moment. Yet, depression and chronic disease continue to rise. Our approach to taking a multivitamin is the same as our approach to wanting a pill to fix every problem we have. It is the pharmaceutical approach but with (mostly synthetic) vitamins and minerals. Ultimately, it is another way for people not to take full responsibility for their health, thinking that a multivitamin pill will give us all we need. You cannot take a pill and expect to have vibrant health. Instead, you have to prepare your own food, eat lots of vegetables and fruits, and avoid toxins. This requires taking responsibility.

Let's be clear though. Taking a multivitamin is not a bad thing. It is just meant to *supplement* already existent good health, not replace or make up for it. What I am saying is that the mentality that is behind many people taking a multivitamin pill negates taking responsibility for health. This approach isn't working to reverse depression and chronic disease because our mentality behind it hasn't changed. What we project into our drugs (that this pill will cure or heal us), we project into our supplements and responsibility is largely left out of the equation.

When you look at the back of the common multivitamin products that exist, you will see the contents of certain vitamins present that give the person taking it thousands of percent of each vitamin. One would think that by getting 10, 20, or 30 times what the recommended daily amount is, we would be healthy and disease free. Yet, it must be understood that these are synthetic vitamins. Synthetic vitamins are vitamins that are made in a laboratory and don't actually come from nature or food. It is safe to say that we were created for things that come from nature (actual food and herbs), from the earth and not from synthetically made vitamins in a laboratory.[113] It is unclear how synthetic vitamins are absorbed by the body and how they are utilized in comparison to the real vitamins and minerals that come from good food.[114]

In vegetables, fruits and herbs, vitamins and minerals are never found in thousands of percents. Additionally, every vegetable, fruit, and herb contains cofactors of other phytonutrients that serve as powerful aids in human health. Phytonutrients (or phytochemicals) are chemicals that are produced by plants to help aid them in survival, thwart competitors or protect them. Humans also use these chemicals to help aid in the absorption of the other nutrients that food provides for us. For example, when vitamin C is put into a supplement it is labeled as ascorbic acid. But this is misleading because ascorbic acid is just one part of the whole vitamin C complex. Vitamin C contains hundreds of different compounds such as enzymes, coenzymes, and co-factors that work synergistically together to produce its desired effects on human health. Ascorbic acid is just one part of the complex. This is only what you get with synthetic vitamin C (ascorbic acid).[115]

Another example would be the consumption of calcium supplements. You can have brittle bones and take a calcium supplement, and see no effect at all in bone density. Calcium needs many cofactors, which are normally present in the same plants that are high in calcium to help it be fully absorbed by the body. The wisdom of plants continues to trump science in this regard. However, that doesn't mean we can't use science to our advantage to create supplements that do help. This is why a whole food multivitamin would be recommended over a synthetic vitamin. Additionally, you have to do the work, take responsibility and actually eat a diet full of vegetables and fruits in order to be healthy. Eating a variety of fruits and vegetables every day will ensure you get a range of vitamins, minerals, enzymes, phytonutrients and other life-giving substances that will provide you with the opportunity for radiant health.

It seems that these days we want a "life hack" for everything, including health. However, nothing in the world of health will ever be able to make up for not having a diet that is loaded with vegetables and fruits. This is such an important point to make that it may be safe to say that 70% of the diet should consist of fresh organic vegetables and fruits. The other 30% can be from clean, non-gmo, organic complex carbohydrates, sprouts, protein (either from animals or plants) and fats. It is critical to know that this is not just the case for already healthy people but especially for those with depression and other mental health issues.[116]

"Good nutrition creates health in all areas of our existence. All parts are interconnected." - T. Colin Campbell, Ph.D

Vitamin And Mineral Deficiencies

When people are not consuming adequate amounts of vegetables and fruits, nutritional deficiencies of all kinds are likely to crop up. This is especially true for those with depression that seek to mask the despondent feelings they have by consuming things that make them feel good like refined sugar, alcohol and fatty foods. In order for the body to deal with the destruction these things cause, it requires even more precious resources, in the form of vitamins, minerals and phytochemicals. Consuming alcohol, sugar and fatty foods can create a dependence while using up even more resources that most people don't have in the USA today.

Across the board, when it comes to even some of the most basic vitamins and minerals, people are deficient. These deficiencies are measured against the recommended daily amount established by the government. As I have observed, these amounts are misleading in that they are minimum amounts, but most often are not anywhere near what someone needs in order to have vibrant health. The recommended daily amount will provide you with a minimum, in order to avoid getting diseases of the past, such as scurvy, but are not enough to prevent cancer, for instance.

Vitamin C

Vitamin C is one of the most well known antioxidants in the world today. It is one of the essential ingredients needed to make collagen. Collagen is a structural protein that is the most abundant protein found in mammals - mostly in tendons, ligaments and skin. Studies have shown that vitamin C reduces the risk of cardiovascular disease, lowers the risk of death from cancer, is needed to make serotonin, reduces the severity and duration of the cold and flu, increases the bioavailability of iron and is a potent weapon for the immune system.[117]

Many existing clinical studies that exist that have measured vitamin C against various health conditions, with results showing that vitamin C was ineffective. However, when you look further at the data, you find that 100-1000mg was used in those studies. It is not surprising that nothing remarkable was found. These amounts of vitamin C are minuscule for what most people need. The government RDA (recommended daily amount) for vitamin C is only 90 mg, which I'm convinced is just enough to prevent problems of old, like scurvy. Evidence supports that we need far more than 90 mg per day to be healthy.[118] Vitamin C is one of the most important things needed for a strong immune system and supports hundreds of other functions in the body. Since the vitamin is water soluble, if you did take too much, whatever is not needed your body will dispose of easily.

Many animals synthesize their own vitamin C. Humans seem to have lost this ability over time. An adult goat, weighing approx. 70 kg, will manufacture more than 13,000 mg of vitamin C per day in normal health, and levels much higher when faced with stress.[119] What if humans need at least 10,000 mgs of vitamin C per day just for basic function and health? If this were the case, 100-500 mg would have little to no effect other than to provide the bare minimum to the body. Linus Pauling, the two-time Nobel Prize winner and brilliant scientist, who spent the last 30 years of his life researching the effect of high amounts of certain vitamins on the body, took 18,000 mgs of vitamin C per day for basic maintenance. In cases of the cold or flu, many easily tolerate 30,000-60,000 mgs per day just fine. I have squashed many oncoming colds/flus in one day using these high amounts of vitamin C.

Vitamin D, Calcium, And Omega 3

Research has proven that many are chronically deficient in vitamin D. In our modern age, people do not spend much time out in the sun on a daily or weekly basis. Growing up as a kid, I remember being outside the entire day. Now, kids spend so much time in front of the television or playing video games that the potential for adequate levels of sunlight, leading to the production of vitamin D, is significantly lower than it used to be.

One study showed that 48% of white preadolescent girls in Maine and 52% of Hispanic and African-American preadolescent girl were deficient in vitamin D.[120] A study of middle aged British adults demonstrated that 60% are vitamin D insufficient, and the number rose to 90% during winter and spring.[121] It is estimated that in the adult population those deficient in vitamin D could be as high as 80-100%.[122] Vitamin D is essential for regulating calcium levels, maintaining strong bones, and helps in the fight against infection and inflammation. If you don't have enough vitamin D, you will not be able to absorb calcium properly. The health benefits of calcium are plentiful. If you don't have enough calcium, eventually your body will pull what calcium you do have from your bones to maintain homeostasis or balance in the body. Bone deficiency (osteoporosis) is at an all time high in the USA today. An estimated 53 million people in the USA have porous bones.[123] Calcium is also a critical part of the immune system, is thermally cold and helps to put out the fires of inflammation in the body. Without adequate vitamin D and calcium, over time, your body will suffer.

Vitamin D helps to pick up calcium from the gut and put it into the blood. Once it is in the blood, omega 3's are needed to push calcium into the tissues/cells. In many ancient Chinese formulas herbs that contain large amounts of calcium are used to cool the body down. Calcium, if it is able to be transported into our cells, keeps things cool and puts out the fires of inflammation. But, in order for calcium to get into our cells, fatty acids are needed to be able to facilitate this. That is why just supplementing calcium on its own has not been shown to help strengthen bones. Green leafy and cruciferous vegetables not only contain calcium and omega 3's, but also the necessary cofactors to make calcium absorbable for the body.

Omega 3's are a powerful tool in the physical healing of depression.[124] They are found in both animal and plant sources. Both dopamine and serotonin, which are key neurotransmitters in the brain, are positively influenced by the presence of adequate levels of omega 3's in the brain. It is also key to know that omega 3 is actually 3 different molecules: DHA (*docosahexaenoic acid*), EPA (*eicosapentaenoic acid*), and ALA (*alpha-linolenic acid*). Each one of these molecules has different functions in the body. DHA is the only one abundant in the brain, keeping membranes flexible and pliable, helping with the transmission of signals. EPA is found on the neuronal level helping with the correct function of dopamine and serotonin, and also is a key component for anti-inflammatory hormones. ALA influences good heart function and doesn't have much of a known effect on depression.

Omega 3's have been implicated in multiple studies to be very helpful in dealing with inflammation.[125] As explained above, while the omega 3's may be helpful in dealing with inflammation on their own, they help to move calcium into our cells. Getting more calcium into our cells has been known in Chinese medicine to be a potent force for cooling down the body and thereby dealing with inflammation. The brain also relies on DHA for proper function, being implicated as an essential nutrient in neurodevelopment, cognition and neurodegenerative disorders.[126] Coronary heart disease is another condition that is directly related to systemic inflammation in the body. Omega 3's have also been implicated in helping to reduce the risk of this health issue.[127]

Dr. Stephen Ilardi comments in his book *The Depression Cure* that, "depression researchers have carefully studied the effects of supplementing with each one (DHA vs EPA). And based on the available evidence, EPA looks like the more potent of the two – by far."[128] This new research also points to EPA as being the most beneficial for regulating mood. He recommends a starting dose of 1000mg of EPA and 500mg of DHA for his patients. Standard Process, Vitacost Mega EPA,

Omegabrite, Nordic Naturals, and Carlsons are good brands.

In general, I advocate more towards getting nutrients from plants, and the same goes for the consumption of omega 3's. One of the most concentrated sources of fatty acids that is easy to keep in the kitchen is flax seed. Oil that comes from flax seed is very fragile because of its unsaturated nature, and many of the flaxseed oil brands on the market are rancid, even though they appear not to be. If you only wish to consume plant-based sources, I suggest purchasing organic golden flax seeds, using a coffee grinder and consuming them fresh every day. Grind two tablespoons of organic golden flax seeds and consume them immediately upon grinding them by sprinkling them onto food or adding them into a smoothie, juice or water. Chia seeds, hemp seeds/hearts, and walnuts are also fantastic sources of omega 3's. Chia seeds also have good levels of calcium and magnesium and are a fantastic food source for athletes and those who love to run.

Be sure to soak walnuts before eating them, so that you can remove the layer of phytic acid, which can cause digestive disturbances if not removed. Soaking the nut helps to remove this acid. Some nuts need to be soaked for longer periods of time, others do not. Look up a soaking chart on the internet to see how long a particular nut should be soaked before consumption. Flax and chia seeds are two of the few seeds that don't need to be soaked ahead of time.

Vitamin B3

Vitamin B3, also called niacin, has helped many people feel better when depressed. The reason why is related to tryptophan and the creation of serotonin in the body. Tryptophan, an amino acid, can be converted into niacin in the body. Tryptophan is also the amino acid that induces states of relaxation and is found in high amounts in turkey, which is why many feel the need to nap after Thanksgiving dinner. Tryptophan is also the building block of serotonin. Many of the antidepressant medications artificially regulate serotonin levels in the brain. A deficiency of niacin has been associated with fatigue, anxiety and depression.[129]

The best niacin supplement to take is the flushing kind. Flush free versions of niacin exist and will be indicated on the label if they are flush free. If you have never taken niacin before and you consume a large enough amount, within 15-45 minutes you can begin to feel very warm and prickly, with your skin turning blotchy red colors for a little while. This reaction is completely harmless and subsides very quickly. Many people find benefits from taking between 100-500 mgs per day. However, personal accounts have seen people needing as much as 1,000+ mgs before an effect was noticed. Most synthetic versions of this vitamin work well.

Vitamin B12

Vitamin B12 is a water soluble vitamin that is crucial for the stability of mood in human beings. Two forms of vitamin B12 that are active in human metabolism are methylcobalamin and 5-deoxyadenosylcobalamin. It is critical to get them both. These are methylated forms of B12 and are much better for the body than cyanocobalamin. It is involved in the metabolism of every cell in the body and helps form the protective covering for nerves for good conduction. It is a must have vitamin if you feel down or depressed. And since it is a water soluble vitamin, it is easily dissolved and excreted from the body if excess occurs.

A recent study in the American Journal of Psychiatry found that 27 percent of severely depressed women over the age of 65 were deficient in B12.[130] Even a slight deficiency of vitamin B12 has been associated with fatigue, depression, poor memory, headaches, and pale skin.[131] Upwards of 40% of the population may be deficient in this vitamin and even more may not be able to absorb it due to digestive complications.[132] Humans can produce B12 in the gut under the right conditions. However, given how deplorable digestive health is in the USA today, most people are not producing very much or any of this vitamin. Additionally, with the low consumption of vegetables, many may not be getting anywhere close to their daily needs. One natural substance that is high in B12 and is great for vegetarians and vegans is Hawaiian spirulina. Clinically, we use Cataplex B12, which is a whole food supplement deriving B12 from natural sources. Another great form of B12 is a supplement called Vegansafe B12. In Florida, many acupuncture physicians are licensed to give B12 injections, and many have found these injections to be very helpful.

Vitamin B9 - Folate

Patients that have depression have been tested to have, on average, 25% lower levels of folate than healthy controls. One study shows how an antidepressant medication was enhanced through the use of simultaneously taking folate. The vitamin alone most likely has the power to make one feel better without the antidepressant and may be important to supplement if one feels depressed.[133] Please be sure to take a methylated form of this vitamin as well. Folate is necessary in the body for the production of DNA, RNA, and metabolizing amino acids. Adequacy of this vitamin lowers the chances for birth defects and works to prevent anemia, as it is needed for the formation of red and white blood cells. When folate has been supplemented, it has been shown to enhance feelings of well being, alleviating depression.[134] Some foods that are high in folate include lentils, asparagus, spinach, broccoli, avocado, mango, lettuce and oranges. Consuming a variety of foods with folate will ensure adequate levels are consumed naturally, and potentiate feelings of well being, while alleviating depression.[135]

SAM-e

S-adenosylmethionine (SAMe) is a naturally occurring compound which affects the function of both serotonin and dopamine. A 2002 review by the U.S. Agency for Healthcare Research and Quality found that SAM-e was more effective than a placebo and equally as effective as antidepressants. A standard dose of SAM-e is 400-800 mgs per day.[136]

St John's Wort

Many have tried and benefitted from St. John's Wort as a way to relieve mild to moderate depression (Vorbach EU et al., 1997; Pharmacopsych 30: S81-5). The only problem that is commonly seen is that many nutritional supplements in stores are made of 10% of St. John's Wort and 90% fillers. Getting only 10% of this is not going to make a difference, which is why many have firsthand experience about how it didn't work for them. Not only are many of the nutritional supplements on the market of low quality, but you may also need a particular amount of the supplement for it to be truly effective. In the clinic, we use Standard Process, which contains very high-quality concentration supplements. Their formula, St John's Wort-IMT, also includes inositol and min-tran, which is a base of calcium, magnesium, alfalfa, carrot oil and kelp. Inositol has also shown beneficial results in depression cases.[137] All these ingredients together help to synergistically support the nervous system. St. John's Wort does have interactions with certain medications, so please be sure to consult your physician before taking it.

GABA

Like the other nutrients listed here, studies highlight how low levels of GABA are found in those with depression. GABA is a neurotransmitter and is mostly inhibitory, playing a role when the body experiences too much stimulation. Essentially, it has a very stress reducing effect on the body. Clinically studies on GABA are largely absent; however, anecdotally many have reported feeling better when taking GABA for certain periods of time. It has the potential to be beneficial for anxiety, depression and sleep disorders. A standard dose is between 200-1000 mgs per day.

Other Nutritional Deficiencies

Selenium, an important micronutrient, has been proven to be critical for thyroid function. One of the symptoms associated with an underfunctioning thyroid is feeling depressed. Selenium helps to reduce the effects of mercury toxicity[138], is critical for thyroid function interacting with iodine, zinc and copper and helps to elevate mood.[139]

Other nutrients that are critical for mood and feelings of wellbeing include iron[140], zinc[141], and iodine.[142] When a wide variety and large quantity of fresh organic vegetables and fruits are consumed on a daily basis, the potential for nutritional deficiencies leading or contributing to lower mood and feelings of depression lessens significantly. On the other hand, when only 10% of the population is getting the bare minimum of the recommended daily amount of vegetables and fruits per day, deficiencies of all kinds are going to be present for those struggling with depression, anxiety and other mood disorders. This not only holds true for mood disorders but also for chronic disease.

Exercise Deficiency

One other notable deficiency that exists among those who are depressed is an "exercise" deficiency. It is worth briefly repeating here how important it is to the overall wellbeing of humans, especially those who feel depressed and anxious. When I was a kid growing up in the 80's, we spent almost every waking minute during the summer playing outside. We got plenty of sun and were exercising in one form or another most of the day. We didn't have video games, cell phones, or computers until I was a teenager. Kids today are more obese than ever and playing outside occurs less and less for them these days. Lack of movement and exercise is playing a huge factor as to why more and more people are depressed and anxious.

Consistent exercise has been shown to be one of the best things to combat depression naturally.[143] People are exercising less than ever before, with only 20% of adults meeting the recommended amount of exercise per week according to the CDC.[144] Getting adequate exercise, next to consuming the right nutrients, could be the ultimate physical anti-depression tool. Ironically, not exercising because you don't feel like it or because you don't have the energy to do it could be relieved by actually doing the exercise.

I have always found that one of two components must be present for me in order to exercise.

1. I have to enjoy it.
2. I love being with other people with whom I enjoy the exercise.

For me, this has always been playing racquet sports such as racquetball, squash or pickleball. In the past, it was playing basketball competitively. In each of these sports, an enjoyment of the activity was present along with company from others to perpetuate continuance of the exercise. If you do something alone, like running, I suggest listening to classical music, your favorite podcast, or audio books as wonderful ways to stay motivated to exercise. If you have trouble putting pressure on your legs or knees, consider using an elliptical machine or another type of device that takes some pressure off your legs.

As a side note for exercise, I would not recommend swimming because of the amount of chlorine that is in pools. Chlorine is a toxin that is only going to make you feel worse over time. Chlorine and fluoride are toxic and are in a family of elements called the halogen family. Iodine is also in this family of elements and competes with these other elements for uptake in the body. Iodine, when combined with tyrosine, an amino acid, makes thyroid hormone. It has been estimated that over 40 million people in the USA have hypothyroidism or an underfunctioning thyroid.[145] For some reason many people's bodies are not making enough. One of the reasons for this could be that thyroid uptake has competition from fluoride and chlorine. One hundred years ago, exposure to chlorine and fluoride was much less than today. We get exposure to chlorine in massive amounts through showering and through swimming pools. The history of how fluoride made its way into our water and personal care products, specifically associated with dentistry is a dark one.[146] Therefore, it is advised to avoid as much exposure to chlorine and fluoride, while making sure you get adequate amounts of iodine from organic sources.

The body has four ways to get rid of toxins - through urine, feces, breath and the skin. The skin is the main sensory organ of the body. It is critical to exercise and sweat. Sweating within 5-10 minutes of exercising is highly recommended. By sweating your body will be able to start ridding itself of toxins. Many people are chronically dehydrated, are constipated and don't sweat. As a result, toxins begin to accumulate in the body, which leads to inflammation and chronic disease. Drink plenty of water, make sure you are moving your bowels 1-2 times per day and sweat at least 3-5 times per week with a good form of exercise.

Professors from the University of Toronto have compiled and analyzed over 26 years worth of scientific research concluding that even moderate levels of physical activity—like walking for 20-30 minutes a day—can ward off depression in people of all ages.[147] The whole point is to find something you love and do it consistently. Other people will help you be more accountable if you play group sports or participate in group activities. The whole point is to get moving. Move, even if you don't feel like it. If you watch an hour or two of television at night, do so with an exercise bike in front of the television. The bottom line is that exercise makes people feel good.[148] Health is a collection of habits, the right habits, done consistently, for the rest of your life, including exercise.

Summary

Depression is a huge problem plaguing many people in the world today. The pharmaceutical model of taking a drug to heal is not what is going to cure people of depression, anxiety or other chronic health problems. The root of most chronic health problems boils down to three things – nutritional deficiencies, environmental toxins, and negative emotions (stress). It just makes logical sense that we cannot continue to expose our bodies to hundreds of toxic chemicals and metals day after day and not expect to suffer the consequences in the future. Children are suffering even more chronic health problems today as well because of the toxins and deficiencies they inherit from unhealthy parents. In other words, we are seeing children get sick much earlier in life. The bank account of health that their parents had is empty and kids are inheriting big health debts today.

People will not be able to heal if they are not eating adequate amounts of nutrients. People know they should eat well, but as we have seen, much of what is consumed and deemed to be healthy is actually very toxic. People also know they should exercise. Yet, people continue to do things they know are not healthy for them. Even after you have read these last chapters, will you completely stop consuming dairy, wheat, sugar, soy, corn, fried food, eggs, pork and alcohol? Will you really be convinced at how horrible these foods are and the damage they are causing in the health of the world today? Will you buy organic skin care products and stop polluting your skin? Will you drink clean filtered water? Will you stop buying bottled water and wasting plastic? Will you find an activity you love to do and consistently exercise? Will you start taking good quality organic whole food supplements to start giving your body a chance to heal? Will you detoxify your life and cleanse your physical body in order to heal from depression and anxiety?

Many people in the world have a good idea about what they should and should not do in life to be healthy. These last couple chapters should have made this much clearer. Yet, will simply knowing this information really make a difference? Will this information motivate you to implement habits to transform your life? Those dying from lung cancer often continue to smoke. Those who are obese are told by their doctors that they need to exercise but still do not. Those addicted to sugar will continue to eat sugar even though they know it is damaging their health.

People transform their lives only through changes in consciousness or being. Consciousness deals with how things are transformed in our life and where real changes get made. Consciousness involves the very core of our being. Consciousness is the container for all our ways of being. Being or consciousness is the sum total of the positive and negative emotions that you hold within. Emotions are our ways of being. You can BE happy or you can BE sad. You can BE afraid or you can BE courageous. Love, joy and peace are states of being that already define who we are and we have access to these states of being at any time, whether we realize it or not.

Human beings learn ways of being and then much of life becomes about repeating these ways of being, even if they hurt or harm us. People may try a diet for a period of time, which works, but then they fall off the proverbial wagon and they go back to old ways of being. People might exercise for certain periods of time only to fall back into old ways of being that created the problem they have in the first place. This is what is meant by ways of being. Where do these patterns or ways of being come from? How do we really transform our ways of being so that we can live life with power and freedom? Emotions or ways of being are what dictate whether we will have lasting or momentary changes in our lives. Transformation and lasting change only happens when we have a change of being, when we surrender in part or whole the emotions that drive us to behave the way we do and maintain our habits. Lasting change comes from the surrender or letting go of the ways of being or emotions that have created the problems we have. When we learn how to surrender our emotions, we give space to have the power to create anything we want in our lives, including freedom from depression.

The third cause of depression and any other chronic health problem is negative emotions (stress) or negative ways of being. The rest of this book is dedicated to exploring how we can transform our consciousness and let go of the negative emotions causing us to be depressed. Once we do this, we can be free from the constraints of our emotions and our past.

PART 2
THE KEY ROLE OF EMOTIONS IN LIFE

4 WE ALL WANT TO FEEL GOOD

"Mental pain is less dramatic than physical pain, but it is more common and also harder to bear. The frequent attempt to conceal mental pain increases the burden: it is easier to say "My tooth is aching" than to say "My heart is broken." - C.S. Lewis, The Problem of Pain

Like the other 39 million people in the USA who suffer under the heavy weight of depression and to the many millions more who suffer and have never sought treatment, answers do exist. It is possible to heal fully. Not only is it possible, but with courage and determination, you can heal in a short period of time.

For 11 long, arduous, and soul-sucking years, I was constantly pushed to the brink of not wanting to suffer and live another day. Not wanting to live was one of the most frequent thoughts I had on a daily basis. I was severely depressed. The world was dark. I felt completely alone. My soul suffered under the agony of what I was feeling. I didn't understand why. I did everything I was "supposed" to do. I went to doctors, took medications, went to therapy, read hundreds of books about healing and pleaded, begged, and prayed to God for answers, but I found none. I gave up after four or five years, basically feeling that I was never going to find answers. I felt dead inside; little hope remained.

That was until I discovered how depression is seen through the eyes of Chinese medicine combined with modern mindfulness tools. For thousands of years, the Chinese have brilliantly understood what ails the body. When Chinese medicine is combined with a modern understanding of how the mind operates, things began to make sense for me. The solutions existed to heal and, when used, 11 years of depression instantly came to an end. Clinically, I have seen this work for many others as well.

The root of depression is not a chemical imbalance as we have been led to believe. The ultimate answer will never be found in a pill, supplement, or a drug. On the physical level, I am convinced, along with many others in the natural healing world, that depression is an inflammation issue. The brain and body are agitated from eating foods that are destroying and killing us. The foods that are killing us are the most commonly consumed foods in the USA today. If you change your diet to include massive amounts of anti-inflammatory foods and cut out all the inflammatory ones, many people experience healing just by doing this. Let me be clear, a drug will never be a sustainable source of happiness, nor will it fix your diet or the inflammatory foods you consume. Diet is so important in the healing process, and has been an integral part of my healing. But, in my opinion, diet is not the ultimate root of depression either.

The key to healing from depression is in releasing negative emotions. It is learning to deal mindfully with present stress we experience and letting go of past pain and wounds that we have suffered. Emotions are the key to being free from depression. Simultaneously, the emotions we carry within are also the primary cause of depression. Your emotional state can instantly change your brain chemistry, in either helpful or destructive ways. It is both the cause and the cure. Most people, including me, didn't realize that something so simple was the answer. When negative emotions release from the body, they instantly are replaced by more positive ones. An even higher understanding of this is that, at the heart of your being, you already are love, joy, and peace and letting go of negative emotions simply allows what you already are to shine forth. The process of releasing negative emotions from the body has gained ground all over the world. It is the basis of this book and was how I healed from 11 years of heavy, suicidal depression.

Anyone Can Heal From Depression

If I had to summarize in one succinct statement what people truly want when they come to me for the treatment of depression, other health issues, or even about life in general, it would be this: People just want to *feel* good.

The power to feel better is an ability that you already have, have always had, and will always have. The only thing that is left to do is unlock this ability, which you were innately born with. Sadly, most people are unaware of how to do this and are continually being held captive to their own emotions. Even after a master's degree in theology, counseling, and psychology, I had never been taught, nor had even heard, that my own emotions were the problem as to why I was feeling depressed. I had no idea how to let them go. I learned to share about how horrible I felt with anyone who would listen, both in a professional setting, and also with family and friends. But talking about how badly we feel is not the same as letting go and surrendering. Most of us don't let our emotions go, we just simply learn to stuff them deep inside. Learning to let emotions go is simple and it is the most powerful way to heal.

All of life boils down to one primal element; we all just want to *feel* good or at least better than we do now. If we stop and think about it, almost everything in life is motivated by emotion. The currency of all of life is emotion. Emotion gives meaning to absolutely everything in our lives. Life would be robotic, static, flavorless, and mechanistic without emotion.

Emotion hits us from the moment we wake up in the morning. How do you *feel* when you hear the alarm clock sound? Do you *feel irritated* that you have to get up?

Do you *feel resentful* when you hear that all too familiar ringtone that wakes you up? Are you *sad* that you don't have more time to sleep? Does the air *feel cold* when you pull the sheets back? Do you *feel exhausted* when you wake up because you had insomnia the night before? Do you *feel tired?* Are you immediately *feeling stressed or anxious* thinking of the responsibilities that the day will bring?

On the flip side, do you *feel excited* because life has so much potential and purpose that you can't wait to see what the day will bring? Do you *feel hopeful* that something great will happen today? Do you *feel contentment, love,* and *joy* when you awake in the morning? Do you feel deeply *committed, purposeful,* and *dedicated* to the person you wake up next to every morning? Do you feel *comfort* when you smell that fresh pot of coffee that is percolating while you are still in bed?

These examples are a diverse range of the raw and powerful emotions, both negative and positive, that we all have the potential of feeling within the first three minutes of every day. The rest of the day holds the same or even greater potential to feel a plethora of different emotions. We all want to feel good, not only momentarily, but also sustainably at all times. Feeling good, centered around experiencing love, is the true state of the heart. Emotions and their subjective expressions, feelings, are the foundation of how we experience all of life. We interpret everything that happens to us in life through the filter of these feelings. Everything we do at the heart and center of our lives was generated because of a feeling or multiple feelings. Feelings are what motivate us to do or not to do almost everything in life.

On the most simple and basic level, we divide emotions and feelings into two camps: positive and negative. It is interesting to note that we largely define our lives by the experiences we have that carry the most negative or positive emotions in them. These are the mountains and valleys of our lives. It is these experiences and the filter of our emotions that are at the heart and center of why we are the way we are and why we have the life we have. The sum total of our emotions indicates how we will show up in every experience. For example, if you have many life experiences from the past that hold worthlessness, you might have a tendency to show up in certain situations with defensiveness and anger in an attempt to protect yourself from the wounds of worthlessness you carry. These emotional experiences, both positive and negative, are the heaviest contributors to our programming in life. Therefore, what are some of the most common experiences in life that we have that have either generated massive amounts of positive or negative emotions that have radically shaped our world, influenced our behavior and have brought us where we are in life today?

"Depression is the most unpleasant thing I have ever experienced. . . . It is that absence of being able to envisage that you will ever be cheerful again. It is the absence of hope. That very deadened feeling, which is so very different from feeling sad. Sad hurts but it's a healthy feeling. It is a necessary thing to feel. Depression is very different."

- J.K. Rowling

The Mountains of Our Lives

Let's consider a sample of the wide range of both positive and negative experiences for a moment.

We buy or adopt a dog because the love it constantly gives us feels good. We feel many wonderful feelings when we arrive home after a long day of work to be greeted by the excitedly wagging tail and joy on our dog's face when he sees us. Our hearts melt for a few seconds as we embrace our precious pet and rustle the fur on its face. The world disappears for a few brief moments. Dogs, unlike humans, just offer us excitement and love. They are amazing. This feels good.

We feel good when we buy things. Do you feel good when you buy a new pair of shoes, a new dress, special cologne, or a new car? And when we wear that new article of clothing and people notice and compliment us, it feels good, really good. We feel special, important and noticed. Those things feel good.

What about the moment that you held your first born child in your arms for the first time? Many have called this feeling "indescribable." The joy is too inexpressible for words. This feels good.

How does it feel eating chicken wings, drinking beer, and watching your favorite sports team win by one point in double overtime? This feels good.

Think about the time you had your first kiss. Perhaps this was a feeling like none you had felt before. It awakened a feeling in you like never before. The passion as it streamed through your veins, the anxious exciting anticipation, and the warmth and softness of another's lips on yours can be otherworldly. The feeling of knowing that someone desires you and you desire them is amazing. Being cherished and desired feels good.

Many have described getting married as one of the happiest days, if not *the* happiest, of their life. All of your closest family and friends gathered to celebrate this sacred union. It is just one huge wave of positive emotion. Getting married, for most, is exciting and feels good.

The sand crinkles beneath your feet. It is warm and feels like a fine white powder that sifts gracefully between your toes grounding you to the earth. Your pores absorb every ray of light from the sun, almost feeling like you are profoundly nourishing a part of your soul. As you lie there with a margarita (or whatever your drink of choice is), you breathe in the salty pure ocean air. You take a few deep slow breaths as your body sinks into the beach chair. This experience is what you have looked forward to for six months, a reprieve from work and the world. After the beach chair molds itself to your body, you pick up an engaging book that takes your mind and imagination to creative, playful spaces. Vacation and the beach feel good.

You daydream back to the moment of your life when the person you love exposed their heart, soul and physical flesh to you and you to them for the first time.

The pure bliss of lovemaking, passionate embraces, rich, colorful kisses all over and the waves of ecstasy that washed over you as you felt the ripping power of orgasmic pleasure. The world melted away. In these moments, the past and future disappear because the sheer pleasure of the moment brings every fiber of your consciousness into the present moment. You and the one you love merge into the oneness of divinity, the lines of self become blurry, and you feel deeply connected. This feels so good.

These are the moments that most of us live for, desire, and covet because we all just want to FEEL good. Feeling good brings life to our bones and health to our bodies. We largely define our lives by the moments, experiences and people that we associate with feeling good. We tell others the stories of our lives by the things that have made us feel good. Who doesn't like to hear a good, heartfelt story? We plan our lives loosely on the next experience that will stir up these good feelings within us. We are all in one way or another after the pursuit of pleasure because pleasure feels good.

In the richest sense, this isn't a narcissistic pursuit of pleasure; it goes far beyond that. We are hardwired to go beyond simply feeling good just for a moment. We are made to transcend feelings altogether to enter the highest states of being of love, joy, and peace. At the pinnacle of emotion lies these states of being that transcend even the richest of feelings. In these states of love, joy, and peace, the world could be collapsing around us, but we are immovable because of this inward strength and awareness we now have. Life is a progression of movement towards these states whether one realizes it or not.

The Valleys of Our Lives

What about the things in our lives that don't feel good? What about the most painful memories and experiences that we have experienced? How do these experiences shape our lives, affect who we are and leave an imprint in our world that greatly impacts us, often for the rest of our lives? What are the far-reaching consequences of such events in our lives? Just as we consider the things that make us feel good, let's consider for a moment the things that do not feel so good in life.

A Broken Heart

Do you remember the first time that your heart was broken into a thousand pieces? Do you remember the overwhelming sense of grief you felt over losing the one person you thought you were going to spend the rest of your life with? The emotional (and perhaps physical) pain that you experienced was almost unbearable—your heart breaking in two. The endless days or months of tears that streamed from your face that seemed to go on forever. Perhaps you were so angry at yourself, the other person or even God for allowing this to happen to you. Perhaps a whole range of fears swept over you, the fear of not being good enough, the fear that you may never find another person like him/her, or the fear that you are not lovable or don't deserve true love. When we break up with someone that we invested our lives in, it feels awful, gut-wrenching, and supremely painful. This does not feel good.

Growing up Without a Mother or Father

Did you grow up never knowing a father or a mother? Did it feel like you have always existed in life with this massive void that was never filled by a father or mother? Or maybe you were adopted, and you have lived with feelings of rejection your entire life? Why didn't they want you? Why didn't they stay? Why don't they want to be a part of my life now? The fear of rejection, betrayal, resentment, and hurt don't feel good.

Failure

Have you ever wanted to achieve something so badly in life and just as you were on the verge of getting it, it just slipped right through your fingers? Perhaps it was the promotion you didn't get or losing the championship game, or not winning the competition you had dedicated your life to? Often we are flooded with feelings of failure and defeat. We call ourselves a failure and from that moment on we struggle to recover and continue to live defeated. Failure and defeat don't feel good.

The Struggle to Lose Weight

Ever since you can remember, you may have always had a weight problem. Just feeling the extra weight around your body does not feel good. The judgmental looks of other people you see in public crush you every day. You feel terrible every time you get out of the shower and see yourself naked. Perhaps you shower in the dark every day just so you don't have to see yourself. You feel numb. You feel like a loser. You are afraid, so you protect yourself emotionally, adding weight to your body over the years. You have tried every diet and exercise program on the planet, yet nothing seems to work. People say, "You just have to eat the right things and do the right exercise or try harder," but it never seems to work for you. You feel hopeless and helpless to do anything about it. This does not feel good.

Physical, Sexual, and Verbal Abuse

Were you abused physically or sexually as a child or teenager? Abuse is much more common than we think it is and, when it happens, the effects are profound. You carry the trauma into the present moment and how this impacted you at such a fragile age. You project these feelings into everyone and every situation without even knowing it. You live every present moment in pain. You go into adulthood carrying loads of shame, guilt, and fear. You feel ashamed to tell anyone. You feel guilty and tell yourself in some twisted way that you must have deserved it. You feel afraid to have a relationship with anyone out of fear that they won't accept who you are or what has happened to you. This does not feel good.

The Pain of Addiction

Have you lived your life with an addiction? The emotions are often too painful and too numerous to mention—considering how it has affected you, your loved ones, and everyone around you. Certain addictions have massive societal and personal consequences; others are more subtle. Having an addiction on a personal level is like an emotional hell. You feel guilty you acted out, you feel lustful to get whatever fuels the addiction, you feel angry with yourself for having it, and you feel remorseful for all of the damage you may be doing to yourself or others. You want to stop, but you don't feel like you have the inner resources to do so. So it keeps destroying you slowly, painfully, and deliberately. This does not feel good.

Living Paycheck to Paycheck

How do you feel about not having any money, living paycheck to paycheck or about pursuing money or things as the goal of your life? How do you emotionally relate to money? Does it control you? Do you not have enough and hate that you have to work like a dog to pay your bills every month? Do you feel depressed when you look at your bank account after paying all your bills at the end of the month? Do you feel fear, worthlessness and anger when debt collectors hound you? Not having enough money does not feel good.

Health Problems

If you have a disease or a health problem, the way that you know something is wrong with you is because somewhere in your body you don't *feel* good. A symptom is your body's way of telling you something is off and needs attention. A collective set of symptoms/feelings is called a disease. Those collective symptoms do not feel good; they feel bad. Disease does not feel good.

What other kinds of experiences in your life have you gone through, that you can look back on and know, beyond a shadow of a doubt, that these experiences or events radically and forever changed you and how you currently relate to the world and others? How much do these events continue to haunt you and affect you emotionally even now? Every experience we have in life is filtered through a lens of how something impacted us emotionally. Every present experience we have in life is also fueled, influenced, or in many cases controlled by the negative emotions we have stored within us from these past experiences. The experiences in life that are the most negative often have the most crushing and long-lasting effects on how we experience life from that moment forward. These events have programmed our present moment relationally, financially, or even physically in the form of health problems. Those emotions mold and shape who we are, what we think, and who we perceive ourselves to be. Negative and positive emotions color, influence, and shape our whole lives.

Feelings Force Us to Pay Attention

Feelings force us to pay attention to our lives. Feelings force us to be aware even if we choose not to be. If we ignore the feelings we have in our lives, the effects can be catastrophic, leading to full-blown, life-threatening health problems or disease. If we numb our feelings with pharmaceutical drugs or recreational drugs, we miss what our bodies are trying to tell us to get us to grow and heal physically, emotionally, and spiritually. Symptoms in the physical body are our teachers if we know how to heed and interpret them.

If we fail to pay attention to the recurring emotions we have in our relationships, we may fail to see what patterns of relating exist within us that may be causing our relational problems. Instead, we just go on blaming our partners and not seeing our contribution to the problem. If we never explore the deepest and darkest memories we have in life and continue to let that negative emotional energy run things from behind the scenes; we may never grow the way we are designed to grow. Instead, we become sicker and feel even worse. In the most ancient of Chinese texts, we learn that emotions are the principal cause of most physical symptoms and disease.

Western medicine is slowly catching up to this as can be seen in the brilliant book *The Body Keeps the Score* by Bessel Van der Kolk, MD.[149] The truth is emotions and feelings are the context of life itself and how it is experienced in every moment.

Narcissism Or Divine Programming?

Seeking positive emotional experiences is not just a narcissistic pursuit of pleasure. While feeling good in the moment is what many people live for, something much more profound and deep within us longs for us to experience love, joy, and peace at all times. What if it were possible to feel love, joy, or peace at ALL times in spite of what is happening to you in the world? What if such a profound change happened inside of you so that outside circumstances didn't affect you as much anymore? Is it possible to experience life from such a perspective, even if unpleasant things you perceive as negative are going on around you?

The love and peace you already carry within can project itself out into the world through you, rather than the world projecting itself into and affecting you. The point of feeling good is missed by many because the ramifications are much deeper than most think. The things that truly feel the best are actually beyond feeling. Instead, they are states of being. Beingness is what you already are. You already are love, joy, peace, forgiveness, and healing. As you learn to let go and surrender you simply uncover your true state. Therefore, you don't have to try to be anything if you already are that. There is nowhere to go and the peace you seek is already a present state of reality. You "become" peace because you always have been and will always be at peace. Identity never changes. You simply fall in line with or begin to recognize your true state.

How does one experience love, joy, or peace as a state of being? Is it possible to experience the world this way? As you progressively surrender negative emotions, your inner beingness begins to express itself more and more in and through you. Love and peace, as a prevailing state of consciousness, are experienced completely by few people in the world today. However, it is becoming increasingly more common as the total consciousness on the planet continues to grow, deepen, and evolve.

It is not only possible to change our emotional makeup, but it is the number one factor influencing how we grow, evolve, and thrive. A pathway exists to guide us inward, changing our inner world so that what comes out of us are increasing levels of love, joy, and peace. We can become love, joy, and peace and experience these states of being in the world. Divine Grace can only initiate these states of being. It happens to very few people, which is why many people think it's not possible.

As a word of note: throughout this book, when a normally un-capitalized word is capitalized (like "Divine Grace," above) it's to distinguish its deeper, inner, spiritual, or divine use from its regular use.

Going Beyond Even Positive Emotions Into States Of Being

The consciousness and spirit of every human being were created to experience these states of being. Those spiritual leaders, saints, and avatars across time, known and unknown, are examples of this. It is being so filled with Divinity from within that all that comes out of you is divine as an expression of your being. This full expression of divinity within is the end of "emotionality" and the beginning of fully experiencing the presence of God within. The pleasure of feeling is surpassed into Beingness and spiritual ecstasy wrapped up in the expression of consciousness as Beingness itself. It is the perpetual state of the full subjective experience of Divinity. It is literally heaven on earth or the kingdom shining forth from within.

In my years of helping people to heal, the one thing I see that is by far the largest contributor to why people have health problems and diseases is due to stored negative emotions and feelings from the past. It doesn't matter if someone has simple arm pain or cancer, an emotional root normally exists that is imperative to understand and release to properly and fully heal. It is also observed that the people who have the most health problems are often those who have been consumed by and continue to hold onto a lifetime of negative emotions. They also have the toughest time knowing how they experience their emotions and feelings within their physical bodies. They are disconnected or disassociated from themselves. Conversely, when negative emotions and feelings are understood and then released from the body, great amounts of physical healing and internal connectedness can occur.

Years of clinical experience and seeing firsthand the incredible effects the release of emotion has profoundly changed how I see healing. Yet, this is often the most neglected, misunderstood, and least explored area of health. It happens to be the most profound area of health that can help someone to heal. Mentioning this comes from 11 years of personal struggle in overcoming the heavy weight of serious depression after having looked everywhere for answers.

The Role Of Chinese Medicine To Heal Emotion

Chinese medicine is the most profound natural system of healing that we have ever had on this planet. It also happens to be far less mystical than previously thought and its foundations are based upon ironclad science. In these systems of medicine, and as written about in the classical pillars of medical texts generated by this incredible medical tradition thousands of years ago, we find it mentioning how emotion is at the heart and center of the disease process. Additionally, we now have scientifically proven ways to show how one can release and let go of negative emotional energy from the body, thereby facilitating the healing process.

Combining this ancient (and still just as valid) system of medicine with modern consciousness practices helps millions to heal their bodies physically, mentally, emotionally, and spiritually. Emotional healing is spiritual healing; they are one and the same. There is no difference. True internal healing is only activated by God, whether we realize it or acknowledge it because higher states of being (love, joy, and peace) are the very character of God, divinity itself. Only the Author of Peace can bring us peace. Emotional healing brings about physical healing, sometimes very quickly.

After 11 years of struggle, reading hundreds of books in order to understand myself, and having countless conversations with professionals, doctors, pastors, and friends—none of which got me very far—I was led into the world of Chinese medicine where I learned that my stored emotions were the source of my problem. It was in this medicine that I found answers. When the awareness came after 11 long years of looking for answers, that my emotions themselves were the cause of my depression, it changed my whole life. Then, when I let go of the negative emotions and experiences that were fueling the depression, it was lifted almost instantly.

Even after a master's degree in counseling, psychology, and theology and reading hundreds of books on therapy and change, it did nothing to alter how I was feeling.

I have discovered that most people also feel like they are at the mercy of their feelings. Both positive and negative experiences just seem to happen to us, rather than us making them happen. My emotions controlled me. Do they control you? What if instead of being at the mercy of our emotions, we could learn to let go of what we were experiencing at any time and experience a feeling of well-being whenever we wanted? It is not only possible but completely doable. Very specific tools that are explained in this book can facilitate this inner emotional transformation.

Clinically, we explore the main negative emotions and memories fueling someone's health problem. Another way to refer to this is the "consciousness" of the health problem. The consciousness of a problem refers to its associated emotions, thoughts and belief systems. After identifying these things, they are released using different tools so that healing can occur. It is quite simple, as healing should be simple on some level and not overly complicated.

What I have found is that while focusing on emotions and letting them go may not be the answer for everyone, it is usually a substantial part of almost everyone's deep healing journey. This book is dedicated to that end. It is to help you understand depression, how to change this reality, so that you can heal and experience radical life-changing transformation. Since emotion is the substrate and foundation of how we experience all of life, it is invaluable to understand how we experience our emotions, how they affect us, and how to release negative ones from the physical body.

Question Everything About Depression

The following questions will be answered in order to explain how this process works:

- How much of an impact do emotions have in our lives?
- Where do the most negative emotions come from in our lives?
- How do different negative emotions manifest into disease and health problems?
- Where does the theory of emotions causing disease come from?
- Is there a tool which can help to identify our emotions and also to help us when those emotions have left the body?
- What tool(s) is/are used to help let go of unwanted negative emotional energy?
- Can letting go of negative emotions help me to grow spiritually?
- How is life experienced when we stop identifying with our mind and emotions?
- What are the amazing benefits of letting go of negative emotions?

If you understand the tools in this book, and if you do the exercises that are recommended, and use the information presented here, your life will open into the possibility of powerful transformation. But you won't just feel good; you will experience a transformation of your consciousness that is constant and enduring, which will positively affect everything in your life.

Releasing negative emotion has the potential to positively affect your relationships, health, job and ultimate path in life. For me and many others, this process has meant an explosion of personal and spiritual growth, well-being, change, and a much deeper sense of self-love and connection to God. Additionally, if you have health problems, you may start healing as a result of using this information. But regardless of whether you want to heal physically or simply just grow and evolve as a human being, the pathway presented here can be very powerful. We all have our own unique path to healing physically and emotionally. My hope and prayer is that the contents of this book will give you the tools you'll need to heal.

A very wise Eastern teacher once said, "The purpose of life is to find your purpose." If you do not know what your purpose is, dedicate your life to releasing every negative emotion that arises in you as you experience it and in due time, your purpose will become very clear.

5 EMOTIONS CONNECT EVERYTHING

"People who seek psychotherapy for psychological, behavioral, or relationship problems tend to experience a wide range of bodily complaints...The body can express emotional issues a person may have difficulty processing consciously...I believe that the vast majority of people don't recognize what their bodies are telling them. The way I see it, our emotions are music, and our bodies are instruments that play the discordant tunes. But if we don't know how to read music, we just think the instrument is defective." —Charlette Mikulka

Imagine for a moment you are in a court of law, and you are being questioned by a prosecutor in front of a jury and judge about your reaction to a disagreement you had with a coworker.

She asks you, "How did you feel about John stealing your donuts from the refrigerator?"

You reply, "I felt angry!"

"How did you know you felt angry?" she rebuts quickly.

Upon hearing her question, you freeze and look at her like a deer caught in the headlights. After thinking about it, you respond, "I don't know how I felt angry, I just was!"

"We need evidence! How do we know you were angry if you can't tell us how you knew that you were angry? Why should we believe you?"

While this is a simple and playful illustration of the nature of emotion, its message is a powerful one. In the last two chapters, we talked about how emotions are the substrate of our entire experience in life. They are the color of our entire life. However, if we try to nail it down, many do not actually know how they experience their emotions.

So how do you experience your emotions?

As in the example above, all of us have felt anger. Some feel it more than others, and some in more powerful ways, as is the case with rage or fury. But we all know the emotion of anger. Other than just knowing we are angry, most of us are not intimately familiar with how we are experiencing anger in the physical body. How do you know you are angry? What does it actually feel like in your body? How do you experience it? Where does the root of your anger come from? Understanding all of these things composes a full awareness of the emotion we are experiencing in the moment.

"An emotion does not cause pain. Resistance or suppression of emotion causes pain." - Frederick Dodson, *Parallel Universe of Self*

What Is Emotion?

When I ask people in the clinic what an emotion is, most of the time the answer I get is that it is a feeling. They're usually stumped by the follow up question - "What then is a feeling?" A feeling is something that you have to feel. Therefore, it is a physical sensation or sensory stimulus that is experienced in the physical body. Feelings are the conscious subjective experience of our objective emotion. Physical sensation is the awareness or perception of a particular emotional stimulus.

If someone comes to me and says "I want to work on my lower back pain," we start with how they know that it is a problem in the first place. How do you know that there is a problem in their lower back? Simply put, one knows it is a problem because one is feeling it. How exactly does this "pain" feel though? Pain in the lower back could be described in terms of a sensation as being weakness, tiredness, heaviness, dullness, sharpness, cramping, constant, achy, etc. The way one is experiencing the feeling is often very important in helping to understand what the pain means and how to let it go.

When people are asked how anger feels, upon actually noticing it for the first time, they may say it is like a *heat* in the head, a *pressure* in one part of the head, a *tension* in the neck or shoulders, their eyes *bulging* out of the sockets, *crushing, pounding,* etc. While certain emotions carry commonalities, they can be experienced subjectively very differently from one person to another. Every emotion is experienced uniquely by everyone. Having an awareness of how one is experiencing themselves and their emotions is a very powerful step towards further self-awareness and emotional/spiritual growth.

Many people have described fear (or anything related to fear) as being experienced in the chest. Fear felt here is significant because the chest is the place of the 4th chakra, which is associated with our heart, thymus gland and with how we experience love or lack thereof. Fear is the antithesis to love which is why many experience much of their fears, anxieties, and worries in their chest. Fear can be experienced as tightness, constriction, pressure, heart racing, or gasping feeling.

Emotions can be experienced anywhere in the body. I was processing through a memory once with someone who was publically speaking in front of others. This person came into the clinic with extreme social anxiety and almost never left the house. The anxiety was rooted in an experience speaking in front of a large group of people. It was disastrous. He had a lapse of memory and his mind went blank. He froze. I asked, "What are you feeling now?" and he responded, "my feet are ice cold right now." His fear literally manifested in his body as cold feet.

We can recreate the past in the present moment because the present is the past. For example, if we went through a painful memory involving abandonment as a child, we may unconsciously recreate the past by living in fear about how others will abandon us in some way. Our memories are always with us in the present moment and are happening to us always as now. We worked through the fear or ice cold feeling that he had in his feet and the rest of the memory dramatically lessened in severity as did his fear of speaking in public.

We even have phrases in society for things like this that are a common experience for many. A common phrase that is used in the context of speaking in front of others, performing in some way or in getting married is, "Don't get cold feet!" This is typically interpreted as "Don't get so afraid that you don't go through with it." These expressions have a basis in physical reality for how we experience our emotions. We don't get cold feet when we feel love, but when we are in a state of fear. "Getting cold feet" is a way of saying that you are feeling fear or a subset of fear such as panic, nervousness, anxiety, insecurity, etc. In this case, it is how we experience our fear when speaking or performing or having to go through with something. Having cold feet is the subjective physical sensation of the emotion of fear.

How do the other emotions feel? How do you experience them? How are they experienced inside of your memories?

Every emotion has a unique feel to it. When we stop resisting the negative feelings we have and allow ourselves to experience them, in due time the energy behind the feeling eventually runs out. This is the process of surrendering the emotion. This is the pathway towards inner growth and the awakening of God or Self within us. The Self, with a capital "S," is the very core of our being, our spirit. It is the essence of who and what we are. The Kingdom of Heaven is within, as the essence of our very being, and the only thing that is not allowing it to burst forth from within us is our inward resistance to it. We continually resist love without even realizing it by holding onto our negative emotions.

"Emotional Intelligence is a way of recognizing, understanding, and choosing how we think, feel, and act. It shapes our interactions with others and our understanding of ourselves. It defines how and what we learn; it allows us to set priorities; it determines the majority of our daily actions. Research suggests it is responsible for as much as 80% of the success in our lives."
- Adele Lynn, Emotional Intelligence Activity Book

What Keeps Us From Experiencing Our True Self?

In short, the answer to this question is ego. The ego is anything that keeps the blinders on and continues to perpetuate our embracing of reality as it is. Our inner resistance is commonly referred to as our ego, or sinful nature (in the Christian tradition). The ego is the expression of being that arises out of our negative emotions. In the health world, there is a common phrase we use that states, "Whatever you resist, persists." For example, as long as you hold onto or resist the fear you have about speaking in public, it will be a fearful experience every time you do it. Your resistance to the fear and the fear inside you are the very source and cause of the problem that you have about speaking in public in the first place. How would speaking in public be experienced if the fears were surrendered? You might like it or derive an inner sense of purpose and satisfaction from it.

What Do Most Of Us Do With Our Emotions?

When people experience trauma or an event that causes one to feel heavy negative emotions, it is usually handled in one of three ways as a coping mechanism to deal with the pain of these emotions.

Repression

Repression is unconsciously holding onto negative emotional energy and not even realizing that we are doing it. It is especially done with memories that we had many years ago. Memories from years past are like the man behind the curtain in the Wizard of Oz, running the show, but we can only see the show and not who is running it! We don't realize that the event that made us so angry 30 years ago is still affecting us just as powerfully today as it did the day it happened, yet we are unconsciously unaware of it.

Suppression

Suppression is *consciously* pushing away negative emotions. We are aware that we are angry and fearful, but we just try to get through something by pushing the emotions down enough so that they are not perceived as a nuisance for us. The irony is that the suppression of negative emotions often is the catalyst that orchestrates experiences in the present that bring these emotions out for us. This is ignoring and learning to live with the proverbial elephant in the room. At times in the clinic, I will ask patients to put their hand out in front of them to give me a "high-five" connecting their hand with mine. I begin pushing and ask them to resist my pressure. As they continue to resist my pressure, their arm will soon begin to manifest this resistance with a symptom in the arm. After a while, the arm will get tired, weak, shaky, or even painful if the resistance continues.

To relieve the tiredness of the arm, all one has to do is stop resisting or welcome my pressure. When they stop pushing against my arm, tiredness, weakness, or pain in the arm goes away. The symptoms, which are the resistance to the pressure, are able to vanish quickly. Likewise, when we are resisting our negative emotions, they can eventually be expressed as a symptom(s) to point us in the direction of what we are resisting or holding onto. It takes a lot of energy to suppress energy. This may be why people are so fatigued these days. The sprouting up of a physical symptom points us in the direction of what is being suppressed.

Escape

Escape is the "go to" for most people. Escape offers a temporary reprieve and elevates our consciousness temporarily or artificially. The reason we all try to escape from time to time is simply because we all just want to feel better. But feeling better is misplaced into temporary escape rather than surrender. We do this every day. We wake up in the morning, and we are an absolute bear until we have our morning coffee. Without it, the "hurricane" will plow through the office that morning. Escape takes so many forms for people in the world today. How else do we escape?

We just want to feel connected, so we momentarily connect with porn to experience the powerful hormones and chemicals such an experience provokes. You work 80 hours a week and become a workaholic to avoid being a terrible father and husband at home. Work gives you the reward of making money and achieving, and it feels good so we pursue it at the expense of our family. You drain a fifth of vodka every night to numb the painful past feelings for a while, only to have them come back with a vengeance the next day, along with a terrible hangover, which doesn't feel good. Or you simply sit and watch television every night, so you can divert attention away from the flood of feelings that you would rather not feel inside when your day finally slows down.

Escaping also comes in many forms such as addiction to sugar, certain foods, alcohol, drugs, cigarettes, approval, or sex. Strangely, it is somewhat positive because it is the very mechanism that points you in the direction of what you are escaping from. If you crave sugar during the day, ask yourself what sugar gives you. You may say, "It makes me feel warm and sweet." Therefore, what in your life is cold and lacks sweetness? "The day my husband died, life became cold and lost its sweetness." Life isn't cold or sour; this is simply *your* inner positionality and projection about it out into your life. The emotions sitting behind the experience of losing a husband of 40 years are loneliness, fear, anger, sadness, and many possible others. You don't have to hold onto those emotions. Would you prefer to continue suffering or would you rather let go of the emotions and be free? All they are doing is causing you to suffer. This is not how God designed us to live. Your addiction can be surrendered when you let go of the underlying emotional context that led to it in the first place.

Emotion, which is suffering, ceases to be suffering as soon as we have a clear picture of it and release it." —Benedict Spinoza

How Do Thoughts Or Affirmations Play A Role In This?

Thoughts are the endless content being fueled by the context of our emotions. Thoughts are engendered from emotions. Trying to change thoughts is almost pointless like trying to grasp the wind. You can say, "I think I can! I think I can! I think I can!" all you want, but if the underlying fear of failure is unchanged within you, doing what you want may prove to be an impossibility. From one emotion hundreds or even thousands of thoughts can arise. Changing thoughts is a big waste of time. But if you let go of an emotion, thousands of thoughts can disappear. Let me give you an example.

A gentleman is sitting in a bar and notices a beautiful woman sitting on the other side of the room. A stirring inside of him is prompting him to want to ask her out. As he thinks about doing it, his mind is bombarded with a ton of different thoughts:

- What if she says no?
- What if she rejects me?
- What if she thinks I'm poorly dressed?
- Did I put on enough deodorant?
- I am not good looking enough for her.
- I am not smart enough for her.
- I am not as successful as her.
- She is way out of my league.
- What will her friends think?
- What will my friends think?
- What do I even say to her?
- Where should we go if she says yes?
- What if I fumble my words and look like an idiot!?
- What if she already has a boyfriend? That will be awkward.

The thoughts we have are almost endless. However, behind every one of these thoughts is one single emotion in this scenario: fear. If you go into the fear by welcoming the physical sensations, memories/pictures, sounds, and smells that are associated with it and let them go, all of the thoughts fueled by the fear will disappear. All the thoughts will be silenced because no fear is fueling them. When no fear is present, with confidence (a positive emotion), you simply walk up to her, say hello, and ask her out. On the inside, you are perfectly ok if she says no and perfectly ok if she says yes. In fact, the likelihood of her going out with you may increase because you are much more congruent on the inside. Confidence is always sexy and attractive. Every woman wants to be with a confident man. Fear is small and constrictive; confidence is large and expansive. Energetically, there is a massive difference in the power sitting behind these two emotions and their expression in our lives.

If she does say no and you are not holding onto the fear of rejection, you won't take it personally. You can tell yourself that it just wasn't meant to be and can go about your business. If you are afraid and stay committed to surrendering the fear, eventually the tide will turn, the scale will tip, and courage will emerge and cause you to act even in spite of the remaining fear you have. In fact, with less fear we begin to see life more clearly because fear is not clouding our mind, judgment, and decisions as it was before. Negative emotions are clouds that fog the mind. Fear prevents us from doing so many things in our lives. By letting go of fear, we give room for courage to expand from within us as a more positive expression of life. Courage is not the absence of fear, but it is doing things in spite of our fears. Beyond courage is acceptance, willingness and love. Love is the absence of fear. But before love comes, courage first moves us to act in spite of our fears. The key to getting more courage is by letting go of your fears or just doing things anyway in spite of our fears!

"Instead of resisting any emotion, the best way to dispel it is to enter it fully, embrace it and see through your resistance." —Deepak Chopra

Content Versus Context

Emotions are the context of life. Context is like the earth beneath us. Content is like the flowers and trees growing from the earth. Most people are so intensely focused on the content of their lives, which is why growth in any area of life may not occur or occur more slowly than it should. Being consciously aware of how we are emotionally experiencing the world will bring to light the context of our existence, which is the most critical aspect of growth and change.

In a counseling scenario a couple comes in because they are having problems. The counselor asks each person to give an account for the basis of their problems. Most of the time, with few exceptions, each person will tell a version of the story which may vilify the behavior of the other person.

The woman may say: "He is so inconsiderate. He always leaves me to do everything around the house!" "He is always watching television and ignoring me!" "He is always working late and we never get to spend time together!"

He might respond: "She does a load of laundry and cooks once per week, and that is doing everything around the house!" "I'm always watching television to get a break from you constantly gossiping about your sister!" "All you do is nag, nag, nag about me working too much, which is why I work even more to get away from you."

From his perspective and hers, this is a conversation 100% based on content. Content is seeing that the other person and their behavior is the problem. We rarely see ourselves as the source of the problem. But it always takes two to tango. And much like dealing with thoughts is pointless, dealing with content only is seldom fruitful in my experience. The context needs to be addressed.

This is getting to the central core of the negative emotions and states of being that are present for each of them. Out of these states of being come the behaviors that are causing problems in their relationship. With curiosity, the following things may arise about context when questioning her.

"How does it make you feel when you do everything around the house?" She responds, "I feel unappreciated, ignored and angry!"

"Why does it appear that you are gossiping about your sister? How do you feel towards your sister?" She laments, "I guess I have just been jealous of her my whole life and secretly want her to fail."

"How do you feel about him working so much?" She responds, "I feel neglected, ignored, worthless, and lonely."

Upon questioning him and his context, we may get the following responses.

How do you feel about her accusing you of not doing anything around the house? He responds, "I feel pestered and inadequate."

Why are you always watching television? He responds, "I feel tired from working so hard and frustrated that she bad mouths her sister all day. I feel lazy and disconnected because I don't want to talk about my day or my feelings!"

How do you feel when your wife nags you? He responds, "I get frustrated, irritated, annoyed, prideful and rebellious!"

In this scenario, is it a bad thing for the husband to consider doing more things around the house, shutting off the television more often and working less? No, of course not. Altering this behavior may be a good thing or a more loving thing to do. Could she stop nagging and gossiping about her sister? Of course. What I have noticed is that people can change behavior in the short run, but if the underlying feelings and how they came into being from the past are not dealt with, long-term change is difficult. Long-term habit forming behavior is driven by emotion and not by thought. How often do habits change in the short run, only to return to the same habits within the next couple months? With each person letting go of their own emotions and the context to those emotions from their pasts, true healing and change can occur.

If the same emotions (context) that are generating the content are not addressed, the content will eventually revert to being the same or very similar. She explores and lets go of feeling unappreciated, ignored, angry, neglected, ignored, worthless, lonely, and jealous. He lets go of feeling pestered, inadequate, tired, frustrated, irritated, annoyed, prideful and rebellious. All of these emotions for each person have a context within their lives, sometimes stretching back deep into childhood. What are the memories for each person that is the original context where these emotions first took real root in their life? This needs to be explored so that we can have the opportunity to let go of each emotion. Context is infinitely more important than content in our relationships. We don't ignore the content, but we must understand and work on altering the context of our lives.

How would the marriage look different if each person took full responsibility for how they were experiencing each other emotionally and letting go of their own negative emotions? We all frequently project and blame others for our emotions. Marriage would look far different because the context fueling the content would be completely different. Changing the context will automatically change the content of the relationship. Both people wouldn't be drawing from the same programming as before. The programming would be different. Both people would be more loving as a result of letting go of their negative emotions. People who are more loving are easier to get along with and relate to. Letting go of the context allows one to alter the content of our lives in a much easier way.

- What negative emotions do you commonly experience within your relationship with your partner?
- What emotional patterns are common in how you experience those that are close to you?
- What are your common triggers?
- Do you find yourself commonly blaming others for how you feel?
- Have you ever stopped and taken full responsibility for your emotions and how you are reacting in a situation?

"When dealing with people, remember you are not dealing with creatures of logic, but with creatures of emotion." —Dale Carnegie

"Our feelings are our most genuine paths to knowledge." —Audre Lorde

The Context Of Emotions At Work

Take a moment and think about how you feel about your boss. Positive things feel good. But what about the negative feelings you have towards him/her. When you let your awareness wander to how you experience your boss emotionally, you may begin to see many emotions that you project upon him/her. Many of us will instantly defend our emotions and say things like:

- "You don't know how horrible my boss is!" (translation: I feel afraid of him)

- "He never listens to me!" (translation: I feel disrespected, unappreciated and undermined).
- "He is always so demanding!" (translation: I feel overwhelmed, angry and guilty for not meeting expectations).
- "She doesn't understand what we go through as employees!" (translation: I feel so irritated and helpless).
- "I can never do anything right for her!" (translation: I feel worthless and not good enough).
- "I get blamed for everything at work!" (translation: I feel ashamed).

The emotions we feel are our full responsibility. We tell ourselves that they are making us feel these things, but we will never heal if we continue to do this. If we continue to blame others for the emotions we experience, we will not grow very much. Taking full responsibility for our emotions is when the magic happens. We are ultimately choosing how we feel regardless if we think we are choosing or not. By owning what we experience, this can be a powerful step towards massive shifts in behavior and initiate internal growth.

> "75% of careers are derailed for reasons related to emotional competencies, including the inability to handle interpersonal problems; unsatisfactory team leadership during times of difficulty or conflict; or inability to adapt to change or elicit trust."
> —The Center for Creative Leadership

My Militant Boss

My second job at the age of 16 was at a restaurant in Grand Rapids, MI called Taco Boy. The manager was a woman that everyone secretly feared. She didn't smile, was super serious about everything, and was...well...militant. My first day of training was a disaster. I was infuriated. This was 1995 and in the foodservice industry, people still worked without using plastic gloves. She told me that every time I touched my skin, to itch, to clear the sweat from my brow, or anything like that, I needed to wash my hands with soap and water. While I worked, she stood there and watched me like a hawk, never diverting her gaze. It felt like she had X-ray vision like an evil Kryptonian.

Over the next five hours, I washed my hands a whopping 43 times! The most dominant things I felt when she was watching me was fear and anger. I was afraid of making a mistake or failing, doing the job right, and losing face in front of the other employees. Every time she told me to wash my hands, I got more and more furious with each passing occurrence. Most of the time, I hadn't even recognized that I had touched a part of my body. I was doing it unconsciously. It angered me that I didn't have enough awareness to know that I was doing that. I went home yelling and screaming that night and told everyone that would listen about the injustices that I had suffered on my first day of work.

I blamed her for all my fear and anger. It was her fault. She was the problem.

I saw her this way because I wasn't taking responsibility for MY context, MY emotions. In my mind, she was "causing" me to feel what I did. However, the reality is she wasn't causing me to feel anything. I was choosing these emotions all on my own. When people don't feel like they have power over their emotions or know how to let them go, they only know to do one thing--blame. Everyone and everything else is the problem. She simply told me not to touch my body and to wash my hands. Such a simple hygienic practice turned into a massive pit of fear and a volcano of anger. She offered me a reflection of myself, a reflection of the fear and anger that already had existed inside of me. This experience with my manager just brought to the surface or revealed what was already inside of me. I just simply didn't know how to let go at the time. So I projected my emotions onto her and blamed her. What else could I do?

- What emotions do you commonly experience at work?
- What emotions do you commonly experience with your co-workers?
- How do you feel about your boss?
- Are you taking responsibility for your emotions or are you blaming the job itself or the people for what you experience?

Taking responsibility is telling yourself that whatever you are experiencing is yours to own. If you want to heal, you can't blame anyone or anything for what you are experiencing emotionally. The word responsibility means "able to respond". You can choose how to respond, either with negative or positive emotion. The best story about such things was written by Viktor Frankl in *Man's Search for Meaning*.[150] He was in a Nazi concentration camp, and he realized that the only thing he could do in the face of unspeakable evil was to surrender his negative emotions and choose how he wanted to feel. He chose to let go and feel love and joy in spite of his deplorable circumstances. If he did it, we certainly can.

Looking at the context of your own life, in full awareness from moment to moment, will allow you to take responsibility for how you experience the world instead of blaming others. Once you have noticed what you are experiencing, you can then shift your awareness to how you are experiencing each emotion within your physical body. The first step towards emotional intelligence is being able to recognize what you are experiencing and how it is being felt in your body. This is the first step towards ultimate emotional and spiritual growth. By recognizing how what you feel and how you feel it, is the first step toward emotional intelligence. The second step is simply learning how to let these emotions go.

"Let's not forget that the little emotions are the great captains of our lives and we obey them without realizing it." —Vincent Van Gogh

6 EMOTIONS ARE POWERFUL

"When awareness is brought to an emotion, power is brought to your life." —Tara Meyer Robson

One of the most difficult things for people to believe is that emotions can be the sole cause of or largest contributing factor to their health problems. The world in which all of us live is one that is completely obsessed with form. By form, I'm referring to physical things, people, substances, and the like. In general, a tendency exists to think that the solution to all of our health problems is something that is in the world of physical form. We see this in the pervasive model of thinking a pill or medication will solve all our health problems. The dream is that cancer, for example, will one day be cured by a pill. Curing cancer with a pill is a fallacy which perpetuates a very lucrative, money generating lie. It ignores the underlying realities as to what the cause of cancer is in the first place. Closely related to this, we also see this plainly with regards to diet, exercise, and the general public perception of what makes one healthy.

A simple internet search of "different diets" brings up hundreds of choices. We have the Atkins Diet, Paleo Diet, Grapefruit Diet, 3-Hour Diet, South Beach Diet, Ketogenic Diet, Best Life Diet, Blood Type Diet, Cabbage Soup Diet, Caveman Diet, Fat Flush Diet, French Women Don't Get Fat Diet, Glycemic Index Diet, Hormone Diet, Macrobiotic Diet, Master Cleanse Diet, Mediterranean Diet, New Beverly Hills Diet, Nutrisystem Diet, Skinny Bitch Diet, Volumetrics Diet, Weight Watchers Diet, Zone Diet, Raw Food Diet, Vegan Diet and many more. Many people secretly throw their hands in the air and say frustratingly, "What the heck am I supposed to eat?!"

Do I eat more meat? If so, should I just eat chicken or fish and not beef? Isn't red meat bad for you? What about all those animals dying? Should I buy grass-fed meat? What if I get toxic eating conventional meat? How do I pay for organic products when they are so expensive? What about the mercury in tuna? Do I eat more complex carbohydrates? Should I cut all the grains out? Should I avoid potatoes because they are so starchy? Do I become a vegan? Do I eat more vegetables? What about the sugar in fruit? Berries are good, but bananas are bad, right? Should I limit my servings of fruit? If I go out to eat, what can I order that is healthy? How many calories should I consume? But not all calories are equal, right?

The questions are endless.

An even more curious question is "What is the emotional energy that is sitting behind the asking of each question?" Frequently, questions are generated from the negative emotions we have stored within. If we let go of the emotion behind a question or stop identifying with it, a knowingness automatically ensues and the questions often are instantly answered.

People are obsessed (negative emotion) with trying to find the right combination of things to eat because many believe that dietary changes will be the magic bullet to healthy living. People also will fiercely defend many of their dietary choices. The meat eaters will staunchly defend meat, while the vegans will passionately defend the ethical treatment of animals, sustainability, and plant-based food. If you suggest to people that they change their way of dieting, you will instantly confront the context or emotional background of their dietary choices. If you suggest to the Midwestern meat and potato eaters that they eat raw food or vegetables, you will instantly be confronted with their internal emotional resistance. If you suggest to a vegan that it may be healthy for them to get some animal meat in their diet, you will also see their internal emotional resistance arise as they confront your suggestion.

For me, following a particular diet has become less and less important over time. What is important is being so in touch with your body that you can tune in, at any time, to listen to what your body exactly needs and lovingly give it what it requires for optimal health, whatever that may be for you. I have convinced many vegans to eat meat because it would greatly benefit their health. Many times I have asked them, "Do you want to feel better? Or do you want to maintain an internal emotional rigidity with regards to what you eat?" Being open to this possibility always includes a certain level of emotional maturity.

As a naturopath and acupuncture physician, I am very well-versed and researched in the ethical treatment of animals. However, I have seen radical changes in people that open themselves up to eating meat. The same goes for getting people to eat more plant food and vegetables. People become exceedingly resistant when it is suggested that they stop eating meat and animal products for a while, and entertain the power of plant food to heal them. I just want what is best for every person to heal. In this, I have learned to let go of my own internal judgments and positionalities.

The majority of people that I see clinically are not getting even close to the number of vegetables they need per day in order to have abundant health. In these cases, decreasing meat consumption and incorporating a heavy plant-based diet can have the same radical changes. Their compliance with eating more vegetables boils down to one thing—internal emotional agreement and compliance. The same goes for getting a vegan to eat meat, if that is what is required to be healthy. The secret to either position is our emotional state. Most of us can make changes in the short term with no problem, but sustaining these healthy choices always boils down to dealing with our internal emotional context. If we don't learn how to be cognizant of and let go of the emotions within that drive us, our eating behaviors may continue to yo-yo and we may continue to have health problems. Our emotions should be one of the first things we start with if we want sustainable, healthy change.

My Eyes Opened To The Importance Of Emotion

I remember seeing how much emotion can impact the physical body vividly in my first year of being a physician. I was testing people for supplements using Nutrition Response Testing (NRT). NRT is an amazing system of being able to test people for the weakest parts of their body, heavy metals, and chemicals, food sensitivities, or pathogens that may be affecting them. It also identifies what whole food organic supplements can precisely deal with these issues. People were tested, started taking whole food supplements, and dietary changes started. In about 70% of the cases, people would make wonderful progress and start healing from all kinds of things. This progress was exciting to see, and of course, patients were pleased. However, for about 30% of the people, it didn't matter what I tested them for or what kind of dietary changes we made, they didn't make much progress.

These circumstances drove me nuts. I was doing everything I could in the physical world. These people were doing everything right too like exercising, getting chiropractic adjustments, and doing all kinds of other things in the physical world to try to improve their health. Some were even doing things into the second level of health such as acupuncture and massage and were not seeing results either. For so many, despite their best efforts to change and do all these things, they didn't heal. Western medicine, or more precisely the pharmaceutical industry, is largely behind this modern-day programming. We are brainwashed to believe that taking a physical pill is the answer to everything that ails us. It seems like a daily occurrence when people find out I am an "alternative" physician that I am asked, "Hey doc, what should I take for x condition?"

I used to get frustrated when I heard this question because it is one that is the result of our very misguided understanding of how the body and health actually work. If a pill, herb, food, or supplement were the answer, we all would be in absolutely amazing health. However, in the USA people are sicker than ever before despite many eating "right," exercising, and taking handfuls of supplements. I am not trying to discourage these things in any way; they are a necessity. Foundational physical health practices are critical, and we must implement them to heal properly. But, so much more about the body/mind needs to be understood. Now when I hear this question, I take it as an opportunity for compassion and to educate people about how Chinese medicine is tailored specifically to their condition and to see the deeper reality behind their health problems—the power of our internal, emotional reality as an expression of our physical health.

The 30% that didn't start healing in my clinic and were not seeing results drove me to find answers for them. They weren't seeing the results they wanted because they were not identifying and releasing the emotional reality driving these physical expressions of health. I had to look beyond Western medicine, even beyond naturopathic medicine, to Chinese medicine. Chinese medicine is a complete system of health, addressing every level of health in the body. In the process, I found answers for my health problems. Diet, supplements, exercise, chiropractic, acupuncture, massage, and other things in the physical world didn't help me to heal my depression. Nor did they do much for some of my patients either. These things have helped so many people and all play a role in the healing I see in my own patients. However, they weren't the ultimate solution for me and some of my patients.

Health is a full expression of physical and emotional practices, not just one or the other. You cannot neglect one over another and be the fullest expression of health. I exercise three to five times per week, avoid toxins, drink tons of water, eat very clean (80-90% organic plant food), and habitually get acupuncture, massage, and chiropractic. Each of these things makes me feel better in various ways; I champion them in my life and in my practice with patients. Yet while these are very important for all of us, they didn't heal depression in me. What if the root of your health issue isn't physical at all?

Going deeper and deeper into the body and seeing positive emotions as the foundation for vibrant health was revolutionary to me and many of my patients. When this world was explored, and patients started to deal with the internal emotional realities of their health problems, things instantly began to change, and very profound healing began occurring. Instead of 70% of patients seeing improvement, this number started to increase to over 90%.

I've seen the most powerful healing responses in people when they exercise, change their diet, take whole food organic supplements, regularly get acupuncture, chiropractic, and massage, *and* (most importantly) learn how to let go of negative emotions. When all of these things are done in concert with one another or when the most important things on each level of the body are addressed, this is the greatest chance for people to heal. Over time I have repeatedly seen how the most important factor in helping someone heal, in the most profound ways, is by teaching them how to let go of their negative emotions.

When you learn how to truly love yourself, eating the right things, exercising and doing other healthy physical practices becomes effortless. It becomes as automatic as breathing. Abundant health becomes effortless, because in a state of love, everything we do in life is effortless. No resistance to eating certain foods can occur in a state of full love. When you are so dialed in, in touch with, and deeply connected to the love inside of you, all healing is effortless, even emotional healing. We have little to no resistance to doing things we love. For example, we can surrender and learn to live from love, even in the face of having to do things the world considers unpleasant (like eating 15 servings of vegetables per day in order to heal). *We can do anything in a state of love.*

Letting go is the aspect of healing that most people are extremely unaware of and don't know how to put into practice. So many people are convinced that they have left the past in the past, but this is rarely true.

The Five Levels Of Healing In The Body

A brilliant medical doctor by the name of Dietrich Klinghardt compiled a chart that outlines the five levels of healing in the body.[151] He compiled this model from ancient Ayurvedic medicine. Ayurveda means "the science of life" and is the ancient healing tradition originating in India. Many people say that ayurvedic and Chinese medicine ultimately came from the same source more than 5000 years ago. Regardless of whether Ayurveda and Chinese medicine birthed from the same place, they share astounding similarities and understand the levels of healing in the body in similar ways.

Dr. Klinghardt's model blends the ancient understanding of the body with the best of natural modern modalities of healing into what I think is the best model of understanding every level of health in the body. This chart gives a summary of each level or "body," along with what we experience at each level, anatomical or conceptual designation, related sciences, diagnostic methods, and related medical treatment and healing techniques.

A couple of things are worth noting about this chart. First, every level that is above the next affects each level below it. For example, if you use a healing technique in the 3rd level, its effects will be seen in that level along with the 2nd and 1st level. If a problem is simply physical, then employing the right healing technique at that level should begin the healing process. However, I rarely see health issues that are physical only. Health problems are normally a combination of physical, energetic, and emotional factors.

If a person's presenting problem is a headache, for example, I must first determine what level is being affected by the presentation of the issue. Every health problem is ultimately physical, electrical, mental/emotional, and spiritual collectively. Just like there are many floors in a building, what makes the building a building is every part of it collectively together.

Let me give you an example of how one issue primarily manifested as a physical issue. One patient came in with nonspecific tension headaches. He had spent thousands of dollars seeing general medical doctors and neurologists. He had MRI's and many other tests done. All were inconclusive. From a Western medicine point of view, nothing in the tests could point to a problem. Essentially, nothing was wrong with him. But yet so many of us know something is wrong precisely because we FEEL our problem. We all know what we feel, and headaches aren't pleasant. When doing his intake, I arrived at the part of the session where I asked about his diet.

I asked him, "How many servings or cups of vegetables do you consume each per day?"

Being a light-hearted, fun loving guy, he responded, "per day?" We both chuckled.

He was consuming only a couple of servings of vegetables per week. I immediately stopped the intake and confidently looked at him and said, "I think I know exactly why you are having headaches and it is a very easy fix." He looked at me confused. He had spent tens of thousands of dollars, and in less than 30 minutes I was very confident that I knew exactly how to help him heal.

I said, "Your brain is starving from years or decades of not getting the nutrients it needs to function without symptoms. We call this "blood deficiency" in Chinese medicine, and it is relatively easy to remedy. You need to start consuming at least six servings of vegetables per day, hopefully for the rest of your life. Also take a Chinese herbal formula along with a few other organic whole food supplements. Removing offending foods such as wheat, sugar, alcohol, and dairy will also help tremendously. Doing these things should take care of the headaches."

I will never forget the incredulous look on his face. This face said to me, "Did you even go to medical school?! That's the silliest thing I've heard all year!" Many times I have seen people who consume very few vegetables have headaches and when they start consuming them, healing occurs in a very short period of time. By following my advice, eating massive quantities of vegetables, and taking whole food supplements, chronic headaches can become a thing of the past.

The Energetic Level Of The Body

But many headaches do not have a physical root. If a headache has an electrical root to it, this is where acupuncture shines. Many think of acupuncture as a mystical "qi" system, but it really is a part of the body's electrical system. Think of acupuncture channels or meridians like electrical power lines in the body. Each acupuncture point is like a transformer that provides electricity to a certain part of the body. If a power line doesn't have 100% electrical flow or is "turned off" to a certain part of the body, health problems can arise. When acupuncture points are stimulated, they encourage the proper flow of electrical energy in the body. When this happens, better blood flow, oxygen, and life-giving chemicals from the brain can help to heal the part of the body being stimulated.

In 2016, I was playing in an outdoor racquetball tournament in South Florida. Between matches, I was reading a book and a gentleman I had never met before started to talk with me. We made small talk for a few minutes before he told me that he needed to run to the car to get some ibuprofen before playing his match. My intuition told me he had a headache and I asked him, "Let me guess, you have a headache?" He said, "How did you know that?" I asked him exactly where the headache was and what the quality of the pain was. He pointed over his left ear on the side of his head, right behind his temple. He said it was about 6/10 in intensity. The electrical channel or power line that runs through this part of the body starting next to each eye is the gallbladder channel. It travels behind the head, down the lateral sides of the body and ends on the 2nd toe. It is one big, long electrical circuit.

He had his shoes off and was wearing socks. I told him to sit in front of me and put his foot directly on top of my knee. I hadn't yet told him I was a physician and he gave me that confused "What are you suggesting to me?" look. I mentioned to him that I was a physician, but that didn't seem to do anything to alleviate his confusion for the moment. Nevertheless, he went ahead and put his foot on my knee. I told him that I was going to try something that is very effective in relieving pain in around 50% of cases. If I located the right acupuncture point and applied pressure his headache should go away in a matter of seconds. I took my fingernail and placed moderate pressure on the acupuncture point on the toe. I looked up after 3 seconds and asked him how his headache was. He was as surprised as a baby tasting lemon for the first time. "My headache is gone! How did you do that?!", he triumphantly asked.

The funny part is that I don't even remember asking him his name. He simply got up, thanked me and went off to play his racquetball match. By stimulating this point, it is comparable to suction being used to unclog a drain. When the electrical energy began to flow better through the circuit, the pain disappeared. This is a very simple example and some people require far more detailed acupuncture treatments over an extended period. But when the problem is electrical, acupuncture works wonderfully.` Some people have had 40, 50 or more years of electrical imbalance, so one treatment is rarely enough these days. If acupuncture is the appropriate healing modality, 5-10 sessions should offer great improvements.

As an acupuncture physician, I have heard many stories over the years about people who have tried acupuncture once and it didn't do much for them. Does this mean that acupuncture doesn't work? Absolutely not. If you have had a chronic health problem for years, thinking that one session of acupuncture will fix everything is unrealistic. It is as unrealistic as going to the gym one time and expecting to look like Dwayne "The Rock" Johnson. If little changes after 6-12 sessions for a chronic problem, it could mean that the problem had a deeper cause, not on the 1st or 2nd level of the body.

Another frequently reported story is how acupuncture has been used to treat headaches. It vastly improves the headaches, but they never seem to go away completely and require ongoing treatment. This is yet another sign that could lead in the direction of the root problem being on a deeper level within the body or the body needs something additional to fully heal.

The Emotional Levels Of Health

One woman came to the clinic one day and had been experiencing a headache for three straight days. Using applied kinesiology, I determined that her headache was a 4th level headache, which is the intuitive or family emotional body. Applied kinesiology is a neuromuscular feedback technique that can be used to determine truth. Problems in this level can arise due to emotions that are experienced within the context of one's family. She had been a patient of mine on and off over the past year, and I had taught her how to process through her emotions using tapping. So my first question to her was, "Did you try to do any tapping on your headache?" She replied, "Yes, I tapped on the headache for a few minutes, but it didn't work. The tapping didn't work."

For ease of understanding, the 3rd level of the body relates to the general emotions that one experiences throughout life. If someone cuts you off in traffic and you get angry, this would be a 3rd level related experience. If you get mad at your mother (family), this would make it an experience in the 4th level. If you get mad at God, it would make it a 5th level, or spiritual emotional issue.

She just needed guidance as to what the genuine emotions were that were driving the headache. Health issues on the 3rd, 4th, and 5th level in the body require patience, curiosity, non-judgment, and good detective work. It is one thing to determine what level a health issue is on, yet another to discover the story driving the issue. So I began doing some digging with many questions.

I began by asking her to give me a rundown of what happened during the morning when her headache started. She stated that she was preparing to host a special party she was looking forward to. Her husband notified her that he had invited his in-laws to attend the party, whom she specifically did not invite because she didn't get along very well with them. Upon hearing he'd invited them, she became agitated and fearful. As time passed that day she began to get more and more resentful about this. She was afraid because she explained how they were judgmental, always second-guessing her, causing rifts between her and her husband, and spreading rumors and gossiping frequently.

The main emotion of the gallbladder channel in the body is resentment. In Chinese medicine, consciousness or emotions are attached to every one of the organs and 12 major electrical circuits of the body. The gallbladder channel runs along both sides of the head. When asked how resentful she was about this, she stated it was an 8/10. The fear was also at 8/10. In her mind—and as commonly happens—she didn't think that this could have anything to do with her having a headache. We tapped on these emotions, and since she had done it with me many times before and had gotten good at releasing emotions from her body, the resentment and fear lessened quickly. In about 20–25 minutes both emotions were released from her body. I then asked her to refocus on the pain in her head; she smiled and said, "It's completely gone!"

She didn't have a physical headache. She didn't have an electrical or energetic based headache. She had an emotional headache and she needed a tool on this level of the body to enable her to heal from this headache. When she was asked about how she felt after releasing these emotions from her body, she gave the answer that I hear almost every day from patients when doing this work: "I feel lighter and more at peace."

Every patient that comes into the clinic with a headache or any health problem is unique and the reasons why they have a headache are unique. This is why it is difficult to do a double-blind study to try to find one thing that works for everyone. This is not to discourage research in any way. It does require us to expand, open and change our paradigm of medicine and healing. Chinese medicine helps you to heal your unique health problem. If ten people come in and have a physical, root headache, what helps each of them may require eighteen very different courses of treatment as seen in this example below.

Chinese medicine is one that discovers the patterns of your problem and then treats the pattern with all the tools available to influence that pattern. A pattern is a collection of symptoms that relate to each other within the foundational principles of Chinese medicine. Those eight foundational principles are hot/cold, yin/yang, full/empty, and interior/exterior. In *The Practice of Chinese Medicine* by Giovanni Maciocia, 18 different patterns exist for the treatment of headaches.[152] Those 18 patterns are as follows:

EXTERIOR
- Wind-Cold
- Wind- Heat
- Wind-Dampness

INTERIOR (Full)
- Liver-Yang Rising
- Liver- Fire
- Liver-Wind
- Liver-Qi Stagnation
- Stagnation of Cold in the Liver Channel
- Dampness
- Turbid Phlegm
- Turbid Phlegm-Wind
- Liver-Yang Rising with Phlegm in the Head
- Retention of Food
- Stasis of Blood
- Stomach-Heat

INTERIOR (Empty)
- Qi Deficiency
- Blood Deficiency
- Kidney Deficiency

All these patterns point to different states of imbalance in the body that we aim to correct. In the pattern of Liver Fire, you see an expression of heat in the body in symptoms such as red eyes and face, irritability, outbursts of anger, migraines and constipation. The principle to heal someone is simply to cool the body down. If something is too hot, we must cool it down. We do this with cold foods, cold herbs, acupuncture points that release heat and doing an emotional release of anger. This will bring balance to the pattern.

In this way, Chinese medicine is very detailed and identifies a health issue as it specifically relates to you, which is why there is not one way to treat a headache. There may be 18 different ways. The job of the practitioner is to first identify the pattern someone presents you with. Very different herbs, acupuncture points, massage areas, exercise and food therapy would be recommended for each pattern. The past or the context of each person's emotional issues are all unique as well. Emotions also are revealed in these patterns as well. Often the source of someone's headache could go back deep into the past, as early as our first memories at the age of 3 or 4. Everything needs to be explored in order to discover and treat the pattern. In Western medicine, a simple pill may be given to most people presenting with headaches, but this rarely deals with the root issue. Chinese medicine gets to the root cause and pattern and treats that very specifically.

These five levels of healing in the body are the best model I have ever seen to explain why people have health issues and how to accurately identify ways to help them. The above examples simply help us to see how a root cause in each level can play itself out in helping someone to heal. Clinically, the best way to help someone is to address health at each level all simultaneously. Changing the diet, taking the right supplements, exercising, getting acupuncture, and dealing with our emotions concurrently is a powerful way to deal with the whole person. A medical structure that has proven ways on all levels to help people heal is the best expression of health and wellness.

Beyond the physical world, the currency of our expression of life is emotion. What we do with emotion will determine how life plays out for better or for worse, especially with health in the physical body. Emotions are both the problem (negative) and the solution (positive) at the same time. They are the key to understanding health problems and healing from them. When the woman with the headache let go of the resentment and fear, love and forgiveness were what healed her. She stepped into the peace, joy, love, and forgiveness that are there for all of us at all times. The key is simply to let go of what is preventing us from experiencing these things.

We all have different experiences. We all have very different thoughts. We all have very different abilities. We all have and lead very different lives. But the one thing that every human being shares is the same emotions. This is our commonality. We all have experienced the same exact emotions. We all can identify with one another in small or large ways because we all experience life with the same emotions. Some experience certain emotions in more powerful or ponderous ways on both sides of the spectrum negatively or positively, but we all experience them the same.

Fibromyalgia Disappeared In One Session

The first major event in the clinic when I realized how profoundly emotions shape us and our physical health was when I saw the effects of them in a patient who came to the clinic for help with fibromyalgia. Jane (not her real name) was a 47-year-old female coming in because she had a very chronic case of fibromyalgia (pain and tenderness all over the body). She also got migraine headaches two or more times per week, couldn't sleep, was very depressed and fatigued. Fibromyalgia is so powerful that people who have it sometimes have trouble even putting on clothes because the clothing rubbing against their skin is too painful. Just 30-40 years ago, doctors dismissed this condition and didn't have a name for it. Patients (mostly women) were shamed and told that "It's all in your head." Her condition had progressed so far that she hadn't held a job in years and was living as a hermit at home, isolated from the world.

At the time, I was just starting to learn that not only are emotions the key to understanding the context of our lives but that they often are at the heart and center of why we suffer from disease. During our second appointment together I had an intuitive sense to ask her one question. Normally I wouldn't have been so forward so quickly, but I just felt that it was appropriate for her and that she was ready. Since she was in a lot of physical pain, I had a suspicion that she was holding onto a lot of emotional pain. Consciousness (and our emotions), over time, can express itself into the physical body as the primary way to get our attention and to let us know which negative emotions are not supporting our life. A very painful physical body is often an indicator of very painful emotional events from the past.

I chose my words very carefully, and I asked, "What's the most painful memory that you ever remember having?" Without hesitation, she replied, "I was molested when I was seven years old." She said it so matter-of-factly that it appeared to come across as cold, callous and disconnected. It was like she knew beyond a doubt that this memory had profoundly shaped and formed who she was. But it was still unresolved within her subconscious. It was festering like a sore that had never healed. She had just learned to coexist with this pain. So how she related to it was in the form of repression, having pushed it down so far that it was mostly "out of mind."

Upon hearing her response, I said, "I'm so sorry to hear that. Would you like to process through this memory together?"

She gave me an exhausted, one eyebrow raised, eye roll when I asked her. In frustration, she said, "I've talked to every doctor, psychologist, psychiatrist, counselor, therapist, pastor, priest, and friend about this memory! I don't want to talk about it anymore!" Her response was very telling. Over the years she had received lots of counseling and therapy and had talked about this memory repeatedly with many wonderful and qualified people. But even after talking about it, the negative emotions in the memory remained virtually the same.

Talk therapy plays a wonderful role in the healing process. However, what I have found is that, at times, it may not initiate any exchange of emotional energy inside us. There may not be a shift in consciousness or a true letting go. You can remain very detached from a memory even as you talk about it, which, in my experience, will not help you to heal from it. In using applied kinesiology or muscle testing, it was determined that this memory was still a 9.9/10 in relation to the intensity within her consciousness. This meant that it was still the most damaging and harmful memory she had compared to all the other memories she had experienced in her life. In spite of many attempts to heal from it, nothing had changed internally about how she held the memory emotionally -- until now.

Thus the look on her face communicated "Not this again! I have talked about this memory so many times! How is this going to be any different?? What is the point of being reminded of all that pain all over again!?" Seeing this in her expression, I was quick to interrupt her thought processes. I told her that talking about something can be very different than actually letting it go. In the process, she would be able to feel the negative emotions releasing from her body as the evidence that it was working. Until you have experienced this for yourself first hand, it can be a little difficult to believe.

With the new understanding, courage in her eyes, and hope in her heart, she suspected this was going to be different. When she was asked again if she wanted to process through this memory, she didn't hesitate and said "Yes."

Before we began to explore this memory together, it was important for me as the practitioner to have a road map of sorts to help navigate through the negative emotions that were in this memory. When memories happen so long ago, sometimes people have trouble identifying exactly what the negative emotions are that are still residing in those memories. In the clinic I have a chart with over 700 negative emotions on it. This chart is used to correctly identify what emotions are present in a memory.

Using Applied Kinesiology (AK), her body was first asked: "How many negative emotions are present in this memory?" The answer was eight. Next, using this chart of emotions, each emotion was identified through the use of AK. After each emotion was identified, the intensity of each emotion was rated on a scale from 1-10. All of these emotions in this memory were a 10/10 for her. Listed below are all of the eight negative emotions that were found in this memory.

- Worthlessness
- Hypertense
- Frozen
- Guilty
- Tormented
- Low Self Esteem
- Fearful

- Rejection

After all this information was gathered, we began processing through this memory using tapping. We addressed not only the emotions in the memory but also the emotions she was having in the present moment about going back into this memory. It was terrifying to her in the present moment to relive these past emotions, which was to be expected. It was the most painful thing that ever happened to her and reliving it *momentarily* was very painful. At each step of the way, she felt a terror or fear about continuing in the present moment through the memory. Therefore, we first dealt with the terror and fear that she was feeling about even going into the past. As she released these emotions, we were able to keep going through the negative emotions in the actual memory one by one.

For two hours, we worked through every one of the emotions in the memory and the emotions she was experiencing about going back into the memory. As each one of the emotions released from her body, she felt more and more relief, and the process got easier and easier. In quantum physics and ultimate spiritual reality, no such thing as time exists. This is hard to process for the linear mind. However, it is an important thing to understand. Even though something happened to you 40 years ago, it is still happening to you right now, because those emotions can all still be felt in the present moment. The past is the present because the present is all you will ever have. Simply by giving permission to bring these emotions up from the basement of the subconscious, most can feel them all over again. This is proof that the past is the present, and this is also the reason why dealing with the memory in the present, literally alters our perception of the past and enables us to see and live a different present.

After processing through every one of these emotions again, using AK, it was determined that the negative energy in the memory reduced from a 9.9/10 to a 2.7/10, about a 72% reduction. A few things remained to be processed through, but our time was over for that day. I asked her how she felt. She said she felt peaceful and much lighter, which is a very common reaction many people have after tapping through tough stuff and letting go. Those memories and emotions are heavy, and when we let them go, the body feels it. You feel lighter. She then left and went home.

"It's amazing how once the mind is free of emotional pollution, logic and clarity emerge." —Clyde DeSouza, Memories With Maya

The Follow-Up Appointment

What happened in our follow up appointment two weeks later was stunning and extremely powerful for me. It allowed me to continue seeing the massive effects that negative emotions and memories from the past have on our physical bodies. I began asking her about her symptoms. As a recap, she had struggled with crippling fibromyalgia and pain every day for years. She had tried drugs, therapy, and numerous other things; nothing seemed to work for her. She had migraine headaches 2+ times per week for years as well. In Western medicine, no cure exists for fibromyalgia, only managing the symptoms with drugs.

I asked her, "How do you feel? How has your pain level been in the last two weeks?" She responded happily, "I haven't had any pain." Since this was in the beginning stages of when I first started using tapping, I was shocked and asked again, "You mean you haven't had any pain in the last two weeks!?"

"Nope!" she responded.

"How about headaches; how have your migraines been?"

"I haven't had any headaches either in the last two weeks."

Flabbergasted, I responded, "Really?! Are you serious?"

"Yes, and I have more energy (5/10, it was a 1/10), and I slept two nights through and that hasn't happened in years."

I was shocked and elated for her. Her fibromyalgia was gone. Seeing how effective processing through this memory had been for her opened my eyes to a new reality of what was possible in helping people with their health issues. Frankly, it was a new world into helping me with the depression I had been struggling with for so long. Using AK to identify negative emotional energy within and tapping through emotions/memories from the past has proven to be remarkable. The best part about it is that anyone can learn how to use it in minutes and once you learn to use the tool with skill, it is a lifelong way to significantly alter your reality.

She wasn't out of the woods yet though. This was just one memory for her. Although it was a very powerful one, she, like all of us, had many powerful and negative memories that had profoundly altered and programmed how she lived, thought, and existed in the world.

You may be wondering at this point if the changes are enduring. The reality is that once emotions release from a memory, they disappear forever. People move forward and not backward because moving forward *feels* good. So in my experience, the symptoms never return. We are such powerful beings that we can recreate them, but this would be foolish.

Due to changing circumstances in her life, we weren't able to process through much more at that time. I didn't see her for more than two years after our initial appointments. However, even after two years when she returned to the clinic, her fibromyalgia symptoms were still gone. This is a testament to the power of the mind we have. Depending upon the inward reality of what we are holding onto, this determines our outer reality, not only in what we experience health-wise in the body but also in our relationships, finances, work, family and our relationship with God. Our experience of everything in the world is dependent upon our inner emotional reality. Like wearing glasses, our inner emotional world influences our perception of everyone and everything, especially the health of our physical body.

This experience was a powerful shifting point for me clinically. Tapping is a tool and the use of the tool grows with a deeper knowledge of the body and health. This tool also can give us an understanding of how the mind works and how we can shape the contents of the mind (emotions, thoughts, and beliefs). I frequently mention to people that tapping is a tool analogous to a paintbrush. A paint brush in the hands of a 3rd grader, versus the hands of someone who is a graduate level painter, elicits a much different painting. The tool is the same, but the person who uses the tool and understands better how to use it will paint a more beautiful or complete picture. The more you use tapping, the more skill you gain and the easier it becomes to let things go. Additionally, If you learn from someone who already paints well (a mentor or coach), you will learn that much faster how to use the tool.

I've spent these last years learning how to use this tool and other tools to help people heal. How the tool is used is almost limitless. Here are some of the ways that I have seen this tool used to profoundly alter someone's internal reality (and therefore external reality).

1. **Pain.** I have seen headaches, knee pain, shoulder pain, foot pain, menstrual pain, lower back pain and pain of all different kinds disappear within minutes or a few sessions. To this day, it continues to astound and amaze me.

2. **Relationships.** One of my favorite sessions was with a woman that lost her husband and was just ravaged by grief she couldn't release. She cried endlessly every day for months. We have all heard the common adage: "Time heals all wounds." However, this is not true at all. Within three sessions, she let go of all the grief and six months later was engaged to be married after meeting someone two weeks after our last session. Any relationship problem or issue has emotional roots to it. Often we blame others, but it is what is inside of us that is largely contributing to our relational problems and what we are attracting to ourselves. Tapping can give a different perspective and initiate profound relational healing.

3. **Work.** "I hate my boss!" one person said to me. We processed through this "hate" together. An association was made as to how their boss reminded them of their relationship with their mother. After a couple of sessions working on this, work took on a whole new joy and vibrancy, and this person started getting along wonderfully with their boss.

4. **Disease.** Diseases like cancer, heart disease, or Alzheimer's have huge emotional components, and people can feel better when the emotional components are addressed.

5. **Emotional or physical trauma from the past**. Healing our deepest memories has a profound impact on the way we experience everything in our world.

6. **Sex.** Sex is a profoundly intimate experience which brings up many internal wounds and issues. For many, sex isn't really a super pleasurable experience. It can be unpleasant due to past experiences, religious programming, or the negative things we feel about our body. When healing these things, sex can become the amazing, glorious, ravishing, intimate, sacred, and connecting experience it was meant to be.

7. **Spiritual growth**. The heart and center of spiritual growth is emotional growth. Author Peter Scazzero said it best: "You cannot be spiritually mature and emotionally immature." They are one and the same. Nothing has more profoundly shaped my spiritual life than dealing with the negative memories and emotions inside of me. Our internal emotional reality dictates how we see ourselves and how we see and relate to God. Emotions are how we relate to God just as we do to any other person or experience. We can read religious books, pray, fast, donate money, worship or do any other religious ritual, but if the overall emotion expression inside of us (our consciousness) isn't changing then it is not affecting our heart (the center of emotion). Many people fill the walls of churches but 10, 20, or 30 years of being inside a church doesn't mean that you have had a change in consciousness/emotion. In fact, for many inside churches today, emotional growth isn't talked about at all. People there learn things about God, but our struggle to become more like God (love, joy, and peace) doesn't happen at all or very little. Our emotional reality is often neglected, which is the principal reason growth is limited.

This list can go on and on. Since emotion is the language of our entire reality, dealing with our negative emotions can impact any area of life. Whatever struggles, hardships, problems, or health issues you have in life, the impact of looking within at how you are experiencing what is happening from an emotional standpoint often is the most critical aspect of shifting or changing it in your life.

While we all experience emotions on a daily basis and have many unpleasant memories that continue to affect us from the past, I have found that many people honestly don't know how they experience their emotions. If you don't know how you do that, then you will never be able to know how to let them go. Therefore, it is critical first to understand what emotion is and how we experience emotions within our bodies.

7 REAPING AND SOWING

The mind, with its thoughts, is driven by feelings. Each feeling
is the cumulative derivative of many thousands of thoughts.
Because most people throughout their lives repress, suppress,
and try to escape from their feelings, the suppressed energy
accumulates and seeks expression through psychosomatic
distress, bodily disorders, emotional illnesses, and disordered
behavior in interpersonal relationships. The accumulated
feelings block spiritual growth and awareness, as well as
success in many areas of life.
—Dr. David Hawkins, Letting Go: The Pathway to
Surrender"

"…a man reaps what he sows." —Galatians 6:7, New
International Version

Reaping and sowing is a concept that is supported in all of the world's major religions in one form or another because it is a universal truth. Whatever you sow, you will reap. This applies to every facet of our lives. It applies to what we see and experience in our relationships, finances, families, careers, and our physical bodies with health or disease. Uncovering this truth and seeing how it applies to our lives is one of the most important things to understand to start healing. Let's look at an example of how sowing and reaping applied for a client of mine.

I had a woman come in with chronic pain in her neck and shoulders. Chronic pain is one of the most common complaints that doctors see people for. This pain had been ongoing for about five years. When asked about what she had done to work on the problem, she mentioned very common things that many people do such as stretching, taking Advil when it got too intense and chiropractic visits, which helped the most but never fully alleviated the pain for good.

For her, the ultimate question was, "Why do I have neck, shoulder and head pain?" After asking questions about the physical nature of why this pain could have started and not learning anything remarkable on her very first visit, I decided to ask her a couple of questions regarding what the neck normally represents emotionally. With a smile, I looked at her in a purposeful way and asked two questions:

1. "What was going on in your life emotionally five years ago when you started getting the pain?"

Every health problem has a context. That context can be at the moment that a problem starts or it can be from something accumulated from much further in the past. For example, some experts say that different forms of cancer take twelve years or more to develop in the body. She answered this question by telling me how she had a terribly emotional breakup with a boyfriend. This seemed like a very likely context as to the cause of her neck and head pain. My next question was almost answered by itself given the response she gave to the first question.

2. "Who or what is literally a pain in your neck?"

The lights came on for her, and in one sense she was starting to see what the problem was. The answer was obvious that her ex-boyfriend was "the problem." Her ex was still in her life for various reasons, and she still felt many negative things towards him that hadn't changed in 5 years.

In Inna Segal's book *The Secret Language of the Body*, she summarizes possible contributing factors to neck issues as:

> "Relationship problems. Inability to communicate feelings. Difficulty making commitments. Feeling stuck, inflexible, pressured, like something or someone is strangling you. Propensity to sweep issues under the carpet, so you don't have to deal with them. Holding on to unresolved issues in relationships, especially with parents, children, or past partners. Often seeing yourself in a negative self-image. Spending too much time thinking and trying to work things out, and not enough time being aware of your feelings by tuning into your intuition."[153]

The neck emotionally represents the idea of flexibility, the ability to see what's "behind" us and being able to see more than one side of something. With regards to her ex, by her admission, she was very inflexible and stubborn with him. She was still carrying around much negative emotional energy towards him all these years later.

Realizing that the problem was the anger, resentment, guilt, nagging criticism, and suffocating feelings she had towards him was a very important step towards full awareness and taking responsibility for her neck pain. Even though she now was beginning to see the emotional energy that was standing behind the problem, by no means did that mean the problem instantly disappeared. After discovering the energy of what was causing the problem, she asked a very inquisitive question that many people ask: "Since he is the "problem," what are you going to do about it?" I told her that first, he is not the problem, the negative emotions are. Secondly, I was going to teach her how to release them, so she could be pain free. She had sown many negative emotions over the years which resulted in a reaping of chronic neck pain. After learning how to release these emotions, her neck pain completely disappeared.

> "Any person capable of angering you becomes your master."
> - Epictetus

Health Principles of Sowing and Reaping

Let's run with this metaphor of sowing and reaping, break it down and see how the truths of it are applicable as we experience health or disease in the body and see what we can learn from it.

Sow = Plant or scatter seed on the earth.

Reap = Cut or gather a harvest – the fruit of sowing.

Based on this metaphor, the following nine concepts arise as ways to understand how sowing and reaping apply with health in the physical body.

1. Reaping doesn't happen immediately, it takes time.

Anyone who has planted seeds knows that when a seed is planted, one does not see the fruit of what was planted immediately. Some seeds take root and grow very fast, whereas others grow very slowly over time. Each seed has its own unique individual expression and growth. One seed, such as corn, sprouts up very quickly, has relatively superficial roots and one can see fruit within months. Another seed, such as an acorn, takes a long time to root itself and grow. Its roots become deep and wide, and the full expression of an oak tree will take decades. Likewise, every problem we see in our lives, especially health issues, can crop up slowly or quickly. Some health issues are massive and complicated, and some are simple and relatively easy to deal with.

If we sow negative emotions in our lives, eventually they can manifest symptomatically in the body. Our body will reap physically what we have sown emotionally. In the clinic I always use the example of a glass of water to explain this. Let's say I hand you a glass of water and ask you to hold it out in front of you and ask you how much it weighs. Most likely, you will say it doesn't weigh much. However, weight becomes relative due to how long you hold the glass. After ten minutes of holding it, perceptually it becomes much heavier. How heavy will it feel after holding it for one hour? Eventually, you will begin to feel soreness and even pain from holding onto the glass for a long period. Negative emotions are like a glass of water. When we choose to hold onto them, at first they don't seem so heavy. But, after subconsciously holding onto them for 10, 20 or 50 years, eventually the body will give you a symptom or set of symptoms called disease in order to point you in the direction of what you are holding onto that needs to be surrendered or let go.

Our bodies manifest physically the emotional energy that we have chosen to hold from our past. What is interesting about this illustration is one thing. What can you do with the glass at any time? You can choose to let it go or set it down! The same is true of our negative emotions. We carry around our baggage from all those experiences that happened long ago. We all need to learn how to let the glass go.

A cold, for example, may crop up quickly, normally remains relatively superficial, and the body usually deals with it in a matter of days or weeks. On the other hand, cancer normally takes years to develop and build within the body. When one does begin to see the expression of cancer in the body, it is no small feat to deal with this health issue. Cancer may be like an oak tree, whose roots are deep and wide and require a massive undertaking to deal with. This can include a total change of lifestyle, dietary habits, elimination or reduction of stress, change in exercise, and other helpful modalities such as massage, chiropractic, and acupuncture to be able to deal with the issue if one chooses to go the natural route. On the conventional side of things, doctors' visits, drugs, chemotherapy, radiation or other forms of treatments are long, taxing and expensive.

The simple reality is that one doesn't expect that when a seed of watermelon is planted, that a huge juicy magnificent watermelon will be ready to eat the very next day. I have heard from so many people how they were healthy, without any symptoms present in their bodies, and then one day it all began to fall apart. Most of the time, this is very confusing for people. They don't understand why something is happening to them now. They may say things like, "I haven't changed anything in my life recently" or "I thought I have always been pretty healthy and now this!"

As just mentioned, one of the most ominous and destructive of all diseases in the world today is cancer. People just live their lives and then seemingly out of nowhere, a Stage 3 diagnosis is given and a prognosis of 6 months to a year is given to live. People are left with massive confusion, fear, anger, sadness, guilt, and many other reactions from hearing such news. For many it completely catches them by surprise. But the reality is that with most cancers, the ground has been fertile, and the roots have been spreading for years or even decades, and now the harvest has come.

Let's take one physical example to convey this point. Pesticides or chemicals are used to keep pests at bay so that a crop can grow unobstructed in the growth of conventional or non-organic food. I grew up for decades consuming conventional food, as most of us have. Pesticides are carcinogens. Carcinogens cause cancer. This has been scientifically proven repeatedly. Our liver, lymphatic system, immune system and other parts of us work tirelessly to deal with and try to rid the body of these substances every day. These systems may have been able to do their job well for 10, 20, or even 50 years. But for many these days, a moment arrives when these systems don't have the resources or capability to help us any longer. It is this tipping point where we will begin to see the expression of certain health problems. We live in a very toxic physical world today (sowing), and people's bodies eventually will pay the bill (reaping). Cancer rates have risen exponentially in the last 100 years.

So you eat breakfast, lunch, dinner, and have snacks every day filled with small amounts of pesticides. Every day these toxins destroy, wear away, and harm your body. The body continues to take this abuse every day until it can no longer defend and protect you. The harvest comes, and the fruit of the harvest can be very destructive. Pesticides are just one example of a toxin or carcinogen in our world today. As we covered in chapter 2, our world is filled with thousands of chemicals today that all do the same thing in one way or another—they destroy health. Even simple things like our shower water, drinking water, deodorant, shower soap, and shampoo are some potent examples of other things that are filled with toxins. It is hard to pronounce the name of many of the chemicals included in self-care products. You cannot consume pesticides and chemicals in self-care products for 40 years and not expect to pay some bill in the future. One hundred years ago, we didn't have these types of chemicals and crops were grown naturally with natural fertilizers.

Please be aware that this is in no way meant to convey guilt or blame. Blaming yourself for unconsciously making these choices is not conducive to healing. Also, feeling guilty or punishing yourself for the choices you made in the past will not foster healing either. We can take responsibility for what we know and can do now in this moment. We can only make better choices when we become aware of something in the present moment. We can become more aware and learn how to cleanse and heal our body today. The seeds we've sown from decades of poor health choices may be finally bearing fruit now.

Lastly, I hear all the time how most people think they are healthy and eat healthy. If 7 out of 10 people in the USA today are dying from cancer and heart disease, 70% or more of people are not eating and living healthy! Most people in the US consume dairy products, GMO wheat, GMO corn, GMO soy, GMO refined sugars, fried foods and alcohol regularly. These foods will all produce cancer in the body. They are toxic, and it is what most people in the US consume today. The chemical companies responsible for making these "franken-foods" really do know how destructive they are for us. Nothing was wrong with the food before they altered it and added chemicals to them. With the number of toxins that we all are exposed to, health is just a misguided judgment by most people in our world today.

"Your perception of me is a reflection of you; my reaction to you is an awareness of me." - Unknown

2. What is sown will manifest as something completely different to the eye in the future.

Two different seeds that look very similar can grow and be very different from one another. Two seeds that look alike, once planted, bear completely different types of fruit. Two people, such as twins, can grow up in the same family, have the same or very similar experiences, eat the same kinds of food over the years, yet have very different health problems in the future. Why is this? It is because we all have a very unique consciousness. By consciousness, I am referring to the emotions, thoughts, and beliefs that one holds within. Two twins, although alike in many ways, have completely different emotions and perceptions they experience. These emotions and the subsequent thoughts that arise from these emotional roots can be seen in very different expressions of health or disease in the future. How do we see this play out in the body?

Every part of the body has consciousness attached to it. For example, one day a woman came into the clinic with a very persistent chronic, achy, sometimes stabbing pain in the bottom of her foot. The expression of this is associated with plantar fasciitis or heel pain. Feet help to move us forward in life. The heel grounds us to the earth when standing or walking. Inflammation is normally associated with some expression of anger in the body. So I asked her two questions "Are you frustrated about not moving forward in a particular area of your life?" and "What is something negative that you started to experience emotionally when the pain started three months ago?"

She started to cry and told me how frustrated she was at work, not getting a recent promotion and questioning her choice to have taken this job in the first place. She didn't know what else to do and was questioning all of these aspects of her life at the moment. We created awareness around what she was holding onto emotionally and then one by one she started to release all the emotions surrounding this whole situation. At the end of her session I asked her to notice the pain in her foot, and to her surprise, the pain was completely gone. Six months later, she still was pain-free, had quit her job and was in a much better situation where she felt like she was moving forward in life.

Every disease or health problem has consciousness attached to it as well. Depending upon the emotional factors that we are holding onto inside ourselves, certain parts of the body may be affected much more than others. For example, the following aspects of consciousness are commonly associated with the skin: protection, breathing in life, self-acceptance, self-image, guilt, sensuality, and being thick or thin-skinned. Skin issues can manifest when something negative is associated with these concepts.

One common health condition which affects many teenagers is acne. According to Inna Segal, acne can express itself in the body due to the following consciousness factors:

"Acne: Feeling uncomfortable in your own skin, insecure, unacceptable, rejected, not good enough, unworthy of love. Holding on to self-hatred. Trying to hurt and punish yourself for past mistakes. Controlling; demanding unrealistic perfection from self."[154]

I have had so many people in my office that have struggled with acne for so long and tried every medical treatment under the sun. When I read this to them and ask them if any of it applies to them, they may begin to nod in agreement or even tear up because of how specifically it describes how they feel about themselves. When everything else has been tried, the one last area of health that is explored is consciousness. It should be first but is often the last. Consciousness will express itself into the body to get us to pay attention to the negative emotions and thoughts we are holding onto that don't support life. It is the built-in mechanism we have to help us grow, change and evolve.

A seed that is sown looks completely different from the seed's fruit. The volcano of anger that we went through when our spouse cheated on us can manifest as high blood pressure years later. The fear of being hurt as a child, which manifests as wanting to control everything and everyone around us, can manifest years later as diabetes. When we seek to control everything, our body may give us something that has historically been uncontrollable. Before insulin and metformin, blood sugar was very hard to control. Our body is simply bearing the fruit of what we are holding onto. Our symptoms are constantly speaking, but are we paying attention? Do we know how to interpret the language of our symptoms?

"It is we ourselves who create stressful reactions as a consequence of what we are holding within us. The suppressed feelings determine our belief systems and our perception of ourselves and others. These, in turn, literally create events and incidents in the world, events that we, then, turn around and blame for our reactions. This is a self-reinforcing system of illusions. This is what the wisest among us mean when they say, "We are living in an illusion." All that we experience are our own thoughts, feelings, and beliefs projected onto the world, actually causing what we see to happen." - Dr. David R. Hawkins, Letting Go: The Pathway of Surrender

3. Things that are sown can or cannot be fertilized and watered throughout life.

Many of us know that we hold onto certain emotions due to things that happened to us in the past. Many also have a deep desire to grow and do many things to grow and change the expression of our consciousness. We read self-help books, do activities to overcome fears, join support groups, attend church or religious activities, pray, exercise, do things that purposely make us feel uncomfortable and stretch us. Either consciously or unconsciously something drives us all inside to be better, and to feel differently. Some of us grow rapidly, and some do not.

Too much "fertilizer" or "water" in life and we can get burned out, wilt and kill ourselves slowly or quickly. Too little fertilizer and we don't grow much at all. We stagnate, and life just always seems to be the same, year after year. How many of us have the same negative patterns, habits, and ways of being that we had 20 years ago? Often, we don't know how to change this stuff in the first place and are fairly unaware of how others actually perceive us. It happens to all of us. Radical self-discovery can be hard and painful, but necessary and rewarding.

Another phenomenon that occurs unconsciously in most of us is a simple principle in physics. Like attracts like and can act as a fertilizer for what we consider to be good or bad. For example, if you hold onto a lot of anger, you see angry people, situations, and reflections of your anger frequently. Depending on how much anger one is holding onto is the degree to which you will perceive it in the world and others. What is held in mind, tends to manifest. We draw more into our world of that which we are holding onto. This is done very unconsciously for most people. It is not until we make the unconscious conscious that we can make a different choice about what to do with it. Another way to say this is to bring the light of consciousness into our internal darkness. Shining a light onto the darkness inside of us is the first step towards being able to grow and change. The next and more radical step is actively to let these things go.

Over the years life will constantly be reflecting our anger (or any emotion) back to us in different events and circumstances until we let it go. Letting anger go, little by little or in big ways, changes our internal environment so that our perception of the outside world changes, including our perception of ourselves. Many people are unconsciously feeding or adding fertilizer to what was planted within them years ago without even realizing it. Becoming aware of what's deep within our consciousness is like realizing what plant was sewn, chopping it down, and removing the roots, which create space for the expression of another seed, something more joyful, peaceful and loving to express itself in and through us.

"We are dangerous when we are not conscious of our responsibility for how we behave, think, and feel." ——Marshall B. Rosenberg

4. A harvest can be seasonal or life long.

We reap or bear the fruit of what is in our consciousness throughout our entire life. At this point, it is important to talk about what growth actually is. One can have tons of book knowledge and be learning things all the time, but yet have zero change in consciousness or real growth. You can be the smartest person in the world but have very little emotional intelligence. This is not true growth. It is essentially growing in knowledge, but not wisdom. Wisdom is a combination of knowledge and good emotional common sense. You can be the same angry, bitter person you were 20 years ago, yet in those 20 years have accumulated Ph.D.'s in quantum physics or rocket science. While learning book knowledge can be important, it pales in comparison to exploring and changing our inner landscape.

One quick way to do that is to learn from our relationships, particularly marriage.

Many people never think that their ex-wife or ex-husband, who is the "worst" person on the planet, could perhaps be the very best person to reflect to them things that no one else could. We don't see them as blessings, but secretly they are if we can reorient and recontextualize our responses to them. They are divinely put in our lives for our emotional growth. Many fail to learn from these opportunities because we are too busy blaming them and being a victim. We may blame, say it was "their" fault and fail to see the energy that we choose to hold onto that contributed to the problem.

Our parents, spouses, children, co-workers, relatives and everyone else in our lives are constantly offering us a reflection of us. Those closest to us generally offer us the hardest but best reflections because they know how to best push our buttons. When you feel negative emotional energy arise within you as you encounter someone, one of the best questions to ask is, "What do I feel as I experience them?" "What do I need to let go of?" If we continually sow anger, we reap angry people, events, and even health problems that are associated with anger. If we sow kindness, we will frequently be kind to others, and others in return are generally kind to us. This does not mean that we will never go through things that seem perceptively negative. But if what is sown within us is mostly kind, even in stressful, aggravating, or negative circumstances the expression of consciousness in those moments will be mostly kindness. We bear fruit or a harvest of that which is the expression of what is planted, growing, and expressing itself through us. This can be mostly negative, positive or an interesting mixture of both to some degree. We will continue to bear fruit our entire lifetime. What types of fruit are you committed to bearing within you?

"To forgive is to set a prisoner free and discover that the prisoner was you." - Lewis B. Smedes

5. Crops constantly need tending.

Mindfulness allows us to see the kind of crops that are growing within us. Without tending (mindfulness), weeds (unwanted emotions) abound.

My father grew up farming in Nebraska, and recently he decided to work in a greenhouse in Michigan for the summer. He planted five greenhouses full of tomatoes. Planting the tomatoes was relatively easy, but tending to the crops is a constant task. Every day he constantly had to string and restring the vines up. He also has to pull weeds on a daily basis. If he does neither of these things, the vines will go everywhere, and weeds will abound. It would be a chaotic disorder in very little time. Growing tomatoes would be that much harder in a chaotic environment. But by daily tending to these crops, they can grow healthy, unobstructed and express their full potential.

Our minds are constantly experiencing the fruit of our past programming and the overall emotional context of our lives. Our continual and habitual emotions, thoughts and behaviors are the fruit of our consciousness and its expression into the totality of our life. We can choose to go through life mindfully, or we can do so mindlessly. What is a sad reality is that even after teaching tapping or The Sedona Method to patients in the clinic and seeing very good results from using these tools, very few will continue to carve time out of their day to tend to their mind. Less than 5 out of 100 will take the time out weekly for an hour to sit with the contents of their mind and release what comes up.

It seems like only when the weeds have gotten so thick and an annoying problem persists for us that we finally and begrudgingly turn to deal with the contents of the mind. Why wait to do this inner work though? I usually see people in the clinic when a health problem has escalated to such an extreme point that they know something needs to change. Many of us wait until we actually have a problem to change things and deal with the weeds in our lives. Cancer, heart disease, or diabetes are the fruits of years or decades of poor health choices. What drives our daily lifestyle choices at the deepest level are our inner emotions. Even when things have progressed this far, many are unwilling to really change their lifestyles or deal with their inner world or are unwilling to realize that healing can occur outside of Western medicine. Disease has an emotional context. It has roots in the past experiences and habits of our lives. We can read or pray about how to do something, but doing the grueling, hard, inner work required by fully facing ourselves as we are within can be that much more profound. This is no easy or small task.

We must be mindful or aware of the past and how exactly we continue to experience it in the present moment to be able to do something more productive about it. All of this is done with a constant reminder that God sends the rain and is the catalyst for all growth inside of us. It is only by grace that we can surrender in the first place. We are mindful of this as well, knowing that it is foolish to believe that we are the ones who cause something to grow, change, or flourish within. But it is our responsibility to use the tools life has given us to tend to our mind in the best way so that we set up the best conditions for growth to occur.

> "Your task is not to seek for love, but merely to see and find all the barriers within yourself that you have built against Love." - Rumi

6. To change what one is reaping, what is sown must change.

We just touched upon this very subject in the above paragraphs. The root of the problem must be uncovered and removed completely. This is surrender or letting go. Often, I joke with my patients, who normally are in full agreement with me that letting go seems to be very difficult. At times I have commented about what I would say if Jesus suddenly came back and was standing in front of me. I used to ask in my mind, "Jesus, you told us to forgive (let go), but you never told us how to do this?" I'm not asking this question anymore, but when I mention this to people I care for clinically, this question almost always resonates with them too. How do we really let go?

How do we change as humans? How do we alter behaviors that we have had our entire lives? How do we overcome the negative things we know we experience inside of us?

We must completely cut out the roots for radical change to occur. Chopping off leaves will lead to good but only small changes in our lives. But leaves always grow back. Chopping off branches will lead to even more profound changes in our lives. But branches grow back too. Chopping off a trunk of a tree can have very deep and profound changes in our lives. But a tree can even regrow from that. To fully, completely and radically change, we must understand, dig up and remove the entire root of what has been sown and planted.

Certain emotions, thoughts, and behaviors in our lives have superficial roots and are relatively easy to release and surrender. An hour or two may be sufficient for surrendering something. That may be analogous to pulling up a stalk of corn, whose roots are not very deep and can be pulled up fairly easily. At the same time, let's say we have an oak tree of a problem in our lives. God can certainly change our consciousness in a way that this whole tree could be unrooted instantly. However, this is not the case for most people. For most people, the process of letting go would be much like it is done in real life when removing an oak tree from the ground. It must be done branch by branch and limb by limb. The trunk and the roots can take time to fully dig out and be pulled from the earth. Some problems in our lives have deep roots and require constant awareness and surrender.

Clinically, people see this in vivid ways when it can take an entire hour to let go of just one emotion that wasn't all that intense. A vivid realization hits them that dealing with the really deep and profound things of their lives may take intense dedication and constant daily work to fully surrender. We live in a culture where many are programmed to think that consciousness is like Burger King – "My way right away" – but this is rarely the case. Normally, this is just an excuse for not wanting to do the hard work of really digging up the roots of these oak-tree-sized issues in our lives.

Some people have a very real sense that all the emotions buried deep inside of them feel like an ocean or a mountain of things to deal with. The thought of using a mindful approach to life and fully surrendering at all times can seem very overwhelming considering one's vast life experiences and limited time to deal with it. Others have expressed how they are very afraid of truly digging up the past. They are worried that if they bring this stuff up from the basement of their consciousness that the emotions and the pain would just be too much to handle. The irony is that the cancer, a full-blown autoimmune condition or another difficult health problem can be the body's way of expressing itself into their awareness even if that is not what we want. Eventually, you may not be given a choice. Disease has a remarkable ability to force us to pay attention.

Your body may force you to pay attention if you want to or not. Cancer or whatever other difficult health problem can be the oak tree that needs to be cut down and uprooted so that you can truly heal. You have waited 40 years to face this part of yourself, and your body has been keeping score.[155] Would you rather bring up all these things, and let them go, with a potential to be healed or would you like to continue to suffer under the weight of a serious health condition and manage it only with medication and surgery? The courage to face ourselves always arrives when we are truly ready.

> "An illness is merely our consciousness calling attention to something that needs to be looked at within us. There is something about which we are feeling guilty, fearful or other negative emotion. There is a belief system we are holding that has to be let go of and canceled. There is something that has to be forgiven, and something within us that has to be loved, so we thank whatever it is for bringing it to our awareness."
> - Dr. David Hawkins, Healing and Recovery

7. To have a new kind of crop or harvest, a new kind of seed needs to be sown.

When we let go of our negative emotions, the "soil" of our mind changes. These changes support an entirely new crop or expression of life in and through us. When we let go of the negative, it gives room to the growth of the positive in our life. When we sow death (negative emotions), we reap death. When we sow life (positive emotions), we reap life. When we let go of the negative, we allow our true nature to express itself more fully. The fruit of our true nature (Spirit) is love, joy, peace, patience, kindness, gentleness, faithfulness, and self-control. We don't have to do anything to get these things; they are already what we are. By letting go of the negative, we simply reveal our true nature. In the revealing of our true nature, we more fully express this nature into every aspect of our lives. It is expressed into the physical body, our relationships, everything.

If you want to be loved, give genuine love. Genuine love is not expecting something in return. So if you get angry or frustrated because you are giving and giving and not getting in return, this is not genuine, unconditional love. If you want people to be kind to you, give genuine kindness to others. If you want to see peace in the world, be peace first. The more peace you feel inside will correspond with a lessening of the negative emotions that you experience within. The lessening of negative emotions that one feels on the inside corresponds with a radical commitment to surrendering each emotion to God as it is experienced. Even the positive emotions are eventually surrendered as well. When you transcend all emotions, only peace as stillness, beingness, and allness remains.

This is why it is critical to deal with these emotions as they arise in our awareness during every moment of our lives. If we are not aware of how we are experiencing every moment, which is rare for most people, then how will we be able to surrender into peace? If we become aware, and through grace can surrender, peace will become the automatic consequence of surrender. Those who see the most growth in their lives are the ones who commit to let go of every unpleasant sensation, emotion, thought, and belief that arises in every moment of their lives. With this surrender, a new crop or experience of life automatically arises in our life. Everyone is searching for happiness. The irony is that true and lasting happiness (joy) is ever present within waiting only to be discovered. The Kingdom of Heaven is truly within.

"The remarkable thing is that we really do love our neighbor as ourselves. We do unto others as we do unto ourselves. We hate others when we hate ourselves. We are tolerant of others when we tolerate ourselves. We forgive others when we forgive ourselves." - Eric Hoffer

8: Transcend the sowing and reaping cycle completely.

The end of the road in the journey of surrender is realizing that one can transcend sowing and reaping, cause and effect, and the world of duality. It is a profound realization that the mind can altogether be transcended. It is when all thoughts, beliefs, judgments, perceptions, opinions, and emotions stop, that the mind is transcended. This is what peace is. A crop is sown in the world of form. The world of form is the force of all human attachment and suffering. Reality (with a capital R) is outside of the world of form. It is formless. We see Adam and Eve being characterized in the Biblical story in a world of non-duality, a world that existed outside of perceptions of time, right versus wrong, good versus bad, us versus them (dualities) and even form, though they existed in the world of form. They were expressions of Oneness. They had a shift in perception into duality (good and evil), which is where suffering arises from, when they ate of the fruit. The world has been progressively moving from the world of suffering and attachment of form into the world of total peace and the formless (non-duality).

We see the experience of non-duality in all of the beings with the most advanced states of consciousness the world has ever known. This difference of perception or non-dual reality can be seen when Jesus asked the question about who his mother and brothers are. He was fully surrendered into not needing to ascribe egoic attachment to form as MY mother or brothers (because everyone, in reality, is his mother and brother). In the world, people say things such as they would die only for THEIR family or they "love" their kids more than the destitute children living on the street. What is being done is that specialness and value (duality) are egoically given to your children over every other child in the world. This is attachment. Attachment is suffering.

We would suffer (experience much greater negative emotions) if our children were to pass away, but we would feel mostly nothing if we found out John (insert any name) from the other side of the world passed away. From the divine non-dual perspective, there is no "my" child or brother. God would never ascribe more specialness to one person over another. This is what makes love unconditional. And if we surrender into this state ourselves, we will also see the world this way and will love everyone the same, even our enemies. Using the word "my" is only attachment to form, ego and suffering. From the divine perspective, everyone is equally a brother and sister. No separation exists. No attachment to form, possession (my brother) or specialness is present; it doesn't exist in the pristine state of non-duality. When we love someone more than another, this is attachment. We must realize that this too must be surrendered. Unconditional love ascribes no specialness to anything or anyone and loves all equally, because God loves all equality and all are special, regardless of their behavior.

Some may argue this state of consciousness is not possible in this dimension or during this lifetime. It is possible, but so few experience it, which is why it is rarely experienced or even talked about. When the full force of divine love is present and expresses itself as your very essence, because it is your very essence, then you can unconditionally love even your "enemies." Who normally are our enemies? They are people that we feel the very most intense negative emotions towards. In the pristine state of non-duality, the rapist and murderer are loved equally as if they were your brother or sister because, in Reality, they are. In this state, you only feel love towards everything and everyone. Love spills out of you like a well bursting from the ground to everyone and everything. It is non-discriminate, it is non-dual.

No separation truly exists in the fullness of non-duality. It is only the enslavement to the mind and ego that gives us the illusion of separation. A you and me separation disappears just as one would not see the hand as something separate from the fullness of the body. The body is seen as one unit and expression of consciousness, just as every person is a part of the complete whole expression of divine consciousness. We may think our hand is separate, which is what most experience, but this is only an illusion.

It is the mind that dualizes everything. It is programmed to separate (this vs. that), see division (us vs. them), make judgments (better vs. worse) and opinionate (mine vs. yours) about everything and everyone. This is just how the mind works, which is why it can and must be transcended. Without this, the fullness of peace cannot be experienced. In a full state of peace, love, and joy no separation is seen as actually possible. All opinions, judgments, perceptions, thoughts, belief systems, and emotions cease to be identified with. When this occurs, the mind goes completely silent, and the internal chatter stops because Silence is the backdrop or ground of all Reality.

When separation dissolves, it is this wild moment in which we realize that WE just ARE. I am. You are. There is nothing to do, and all is perfect because we have melted into the perfection of Life itself. Our life is hidden in or fully becomes a part of the Totality. It is a complete shift of internal perception. This is the place where the mind is transcended. No crops, ground, soil, seed, or world of form even exists.

It was all just a very persistent illusion generated by the mind or ego. We realize we are the Witness, and no longer that which is being witnessed (the mind and body). Beingness, which is who and what we are, that we are surrendering into, is the fullness, completeness, and allness of all of life. We are that.

Even right now, you may be confused, and not understand what was just said, as if you can't wrap your "mind" around it. Could you just let go of needing to understand it and just be that? Could you let go of needing to argue a different point of view or perception? Or of needing to be right and thereby making this wrong? Seeing the world as right and wrong is duality, and consequently enslavement. How can formlessness be understood with form? How can the mind with its thoughts and emotions try to understand something that is devoid of thought or emotion and is greater than and beyond the mind? Ultimately, it cannot. Knowing about something is very different from Being it. It just has to be surrendered into. A dog doesn't try to understand its dogness; it just is a dog. What's left to know, when one surrenders into the all Knowingness?

"The key to growth is the introduction of higher dimensions of consciousness into our awareness." - Lao Tzu

9: Transcending the cycle of sowing and reaping

People always wonder why bad things happen to good people? It is important to understand that good vs. bad is just a construct and judgment coming from the mind. Money can be used for good or bad. Gunpowder can be used for fireworks or to blow things up. The mind is the only thing that ascribes meaning to things. One can learn how to surrender and let go of all judgments, positionalities, opinions, emotions, and thoughts – the products of the mind. The mind can be transcended. In fact, our natural state of Being is already that reality beyond the mind. We are all simply in the process of uncovering or becoming more aware of it.

Someone gets cancer and asks, "Why me, God?! I have been a good person and do good things?" Both the context of the question and the health problem must be explored with curiosity. What emotion is behind the asking of the question in the first place? Is it confusion, sadness, fear or anger? The thoughts being generated from these emotions could be so numerous even to count. When people hear the diagnosis of having cancer the fear they experience is overwhelming for many. Where are all of these emotions arising from? They didn't just suddenly jump inside of us the moment we found out about cancer. No, they were already there before, having been sown deeply into our consciousness in our past at some time. The health problem we have could be the necessary catalyst so as to clearly see these emotions. They are reflected in our awareness at that moment so that we can let them go. This isn't about blame; it is about taking responsibility for what has been sown. Whatever we experience emotionally in our perception of bad or good is God's way of inviting us further into our own redemptive story.

If we are honest, unless life gives us pressure, most of us avoid doing this internal work and growth. Stress is what forces us to grow. A health problem is a wonderful catalyst into the surrender of our emotions. Cancer could be the very best thing that ever happened to us. It is only the mind which labels things as good or bad.

Cancer may stretch and grow us in ways that nothing else could. When you let go of the emotion(s) sitting behind why you are asking the question, "Why me?" you will find that the question starts to disappear. Often, with the surrender of <u>all</u> of the many complex and deep-rooted emotions that arise in every moment of life when faced with a health problem like cancer, we give our physical bodies the best chance of healing.

Sowing and reaping aren't about blame, guilt, or questioning why anything is happening to us. It simply is the truth of how the universe is wired. When we see the purpose behind why things are this way, we realize that it has always been God's creative way to help us to see reflections of our consciousness so that we can surrender into love and be free. Freedom in this sense is total and complete peace. Peace is what we were all made for because it is what we already are. Peace is waiting for all of us within and is accessible at all times because it is what you already are.

We reap what we sow, and life is a constant reflection because God cares tremendously about us growing and being more like Him. What would happen if you were aware every second of your life of what you are feeling emotionally on the inside? What would happen if you constantly were letting go of and forgiving yourself for feeling negative emotions that don't support your life or growth?

Will you commit to deeply reflecting on your past and present to make a very concerted effort to let go of your negative emotions? If you choose to journey down this road of self-discovery and letting go of the negative within you, your consciousness can change very quickly, and as a consequence, love, joy, and peace can be experienced more every day.

PART 3
THE TOOLS

8 CHINESE MEDICINE DEMYSTIFIED

"The first practitioner of energy medicine is you, the one who inhabits the body being cared for. Using the principles of energy medicine, you can optimize your body's natural capacities to heal itself and to stay healthy. You can bring renewed stamina to a tired body, fresh vitality to a weary mind, and new bounce to a sagging spirit. You can manage your energies to more effectively meet stress, reduce anxiety, and free yourself of many ailments. And you can apply what you learn for yourself to benefit family members and other loved ones."
- Donna Eden, Energy Medicine

"The crux of holistic integration is simply this: reductionism (western medicine) treats disease; holism treats patterns." - Christian Nix

Seeing and taking responsibility for my emotions brought me a very fresh understanding as to why I was struggling with depression. Chinese medicine helped me understand my emotions in the context of my whole body. The Chinese have known for thousands of years exactly why people struggle with depression and have incredible solutions to this problem. Chinese medicine doesn't see a symptom and tries to treat it. Chinese medicine reveals patterns of things that may seem unrelated to each other, but are part of the same pattern on physical, energetic, and emotional levels. When the pattern is discovered, it can be treated from the vast reservoir of knowledge and tools from thousands of years of brilliant medicine.

In the clinic, I frequently will get phone calls from people wondering if I can help them with a particular health problem they have. When we go to a Western doctor, we go because we automatically assume that they can help us with whatever we are dealing with. The same is true for Chinese medicine. In some way, I have been able to help every person that I have treated in the clinic. Chinese medical doctors can help with any health problem under the sun, even the ones that are the most untreatable and unmanageable from a Western perspective.

The Chinese medical philosophy understands the body in an amazing way that facilitates healing through natural means and restores balance to the body. Acupuncture, one of the branches of Chinese medicine, is good for anyone at any time with virtually any health condition. It doesn't matter if it is something as simple as scrapes and bruises, female issues, back and neck pain, or chronic diseases such as cancer, diabetes or Parkinson's. These same diseases and problems were around thousands of years ago, and the Chinese successfully dealt with them then and can successfully deal with them now. All these issues fall into very specific treatable patterns.

Every Westerner should learn about Chinese medicine and the precepts behind this medicine. I am convinced that if everyone was taught and followed the healthy ideals of Chinese medicine we could eliminate 70% or more of all disease and health problems in the world today. That is how powerful this medicine is. If we combined this integratively and seamlessly with the best of Western medicine, this world would be a much different place. In China, you can go to many hospitals, and there is both an Eastern and Western wing. Many of the doctors are fully trained in both disciplines. When a patient comes in, it is determined immediately whether Eastern or Western medicine (or a combination of both) would be best for healing. This model is amazing and combines the best of both worlds. Think of the possibilities! What are some of the main precepts of Chinese medicine?

It Gets To The Root Cause Of The Problem

Don't get me wrong; I think aspects of Western medicine are great. As just mentioned, I think we should combine the best of Western and Eastern here in the USA in an environment that isn't driven by profit. This would be an incredible system of medicine working synergistically. However, what I have observed is that frequently Western medicine does not treat the root cause of most health problems. Most drugs and surgery just manage the symptoms of disease. Drugs, in particular, are designed to be very profitable for the companies who make them, oftentimes and arguably at the expense of the people they're supposedly helping.

If your thyroid is underfunctioning, in Western medicine, you will be given a synthetic drug to take for the rest of your life. What about finding out the reasons for the imbalance in the first place? What about answering the question why the thyroid is not making hormones the way it is supposed to? I have always been a very curious person. When I was diagnosed with hypothyroidism at the age of 17, I remember the doctor handing me a prescription for Synthroid, and telling me that I would have to take it for the rest of my life. I asked him what caused my thyroid to underfunction in the first place. His response was, "We don't know." And that was that. I find most Western medical doctors don't know much about what causes the thyroid not to function correctly. Because they don't know why it underfunctions, they don't look for or know real natural solutions. But an underfunctioning thyroid has very specific causes and proven natural strategies to heal.

Hearing that I would have to take a drug for the rest of my life did not sit well with me. Upon taking the medication, I felt much better, but the medication did not fix the underlying problem. It simply covered it up. We should all be intensely curious and take our health into our own hands. What about inflammation? What about a viral factor affecting the thyroid? What about foods that cause inflammation? Perhaps you need more iodine or tyrosine in the diet? Perhaps your thyroid needs to be cleansed from heavy metals and chemicals? Maybe your liver is not converting T4 to T3 properly? Maybe the rest of your endocrine system is not functioning well for some reason? What if there are emotional causes and an imbalance to your 5th chakra? If your thyroid is damaged from exposure to heavy metals and chemicals, the root cause would not be addressed by taking synthetic hormones, would it? Ask questions, be curious, get responses and be your own detective.

I took medication for over 12 years. Now, since I see this in the clinic as the most common issue to treat, I have done considerable reading, investigating and implementing strategies with people that discover and correct the underlying cause of the problem. When you address the underlying causes, the need for the medication will go away, and you can be restored to balance. Balance is the goal of Chinese medicine. Your body has the remarkable ability to balance itself when the correct things are addressed. I don't take the Western medication any longer, because it's not necessary. This is the heart of Chinese medicine. It seeks to understand all of the causes as to why your body may not be functioning properly by seeing the patterns that created the problem.

Restore Balance To The Body

Chinese medicine is about balance. Disease and health problems are reflections of unbalance. Therefore, any treatment in Chinese medicine is about restoring balance. Chinese medicine doesn't cure anything. It helps restore the body's own ability to balance itself.

One of the main guiding principles of Chinese medicine is the idea of Hot vs. Cold. For example, if someone is extremely constipated and has a burning sensation in the abdomen and sphincter region, these signs could reflect internal heat in the large intestine. If you leave cookies baking in the oven for too long, they will burn and dry out. If you are consuming foods that have a hot or warm thermal quality, such as alcohol (very hot), over time continued consumption creates an imbalance. This is especially true if equally cold things (vegetables) are over consumed.

If a fire was burning, what do we reach for most of the time to put the fire out? Water. So the concept to restore balance in Chinese medicine would be to cool down the large intestines and bring moisture to this area. There are acupuncture points, herbs, prescriptions for food therapy, qigong (which is movement, breathing, and meditation that cultivates life-healing energy), and other things that can expel heat from this part of the body, cool it down and restore moisture, thereby facilitating healing or restoring balance.

In this case, each modality that is present in Chinese medicine can serve in some way to "put out a fire." Chinese medicine is brilliant and, while the medicine can seem quite complex, the guiding principles are very simple. If something is cold in the body, heat it up. If something is hot, cool it down.

Chinese Medicine Treats The Whole Person: Body, Mind, And Spirit

If you just treat the body and leave out the mind and the spirit, healing is incomplete. Unfortunately, Western medicine focuses mostly on the body. Identified in ancient literature as one of, if not the most important causes of lack of harmony in the body are the seven internal "demons." These "demons" are the seven primary negative emotions: anger, fear, worry, pensiveness, excessive joy, grief, and sadness. Emotions are a part of the mind. Considering them must be a part of the total picture when helping someone to heal their whole person. The internal negative emotions and experiences in the past must be dealt with to help someone truly heal on all levels. When someone gets a serious health problem, this is usually just a reflection that there has been disharmony of unresolved internal conflict in someone for a long time.

Chinese medicine also does not treat disease. It does not treat cancer, diabetes, arthritis, or any other Western named diseases. The Chinese didn't think about cures, but balance and harmony. However, all the diseases mentioned earlier (and more) were described in patterns that the Chinese saw reflected in the body. For example, if someone has lower back pain, this may be called Kidney Yang deficiency in Chinese medicine. If you have a deficiency, the guiding principle in Chinese medicine is to tonify or build up. If you have excess in the body, the principle is to reduce. The goal, in this case, would be to tonify Kidney Yang. There are many ways to do that.

If someone has a cancerous tumor, for example, this may be a pattern called damp phlegm (cancer can present as many different patterns). If you jumped into a lake with all your clothes on and then got out, your clothes would feel heavy on you. Internal dampness would be like wearing heavy clothes on the inside. When things are heavy, the internal tendency is that things slow down. Blood, electricity, and other body processes need to keep moving to maintain balance. If there is an internal state of dampness, this can slow things down. After years and years of internal dampness, lack of balance reflects itself in the body symptomatically. If things slow down too much, they can become a substantial mass of phlegm, which the Chinese call a nodule (tumor in Western medicine).

So the principle in this case is to drain dampness and break up phlegm in the body. Many drying (for dampness) and moving herbs (for phlegm) are part of the Chinese herbal pharmacopoeia. The Chinese saw these patterns and used the guiding principles to bring balance and harmony to the body through natural means. It is not in the Chinese medical vernacular to say someone is cured of anything, but it is a part of this medicine to say balance has been or can be restored. Lack of disease is balance. ALL symptoms in the body fall into very particular patterns in Chinese medicine, and any pattern that presents in the body can be treated. The key, in this case and in any case, is to restore balance before phlegm (tumor) appears. Prevention is much easier on the body in the long run.

Activate The Body's Own Healing Mechanism

One thing that Chinese physicians talk a lot about is qi (pronounced chi). While qi is described in many ways, perhaps one of the best translations is that qi is oxygen[156] or even electricity.[157] Qi can take many forms and do many different things. Qi is so many different things, but it has also been described as our life force or spirit. Our spirit is what makes us alive; it is the animating principle of life in the body. A television without electricity is just plastic and other inanimate parts. But with electricity, it comes to life. Without spirit, we would just be a pile of flesh and bones, dust. Without qi, the body is just flesh and bone. Oxygen and the electricity running through the nervous system and acupuncture channel system is the qi that has been described in ancient terms. Qi is not some super-mystical substance, but a scientifically measurable and palpable thing.

The best book that discusses how similar Western medicine is and how acupuncture can best be understood is called *The Spark in the Machine: How the Science of Acupuncture Explains the Mysteries of Western Medicine* by Daniel Keown, (who is an acupuncturist and medical doctor in the UK). This is why upon putting a needle in a patient and stimulating (twisting) the needle, an electrical sensation can be felt by the patient. Have you ever rubbed your feet on the carpet and then touched someone and felt a discharge of static electricity? This is what some people experience with acupuncture. The good thing about acupuncture is that we don't have to twist the needles for it to work. We can simply insert the needles, which are virtually painless and let them balance the body without feeling this electrical sensation. By balancing and regulating electrical flow in the body, oxygen, blood, and pain modulating chemicals from the brain can be delivered to the areas of the body that need it the most. Science, using the understanding of embryology, is finally able to explain how acupuncture works.

One of the main ways a Chinese practitioner works with qi is through the qi channels of energy. These channels correspond perfectly with connective tissue divides in the body. Connective tissue is piezoelectric, meaning that it is a great conductor *and* generator of electrical energy or qi. The qi that is in your body can be likened to a huge river, and this river just happens to be a river of invisible electric energy. While we may not be able to see qi, qi energy can be felt in the meridians and you can feel it flowing in the body with learned sensitivity. You can't see electricity in the power line, but if you come near it or touch the power line, you will definitely feel it. Anyone can learn to feel the electrical qi that is in the body. Modern science has proven this energy exists and we now can measure it with advanced scientific equipment. We use very advanced equipment to produce an electrocardiogram, which allows us to measure the electrical activity of the heart. The heart is the electromagnetic center of the body, which is also why the Chinese called this organ the emperor.

The electrical river of qi is divided into 12 major sections or channels that correspond to the 12 different organs. This energy flows down the arms and back again up to the head, from the head to the feet, and from the feet back to the chest or head area again. These meridians are associated with organs because every meridian or connective channel division of energy connects through a primary organ and has a significant impact on how that organ functions both physically and energetically. Organs in Chinese medicine have physical, energetic, and consciousness qualities. These meridians, channels or sections to the river of qi energy run through every part of the body from bones to muscles, all the way up into the skin.

In a very simple way, if you want to understand how health problems occur, it can be understood by using this same river analogy. If a blockage occurred at any point in a river, what would happen to the foliage downstream that is now not receiving the same amount of water? It would lose the life-giving energy of that water to grow, be healthy and proliferate. The same is true in the river of qi of the body.

For example, the stomach channel runs from north to south, from the face to the feet, and it passes through the stomach on its way down. Blockages in the energy system can occur for many reasons such as eating the wrong foods, not exercising enough, holding onto negative emotions, getting attacked by a virus or bacteria, etc. If a blockage occurred anywhere on this meridian, what symptoms would you expect? Any symptom that relates to Chinese stomach dysfunction could be things such as nausea, vomiting, belching, acid reflux, GERD, esophageal or stomach cancer, etc.

Let's say the blockage occurred at a point along the channel right next to the belly button. If a blockage occurred on a regular river, we would, of course, go to the site of the blockage and do what is needed to free up the flow of water. Inserting a needle in the place of a blockage along this channel will have the same effect and allows oxygen, blood, and electricity to flow unimpeded once again to that area. Once the channel is flowing freely again, balance is restored, and symptoms may then disappear.

Free flowing qi nourishes tissues, cells, muscles, organs, and glands, which is why it is so critical that there is enough of it and it is flowing where it needs to. The expertise comes in knowing where to put the needles and where the imbalance is coming from. Some people have so many imbalances that they need many sessions to correct it. Also, most people have been living with some form of blockage for years, even decades. Some imbalances can be corrected in a few treatments, but some require extensive, multifaceted treatment. In China, if a case of serious imbalance occurs (such as the presentation of a very chronic disease) one will go everyday or every other day for weeks or even months to receive acupuncture treatment. Imbalances occur everyday in our "electrical" system, some being small and some very large. This is why I am a huge proponent of getting acupuncture regularly for life, as it's a simple thing to do with potentially incredible benefits.

Prevent Health Problems With Chinese Medicine

By getting regular acupuncture treatments, receiving constant guidance from a Chinese physician about food and herbs, and living in harmony with nature, you can prevent most diseases, be happy, and live a full life. Chinese medicine was designed to deal with imbalances long before they turned into chronic disease patterns. Imagine if we were raised from the time we were infants learning about how to have a sound body, mind, and spirit—life would be fuller, and we would all suffer less creating a much more peaceful world.

Now that you have some understanding of the principles of Chinese medicine, in this section, we'll examine some of the other tools the Chinese used to help people restore balance to their bodies.

Herbs

In many ways, the Chinese were the first pharmacists, using an extensive list of natural substances to help restore harmony to the body. In fact, many of the drugs used by pharmaceutical companies today are isolated substances that are found in numerous plants and herbs. Isolating a substance and using it in large quantities can often lead to imbalance, but using the whole herb rarely causes imbalance when used properly. The Chinese pharmacopeia consists of hundreds and hundreds of herbs that are used for every health problem and pattern found under the sun.

An interesting quality that the Chinese discovered thousands of years ago is that every herb enters into very specific channels and organs in the body. For example, if disharmony were found in the Stomach channel, one would want to use an herb that brought about an action that affected that channel/organ. Knowing how to use herbs is, in my estimation, the most powerful and most complicated aspect of Chinese medicine. This is why we are board certified to use them.

Herbs are categorized according to their main actions, hot and cold properties, taste (acrid, sweet, salty, bitter, toxic), what channels they affect, and how well they work with other herbs. Herbs are extremely powerful in dealing with almost anything, from simple things like a cold to complex things like chronic degenerative diseases. Some herbs need to be consumed for a longer period and some for shorter. If a health problem took 20 years to develop, taking herbs for months or longer may be required to heal.

Food Therapy

Foods are used much the same way herbs are regarding their energetic qualities and what organs/channels they affect. After a long winter and wanting to cleanse the body (spring cleaning), bitter herbs and foods may be used to help the body cleanse. Dandelion leaves and kale may be used to accomplish this. If the body is cold, spices such as cayenne pepper, cinnamon, nutmeg, or curry may be used to warm the body.

Certain foods are used to balance many different conditions in Chinese medicine including dampness, qi deficiency, yang deficiency, yin deficiency, and blood deficiency. They are also used to target specific organs such as building kidney essence, soothing the liver, or strengthening the spleen. Food can be used to strengthen any part of the body. The Chinese knew thousands of years ago about the energetics of food. I see 19 out of 20 patterns in the clinic today related to blood or yin deficiency, so I rely heavily on food, herbs, and acu-points that strengthen blood and yin, especially dark green leafy vegetables and foods that are red in color.

Tui Na

Tui Na is more than just massage. Some people think that Tui Na was the original form of chiropractic, helping the body to realign structurally. Tui Na uses the hands to stimulate the flow of electricity through the meridians. A Chinese practitioner understands where the flow of energy goes in the body and works with that flow to restore balance.

Moxibustion

Moxibustion ("Moxa" for short) is the dried leaves of mugwort that can be placed on the ends of needles or used separately to be burned over the body. It is used especially in cases of cold in the body or when we desire more blood flow to certain areas. This warmth stimulates the body to restore proper qi and blood flow.

Cupping

Glass, plastic or bamboo cups are used to create a vacuum on the skin, which increases blood flow and circulation. If you watched the last summer Olympics, many of the swimmers had red or purple circles around their shoulders. In Chinese medicine, when someone has pain in the body, this is often referred to as blood stasis. This means that blood is not flowing properly to or around a particular part of the body. By using cupping, blood is forced to move so that fresh blood can circulate through an area. When fresh blood comes to a part of the body where it has not been flowing well, pain generally decreases. Most people love getting cupping done on them.

> "...Emotions...become causes of disease. Of course, affection and emotions definitely affect all the other organs too (energetically and physically), but it is only the Mind that actually recognizes and feels them. For example, anger affects the Liver, but the Liver cannot feel it because it does not house the Mind. Only the Heart can feel it because it houses the Mind, which is responsible for insight. It is for this reason that all emotions eventually affect the Heart (in addition to other specific organs), and it is in this sense that the Heart is the 'emperor' of all the other organs." - Giovanni Maciocia, Foundations of Chinese Medicine[158]

Qi Gong, Tai Chi, and Meditation

Qi Gong, Tai Chi and meditation work on the mental, emotional and spiritual aspects of Chinese medicine by utilizing breathing exercises and specific movements to become more aware of the body. Most people are not as aware of their bodies as they think they are. Qi Gong and Tai Chi provide substantial benefits to health. For example, throughout any given day, how many times do you actually take a deep diaphragmatic breath? Most don't take even one. Most spend their entire day taking very shallow breaths.

Modern science has proven how powerful breathing promotes health. In addition to taking deeper breaths, the added element of staying singly focused on the breath is a practice of meditation. The goal of meditation, among other things, is simply to pay attention. It is also encouraged to foster awareness of the peace we all carry within. Try to sit and meditate and not think of anything, focusing only on the breath. Most people can't go 5 seconds without their mind wandering and thinking about something else. We have so much difficulty quieting the mind in our chaotic world today.

> "If one is calm, peaceful, empty, without desire, then true qi follows. If essence and spirit are protected inside, from where can illness come? If one is

at rest and there are few desires, the heart is in peace, and there is no fear." - Huang Di Nei Jing Su Wen[159]

By meditating we realize how much of a slave we are to our minds and the constant barrage of thoughts we have. Inner peace and stillness are about what the Chinese have called "no mind," which is the same as the "peace that passes understanding" within Christianity. "No mind" is the same as "be still and know that I am God."[160] How can we experience the divine essence within if our mind is constantly chattering? The stillness within us is God. God is not the barrage of thoughts. God is peace, tranquility, and the utter stillness between our thoughts. God can be "found" more within as the mind goes silent. How many of us would love to be able just to shut off our minds? I know many people who have problems sleeping and would love to shut their mind off.

"Those who keep their minds unimpaired within, externally keep their bodies unimpaired…." - Nei Ye, Original Dao: Inward Training[161]

Meditation is comparable to learning a new sport. At first, you might be horrible at it. You don't become the number one player in the world in a certain sport by playing once a month. Athletes train every day for hours to become the best at what they do. Meditation is exactly the same. It must be practiced, constantly and continually, for full benefit. The paradox is that you are practicing to not do anything, but simply to be aware of Being itself. Luckily, if you meditate for an hour per day for 60 days, you can start to see huge shifts within a very short time.

"To live long, people should take care not to worry too much, not to get too angry, not to get too sad, not to get too frightened, not to do too much, talk too much or laugh too much. One should not have too many desires nor face numerous upsetting conditions. All these are harmful to health." - Su Si Miao, 7th Century Daoist Doctor

Using qigong, a Chinese practitioner can use his or her intention to guide the flow of energy in someone's body. Through deep meditation, one can actually feel, see and be able to direct the electricity inside them. They can even learn to project electricity from their own body to another's body. This may seem strange because it is not a part of what we normally see in medicine, but quantum physics has more than proven that this is not only possible, but we can learn to direct energy with our minds and intention. People can be taught to not only feel the flow of electrical qi in the body but also, by understanding this flow, can be directed by a person to help restore balance within themselves. A modern form of this is called Quantum Touch.

Herbs, food therapy, cupping, moxibustion, Tui Na, Tai Chi, and meditation cover many of the different modalities that the Chinese have used to maintain incredible health for thousands of years. I began by stating that if we all employed what the Chinese knew to be good practices for thousands of years, we could reduce disease and suffering in amazing ways. The best of Chinese medicine combined with the most useful aspects of Western medicine in an environment not driven by profit, but by actual patient care, would revolutionize health.

This chapter was written for those who are not that familiar with Chinese medicine. It is truly one of the most remarkable systems of natural healing this world has ever known and has changed my life and how I understand the body. I hope that some of the mystery surrounding this medicine is clearer to you as well.

"All acupuncture methods must find their root in the shen (spirit)."
- Mi Huang Fu[162]

9 HEALING FOODS, HERBS AND FUNGUS

"Today, after several decades of suppression and neglect, psychedelics are having a renaissance. A new generation of scientists, many of them inspired by their own personal experience of the compounds, are testing their potential to heal mental illnesses such as depression, anxiety, trauma, and addiction. Other scientists are using psychedelics in conjunction with new brain-imaging tools to explore the links between brain and mind, hoping to unravel some of the mysteries of consciousness."
- Michael Pollan *How To Change Your Mind*

At the age of 17, I was told that my thyroid wasn't producing thyroid hormone and that I would have to take medication for the rest of my life. This did not sit well with me. When I asked what was causing my body not to be able to produce this hormone on its own, my doctor told me he didn't know. I have found this to be the answer that most physicians give, and they are being very honest. What if it was our crappy inflammatory American diet, heavy metals and chemicals, the uprising of opportunistic pathogens, and serious lack of nutrients that are at the root of thyroid problems and depression? When I took the thyroid medication, I felt better but I still was never back to normal. Often, medication is a band-aid, and if the underlying issues are not addressed, it will get worse over time. If you have a thyroid issue, things can be done to heal naturally.

Many who suffer from hypothyroidism or Hashimoto's thyroiditis feel depressed. In fact, the reason why many people are depressed is that they have an undiagnosed or underdiagnosed thyroid condition. Hashimoto's thyroiditis is considered an autoimmune condition where the immune system is confused and is attacking the thyroid. This idea has never sat well with me as an explanation for autoimmune conditions. The body is far too intelligent to attack itself. However, your immune system is most likely attacking a pathogen (virus or bacteria) that has taken up residence in the thyroid.

Anthony William, author of *Thyroid Healing*, has a very unique view on thyroid issues indicating that the culprit for most thyroid conditions is the Epstein-Barr Virus (EBV), which is the virus implicated in a mononucleosis infection.[163] EBV is a virus in the herpes family of viruses and causes glandular fever. Common symptoms are "flu-like" including fever, rash, fatigue, inflamed throat, swollen lymph nodes and enlarged spleen and liver. It is everywhere and can be implicated in innumerable conditions today. Western medicine is starting to realize that this virus may be the culprit behind many different health conditions today. However, for the time being, this virus has not been understood or studied enough.

Have you had a diagnosed mononucleosis infection? Have you had these flu-like symptoms mentioned above? If so, you may have an EBV infection. If your thyroid antibodies are elevated, your immune system is doing its job, trying to deal with the pathogen creating inflammation in the thyroid. EBV feeds on heavy metals and chemicals in the body. The average person in the USA today is so toxic and full of metals and chemicals which is why this virus has gotten so out of control today. My own TSH levels were over 60 (should be around 1-2) and thyroid antibodies over 1000 (should be under 2). I brought them back into normal range with a very specific nutritional protocol, detoxification and powerful supplements that can cleanse the body and deal with this viral factor.

While we haven't spent much time on the role of healing the thyroid in depression, physically speaking, it may be the most critical thing you do to heal from depression. This cannot be understated. Two books have tremendously shaped how I see thyroid health. One book approaches the thyroid from the best of medical studies that the western world has to offer today. This book is called *Hashimoto's Thyroiditis* by Dr. Isabella Wentz.[164] These books do not agree on some key issues, but both of them suggest all-natural ways to heal. Try one or both as they are both exceptional books.

Liver Qi Stagnation

Most literature in Chinese medicine points in the direction of liver qi stagnation as the first or primary cause of depression or the most significant factor leading to deeper depression over time. Very simply, depression is stagnation, meaning that something has slowed down and isn't moving well. In The *Practice of Chinese Medicine* by Giovanni Maciocia states, "In Chinese medicine, stagnation and mental depression are almost synonymous, implying that all depression is due to stagnation. This is obviously not true in practice, as there are many deficiency conditions leading to depression. However, it is true that all emotions, even those that initially deplete qi, lead to qi stagnation, thus the first effect of emotional stress is some qi stagnation."[165]

While emotions affect the whole body, in the case of qi stagnation, the organ that is most responsible for making sure qi is circulating properly in the body is the liver. The heart and the lungs also are affected by qi stagnation, but not as frequently as the liver. The main pathological emotion of the liver is anger and all of its subsets such as resentment, frustration, annoyance, hatred, rage, and fury. This is one of the main reasons that when I see people with depression in the clinic, my first question often is: "What are you most angry about in life?" The consciousness aspects of the liver have to do with inspiration, creativity, ideas, plans, life dreams, and aspirations. When liver qi is stagnant, these aspects in life suffer. As the health of the liver improves, all of these aspects start coming to life again.

In Chinese medicine, several factors contribute to stagnation or depression including an irregular diet, overwork, and constitutional weaknesses. In the diet, the bad foods we already discussed create inflammation and lead to the body producing phlegm. Phlegm is gooey, sticky and slows things down. These things lead to qi stagnation.

When the body is overworked, it can eventually lead to deficiencies in the kidneys, which are the organs responsible for providing us with willpower, or the drive to engage fully in the world. Constitutional weaknesses may refer to general genetic predispositions that have been present since birth or general weaknesses that present themselves with the onset of depression.

Twelve different patterns related to depression are found in *The Practice of Chinese Medicine* by Giovanni Maciocia. Western medicine has led us into a one-pill-fits-all mentality. This is not at all like Chinese medicine. Depression can be treated dozens of different ways because one person may have one pattern and someone else a completely different pattern. Yet, both are depressed. Patterns are treated very differently. Chinese medicine takes into account your specific individuality. Therefore, out on the street when meeting people, I frequently get asked, "Hey, what should I take for _____?" My normal answer truthfully is, "I have no idea!" This isn't because I don't have adequate responses, but I would have to explore one's health history to see what the pattern is and then treat the pattern accordingly.

In each pattern we can determine the emotions contributing to the problem and the organ(s) most affected by the condition. Next, you can use diet, herbal medicine, acupuncture, massage, and forms of meditation to release emotions from the body. We form a treatment plan specifically designed for you and your pattern. This is what makes Chinese medicine so brilliant not only for depression but for any condition with which one struggles. It is a complete system of medicine, and any symptoms people have fall into patterns that have been treatable for thousands of years.

The twelve most common patterns related to depression in Chinese medicine are:

- Liver-qi stagnation
- Heart- and lung-qi stagnation
- Stagnant liver-qi turning into heat
- Phlegm-heat harassing the mind
- Blood stasis obstructing the mind
- Qi stagnation with phlegm
- Diaphragm heat

- Worry injuring the mind
- Heart and spleen deficiency
- Heart-yang deficiency
- Kidney- and heart-yin deficiency,
- Empty heat blazing, Kidney-yang deficiency.

Each of these patterns presents with different symptoms. Depression can uniquely be a part of each of these patterns.

Food In Chinese Medicine For Reducing Stagnation

In Chinese medicine certain foods can help reduce excesses or stagnation in the liver. Food is a powerful ally when dealing with stagnation. Stagnation, at least initially, is seen as an excess. It may turn into a deficiency over long periods of time, and then an entirely different group of foods will need to be consumed. Therefore, if you have a question as to whether these foods would help you, consult with an acupuncturist or Chinese medical doctor. Due to negative emotions (especially anger), toxins, and nutritional deficiencies, the liver can run hot and get inflamed. The foods listed below are some of the things that can help the liver.

Foods that calm and soothe the liver, reduce excess, and stimulate the liver out of stagnancy are:

- Vegetables
- Legumes (beans and lentils)
- Sprouted foods
- Raw organic unfiltered honey mixed with lemon juice
- Citrus peel
- Romaine lettuce
- Asparagus
- Alfalfa
- Chamomile tea
- Amaranth
- Quinoa
- Onions
- Garlic
- Leeks
- Scallions
- Chives
- Watercress

- Mustard greens
- Ginger
- Black pepper
- Horseradish
- Turmeric
- Basil
- Bay leaf
- Marjoram
- Cumin
- Fennel
- Dill
- Rosemary
- Mint
- Lemon balm

Acupuncture For Reducing Stagnation In Chinese Medicine

All of the above mentioned twelve patterns have various acupoints that are specific in dealing with each of those patterns. Acupuncture also has an amazing ability to decrease inflammation in the body. Many points on the body not only treat specific organs but also soothe stagnation, release heat, reduce phlegm, strengthen deficiency and calm the mind. While these points will not be discussed here, I highly encourage you to try acupuncture if you are battling with depression. It may not be the final answer for you, but most likely it will very positively contribute to your feeling better.

Herbal Medicine For Reducing Stagnation In Chinese Medicine

Herbs have been used for thousands of years around the world as the world's first "pharmaceuticals". Multiple herbal formulas exist for all 12 patterns that can be extremely beneficial in dealing with depression. I am convinced that formulas used beyond 50 years ago were experienced more powerfully than today. This is not because the herbs are any less powerful, but because health is so much worse in the USA today than it has ever been. We have never had so much excess from sugar, dairy, and genetically modified pesticide-laden wheat products. These excesses are far more pronounced than they were just 50 years ago. Herbal formulas need to be used for longer and especially in combination with detoxification and other serious lifestyle changes to help people heal most effectively.

The most wonderful part about properly prescribed foods, acupoints, and herbal formulas is zero (or very minimal) side effects. Over 100,000 people die each year from properly prescribed pharmaceutical medications. Millions of other people feel powerful side effects from the medications they take on a daily basis. Unless it is a life-saving medication, like insulin, Chinese herbs exist for virtually every health problem known to man. Even in the case of type 1 diabetes requiring insulin, with proper diet and lifestyle modifications, Dr. Gabriel Cousens MD has proven that even the need for insulin can be reversed and the patient healed. When truly healthy, the body has the potential of producing insulin on its own again. I never advise my patients to come off medications, as this is a violation of my scope of practice. However, when some become truly healthy, the need for medication can diminish or disappear for many.

Meditation For Depression In Chinese Medicine

Historically one of the primary ways used by Chinese medical doctors to help deal with emotions in the mind was through meditation. Tapping and other consciousness based tools expand upon this practice and make it even better and more direct in dealing with a health problem. *Full Catastrophe Living* by Dr. Jon Kabat-Zinn is the modern bible with regards to meditation.[166] In this book hundreds of studies are cited as evidence from a scientific perspective that meditation has a profound and lasting effect on helping people feel better. As a part of his work, he has recorded many guided meditations which you can purchase, listen to and follow along with. These guided meditations will teach you how to meditate. I highly recommend them. The guided meditations of Kelly Howell are also very useful.[167]

The Benefit of Psychedelics

Psilocybin, the psychoactive component found in over 200 species of mushrooms, is now being hailed to be for psychiatry and mental illness, what antibiotics were for medicine. Psilocybin, along with LSD, Peyote, Ayahuasca, Iboga, and DMT, are also known as psychedelics. The word psychedelic means "mind manifesting." Another term that is frequently used when describing these substances is entheogen. Entheogen is a term that means "bringing forth the divine within" and has been used due to how powerful and life changing experiences are with these substances and the ability they have to affect mystical spiritual experiences.

In 1962, Walter Pahnke, a minister and psychiatrist, set up an experiment using psilocybin that would later be called the March Chapel Experiment.[168] This experiment was run at the Harvard Divinity School and almost all the participants were graduate divinity students. One of the participants, Hudson Smith, described his experience as, "the most powerful cosmic homecoming I have ever experienced."[169] In a 25-year follow up to this experiment, all subjects described it as a "genuine mystical nature and characterize it as one of the high points of their spiritual life."[170]

How psychedelics are able to offer the life changing experiences users describe is not completely clear yet to science. However, new research is pointing the way into our experience of something that has been called our default mode network, a group of areas in the brain that seem to show lower levels of activity when we are engaged in a particular task like paying attention, but higher levels of activity when we are awake and not involved in any specific mental exercise.[171] It is the part of us that is commonly referred to as our ego. Our ego is essentially a survival mechanism that evolved over time to keep us alive. However, if we take the standpoint from a more spiritual perspective that actual death and life are not possibilities and that we *are* always, then as awareness and consciousness increase, less of a need for the ego exists. Having said this, psychedelics have been proven to turn down the use of this network and expand the areas of the brain related to consciousness itself. Thus, many users have reported experiencing extreme feelings of love, joy, peace, and oneness with everyone and everything. It could be the default mode network that is too active in the brain with those struggling with depression, which is why science is proving how effective it is, even if done one time for someone struggling with this health issue. The following study demonstrates how remarkable, long lasting, and relieving psychedelics can be at healing those with depression.

At Johns Hopkins University in the department of psychiatry and behavioral sciences research is being conducted on helping late-stage cancer patients deal with depression and anxiety by using psilocybin.[172] In a study of 51 patients that were given a single large dose of psilocybin, in a six month follow up, 80% showed significant decreases in both anxiety and depression, with 60% going back into normal range. Of the participants, 70% rated this one experience as being in their all-time top 5 most spiritual experiences. Results of this were published in the Journal of Psychopharmacology.[173]

Another study of 29 patients with depression and anxiety were given psilocybin, and the results speak volumes about the effectiveness of this substance in helping people with this issue:

"…Psilocybin produced immediate, substantial, and sustained improvements in anxiety and depression and led to decreases in cancer-related demoralization and hopelessness, improved spiritual well-being, and increased quality of life. At the 6.5-month follow-up, psilocybin was associated with enduring anxiolytic and antidepressant effects (approximately 60–80% of participants continued with clinically significant reductions in depression or anxiety), sustained benefits in existential distress and quality of life, as well as improved attitudes towards death. The psilocybin-induced mystical experience mediated the therapeutic effect of psilocybin on anxiety and depression."[174]

In other studies, participants reported that consumption of LSD in the right set and setting was found to be one of the most profound and life-changing spiritual experiences they have ever had.[175] Many others who have ventured to Peru to participate in an ayahuasca ceremony report very similar radical life-changing experiences. Ayahuasca is a visionary psychedelic decoction that has been used in Peru for thousands of years and is protected because it is part of a long religious tradition. When done in the right set and setting, ayahuasca is very safe. I have spoken to many people that have had similar radical life-altering experiences with this substance.

In one such case in December of 2017, I spoke to a woman who had just completed her second ayahuasca experience. I asked her how her first experience was and her response was characteristic of many people I have asked about this. She said, "It is indescribable, really. I can't begin to tell you what it is like because words would fall very short of being able to tell you. However, I can tell you what affect it had on me." She went on to say that she had been a hopeless heroin addict for the past 10 years. She took the ayahuasca and after one night, she never touched heroin ever again. She said she felt so much love from the Universe (what she referred to as God), realizing that this was no different from the essence of who and what she was. In her words, love is what healed her from the addiction.

LSD, magic mushrooms and psilocybin are categorized as Schedule 1 drugs, which are those that are found to be highly addictive and have no medicinal value. I think the pharmaceutical companies saw how powerful and effective these substances were and knew that they couldn't profit from them, so they decided to lobby against them making them illegal. Imagine taking one dose and having an experience that was so powerful that your depression and anxiety lessened significantly or disappeared completely? If so, that wouldn't be good for these companies' business and wouldn't force people to take drugs for years or even an entire lifetime.

Although psychedelics are wonderful, it is very important to use them wisely. In *The Psychedelic Explorer's Guidebook*, written by psychologist James Fadiman, he mentions that "set and setting" are the most important aspects to have before beginning a psychedelic journey.[176] What this translates to is being with people that you explicitly trust, who will take care of your every need lovingly in a very safe environment with minimal to no distractions. It also means using the substances with soothing and inspiring music (such as classical). In cases where people were confronted with fears or challengers, someone was there to help them to let go of the resistance to the experience. It is when these conditions are not present that people can have bad experiences. Having the proper dose is also critical due to the intensity that the experience can afford someone. People may panic, become anxious, confused, and disoriented. It is also not recommended for those with existing psychosis, such as those with schizophrenia.

Psychedelics, such as magic mushrooms have been used in very sacred settings in people groups all over the world for millennia. It is suggested that they be approached with reverence and seen in a sacred light due to how transformative they truly can be.

Just as people are waking up to how incredibly medicinal and effective marijuana can be in its various forms for many health conditions, many are discovering how powerful magic mushrooms, LSD, or other psychedelics can be in helping alleviate not only depression and anxiety but also other health challenges. Just as alcohol and marijuana need to be consumed responsibly, so also should mushrooms be used responsibly.

As of July 2021, it is still illegal to consume magic mushrooms (psilocybin) and LSD. Ayahuasca is legal to consume in various parts of the USA for religious purposes or abroad in places like Peru or Costa Rica. What is presented above is simply informational and is not meant as an encouragement to break the law. However, people suffering from depression want help, answers, and solutions that work. The evidence from recent research shows how powerful these substances are when used responsibly. Additionally, many thousands of people that have tried it recreationally state emphatically how wonderful it is when dealing with depression. You can make a difference by writing to your local politicians and raising awareness about how beneficial these things can be. Recently (November 2020), Oregon was the first state in the USA to decriminalize psychedelics and grant therapists the ability to use these substances in a therapeutic environment legally.

Kratom

Kratom is a very special supplement that has some remarkable uses. It comes from a tropical evergreen tree that is in the coffee family. The leaves of the tree are commonly dried and ground into a powder, taken in powder form, encapsulated, or consumed as a tea. It has four main effects that include inducing relaxation, relieving pain, enhancing mood, and stimulating. Certain strains of kratom are more potent with one or more of these qualities but lack the others.

Many people are drawn to kratom because of its wonderful ability to relieve pain. So many people in this world are in physical pain. I believe fervently that much of the physical pain we see actually has an emotional root that most don't know how to delve into and let go of. However, for those that are still holding onto their emotional pain and still need physical relief without the addictive potential of opiates, Kratom is wonderful. It is a wonderful herb, but in many cases is still just a band-aid. It needs to continue to be used to be effective. One study has shown that kratom does enhance mood and relieve anxiety in some people, while also stating that it is a wonderful alternative for those who have struggled with opiod addiction and has the potential to be mildly addictive.[177] It is something that should be used responsibly.

In the case of depression, certain strains exist that are mood enhancing and stimulating, giving people a very mild euphoric, feel-good sensation. For the person with depression who is just trying to feel better while simultaneously working on other issues to get at the root of the problem, this herb can be very useful.

Kratom was recently in the news because the DEA wanted to make it into a schedule 1 drug.[178] A schedule 1 drug is labeled this way because it is said to have no medicinal benefits and is highly addictive. This is beyond ridiculous. Remember, marijuana and magic mushrooms are also schedule 1 drugs, and they are not addictive. In fact, even though on a federal level (as of May 2019) marijuana is still a schedule 1 drug, many people throughout the USA have realized how wonderful and powerful the uses of marijuana and hemp are to help people heal. The same is happening with magic mushrooms. It is highly medicinal and both have incredible benefits and are not addictive.

When the DEA pushed for Kratom to be made a schedule 1 drug, thousands of people revolted and sent a petition to the White House in protest. The DEA completely backed off because people reacted stating that this was invaluable in helping them deal with their physical pain. It has also been indispensable in helping people wean off heroin and opiate addictions. This was back in 2016, and now, almost a year later the FDA is making the same push to label it a schedule 1 drug. It has been "reported" that it has been responsible for over 36 deaths. This is complete nonsense, and it is amazing to see how far our government will go to protect pharmaceutical interests. Kratom is dirt cheap, works fabulously and helps millions of people. These millions of people may not be pharmaceutical customers, so heavy lobbying and pressure have been made to make it illegal.

I feel the data is being manipulated about it being unsafe and the FDA is not protecting the interests of the people at all. I think they are completely catering to the greedy hands of the pharmaceutical industry. If you are in pain, want a safe energy boost or are just feeling a little blue, give kratom a try. Much information is out there on the internet about where it can be purchased, which strains should be taken for the desired effect and how much to consume.

10 APPLIED KINESIOLOGY & MUSCLE TESTING

"It is through science that we prove, but through intuition
that we discover." - Henri Poincare

"The intuitive mind is a sacred gift and the rational mind is a
faithful servant. We have created a society that honors the
servant and has forgotten the gift." - Albert Einstein

What if a tool existed that could be used to get a "yes" or "no" answer to any question that you asked about anything in the universe? What if this tool existed and it could be used to discover exactly why you had a specific health problem? Imagine finding out the real reason(s) why you suffered from pounding headaches, lower back pain, low energy, depression, cancer, or even AIDS.

Imagine the astounding implications this would have, not only for you and your life, but for the world at large. Imagine getting to the root or truth of an issue quickly and easily. Imagine also that this tool could be used not only for present moment things but also to ask about anything in the past. The questions would be endless, and the implications mind-blowing. Questions could be answered about anything from physical issues to world events, political issues, determining innocence, guilt in court, or even spiritual questions. It would be amazing if a tool like this existed, wouldn't it? If we all used this tool to heal, the world would literally be revolutionized overnight.

Well, a tool like this does exist, and it is used by tens of thousands of people in the world—mostly by alternative health care practitioners as a way to get feedback from the body. It is called applied kinesiology (AK) or muscle testing. In my personal experience, AK was used to discover the experiences and emotions that were contributing to my severe depression.

Before you write this off as new age, a hoax, or something that is simply impossible, please read further and keep an open mind. If thousands of well respected, highly-trained practitioners all over the world use this tool for many different purposes, it's worth finding out why they all utilize it. Moreover, with the advance of quantum theory (the cutting edge of science), a very logical and scientific basis exists that quantum mechanics can explain as to why this tool works.

What Is Applied Kinesiology?

Kinesiology comes from two words, "kinesis," which means "movement" and "ology," which means, "study of." Therefore, kinesiology is the study of movement. Even more specifically, it is the study of the principles of mechanics and anatomy in relation to human movement. Applied kinesiology takes kinesiology and breaks off into something even more specific. AK involves using a muscle in the body that is tested in response to physical, energetic, mental, or emotional stimulus. In the presence of a stimulus, the muscle response when tested will either remain strong or go weak. A weak muscle response is indicative of something that does not support life. A strong muscle response corresponds with something that supports and benefits life. It's that simple.

How To Perform Applied Kinesiology

Applied Kinesiology can be performed using any muscle of the body. Most of the time, the arm (deltoid muscle) is used and is extended parallel to the ground. While the subject is holding out his/her arm, the tester presses downward using two or three fingers just above the wrist with light pressure. The subject is asked to resist the downward pressure. If no stimulus is being tested, the arm will be able to hold or resist the pressure and remain locked into place while the pressure is being applied. When something that is tested is positive or life-supporting, the arm response will remain strong or locked. When something that is tested is negative or life-threatening, the arm response will go weak or unlock.

AK testing is very simple to do, but it takes a lot of practice to feel the subtleties of the muscle response. If you use AK frequently, over time you will find that you apply less and less pressure when performing the test. Dr. John Thie uses "The Rule of 2's" and says that "It is unnecessary to apply more than 2 pounds of pressure…Apply and release the pressure within 2 seconds."[179] When learning AK, I used to put undue pressure on peoples' arms and they walked out of the clinic having gotten a full arm workout! I quickly learned that wasn't necessary. Movement of the arm more than 2 inches is also unnecessary. So in summary, you can use AK and perform the muscle test with 2 pounds, 2 inches, and 2 seconds.

Here is a simple example of how AK can be used. In the clinic, I keep a packet of Splenda handy for testing someone for the first time. Splenda is a neurotoxin and is detrimental to life. The subject takes the Splenda and holds it in their hand or over their solar plexus. With the other arm, the muscles test is performed. When tested the arm instantly goes weak, losing about 50% of its strength. This has been demonstrated with 250-pound football players. They too lose 50% of their strength, even when resisting with all their might. The reason for this is due to the fact that Splenda is artificial and neurotoxic and does not support life, so no one should be using it. In contrast, one could use an organic apple to test someone and the muscle response would be strong, as organic apples are supportive or benefit life. This is the most basic way to use applied kinesiology.

As noted above, AK is not a test of strength though; it is a response of energy to a stimulus. Dr. John Thie says, "The muscle test offers us an immediate, subjective (though objectively observable), and personally meaningful measurement. It provides us access to powerful techniques for effecting change and reinforcing that change in the whole person: physically, mentally, emotionally, and spiritually. We are not measuring the gross physical strength of the muscle, but are monitoring the muscle response as an indicator of changes in energy."[180] Remember, AK is a tool that is used to discover truth. That which is truthful supports life; that which is false does not support life.

How Does Applied Kinesiology Work?

The best explanation that I've encountered to answer this question is found in the works of Dr. David Hawkins. The phenomenon of AK can only be explained through quantum mechanics. He states, "It is a replicable experiential phenomenon that is not explicable by ordinary logic or Newtonian physics. It is made comprehensible by the advanced physics of quantum mechanics in which the intention of the observer/questioner does or does not facilitate a collapse of the wave function (the von Neumann Process 1). Thus, the state of the universe (Schrodinger equations) via the Heisenberg principle is often reduced or not (Dirac process), and therefore, the quantum response is limited to "yes" or "not yes."[181]

There you have it, a perfectly logical explanation of AK. Wave function, the von Neumann Process, Schrodinger equations, and the Heisenberg principle are a part of everyone's language, right? Ok, I'm joking. However, when asked about how it works, I normally fire a question back to people and say, "Do you really understand how your cell phone, microwave, or even your car works on a physics level?" Most respond that they do not. Like me, they don't really care to know how a cell phone works. What I do know is that it does work. AK is the same way for me at least. When certain things are tested, a weak or strong muscle response is noted, in which the difference is easily observed. Quantum physics can explain how it works, but I know from years of clinical experience that it works very well in application. In fact, thousands of practitioners use it to extract unconscious information from their patients/clients and that is what we are most concerned about.

To further expound on what AK is, Dr. Hawkins states:

"That truth makes the body musculature go strong and falsehood results in its weakening was an empirical discovery (Hawkins, 1995). The phenomenon is due to the fact that truth exists as an actual reality, whereas falsehood merely has no substrate of reality. Thus, the muscle-testing response is either "yes" or "not yes" ("no"). The mechanisms are clarified by understanding basic principles of quantum physics by which the Heisenberg Uncertainty Principle itself is the "litmus paper." Phenomena are the consequence of the collapse of the 'wave state' of potentiality to the 'particle state' of manifestation and actuality. These are the result of intention and observation itself. The observer and the observed become an operational unit. Truth has actual existence and therefore collapses the wave function. Falsehood has no reality (nonexistent) and thus fails to get a response (the arm weakens). Thus, like electricity, the wire is either 'on' and carries current ("yes") or it is 'not on' ("no").[182]

Applied Kinesiology For Emotional Stimulus

AK can be used to identify and test emotional states, not only those that are occurring in the present moment but also ones that are past memories. The tester may tell the subject to think about something they love, and then immediately perform the muscle test. The response of the arm will be strong. Then, the tester asks the subject to think of something they hate and then immediately tests the arm response. It will go weak. Love supports life. Hate or any negative emotion does not support life.

With regards to emotional stimulus Dr. John Diamond, M.D. says:

"By testing the muscle, a procedure that takes no more than a minute, it is possible to assess accurately and then to correct instantly the negative emotional attitudes affecting us at a given time. The test is a test of life energy…you will know the specific emotional attitudes affecting you at that moment…and instantly overcome your negative mental attitudes (VII)…For the first time, I discovered that it was possible for me accurately and instantly to find the precise emotional attitudes affecting myself or my patients, and in fact, to pinpoint them for anyone, including my professional colleagues…it was the first time that I or anyone could learn his or her own conscious and unconscious attitudes – accurately and instantly."[183]

Dr. John Diamond discovered that if someone was struggling with some kind of medical issue and this issue was being affected by an unconscious emotion or memory, the emotion could be identified and worked with in order for healing to occur. Out of this understanding, AK was used personally to identify the memories and emotions in those memories that needed to be released. It has been an invaluable tool.

In the fantastic book called *Psychokinesiology*, which uses AK to explore our emotions, it is noted that "Muscle testing is reliable and accurate. In the hands of a well-trained practitioner, quite a bit of valuable information can be brought to the surface in such a way that the client goes through little, if any, emotional cathartic episodes." Later they go on to say, "Muscle testing is the key to unlocking the unconscious process quickly and effectively. With it, you can find out exactly what the unconscious is thinking and feeling about a thought, idea, or a behavior."[184]

Applied Kinesiology For Questions And Statements

Any question or statement can be posed to the subject about anything having to do with them or about anything in the world. The reason AK works with regards to information in the universe is because we are all energetically connected to everything in the universe much like every computer is connected to the internet.

Think of the implication this tool has in the hands of integrous people who really want to know the truth. Through this understanding, Dr. David Hawkins instantly understood its cosmic importance. Never in the history of humanity have people had a tool to be able to instantly know truth from falsehood. All ten of his books were based upon the information he discovered from the use of this tool. Kinesiology exposes truth or lack of it. In a clinical setting, we want to know what is true about the condition of the person in front of us, what is causing their ailment and what their body wants to do about it in order to heal. These responses can be received from someone by using AK and a structure to know which questions to ask.

It is very important to note that this is a test that should be used with integrity. If you are angry and you want to prove if someone lied to you, the test will not work. AK is to be used for integrous means and without personal agenda. If you have an agenda or intention before testing, this will skew the test. Attention rather than intention is what must be used to perform the test. You must have no attachment to the result one way or another. The use of the tool requires humility and adaptability, especially if actual truth doesn't line up with what we believe to be truth.

Clinically, a practitioner must empty themselves of agendas, intention or predetermined thoughts (less agenda and more clarity is more common with those of higher levels of consciousness). If not, they will not be at full attention to make sure that the information received from the person is accurate. A good applied kinesiologist is one who has no agenda but is one who, in a health setting, is open to being attentive to whatever comes up. An example of this would be working on a family member whom you have known your whole life and always appears angry or grumpy. When making a statement such as "Anger is the primary emotion that is affecting his/her emotional state," and then performing the muscle test, it may skew the result because you may want the answer to be yes. It is best to be open to the truth itself. Perhaps the anger on the surface is being covered by a deep sadness over the loss of a spouse ten years previous. The anger is fueled by the sadness. But if you think you know better than that person's own subconscious, you will not get an accurate answer. You need to be open to truth itself and not just your opinion.

How To Use Applied Kinesiology To Help Someone With Depression

Any health problem has a primary or main category in which the problem exists. If someone comes in and they say they are depressed, the first set of statements I make and test in this process using AK is to determine on which level the bulk of the issue is in. It is great to know if the problem is primarily physical, energetic, mental/emotional, family emotional, or spiritual. Depending upon the muscle response, helping someone to find relief for their depression is approached very differently depending upon where the source of the problem is.

To see how this would be done, consider the following example made with statements where AK is applied. After each statement, the AK test is immediately performed. Either a strong or weak response will occur after each statement is read aloud. Only one of these statements will test strong.

- The depression is primarily physical. Test. Strong/weak.
- The depression is primarily energetic or electrical. Test. Strong/weak.
- The depression is primarily a general emotional issue. Test. Strong/weak.
- The depression is primarily a family emotional issue. Test. Strong/weak.
- The depression is primarily a spiritual emotional issue. Test. Strong/weak.

The approach to healing physical depression is very different from healing from emotional depression. If the problem is physical, then a change in diet, nutrition, supplementation, exercise, detoxification and things in the physical world should bring about very positive results. If depression is emotional in nature, this doesn't mean that physical changes won't help. In fact, they often help quite a bit. However, to fully release the problem, the memories and associated emotions to the problem need to be released before complete relief can be found.

My first experiences with helping people and using AK were simply limited to the physical realm. I used a technique called Nutrition Response Testing (NRT). NRT is a physical testing framework that uses AK and can be used to discover many things. NRT can be used to discover which toxins are causing problems in the body, where specifically they are causing problems, which parts of the body are the weakest and need the most support, and what exact whole food supplements can be used to support toxin removal. NRT is a physical testing structure that uses AK as the tool to get feedback responses. Using this tool with someone who has a physical expression of depression is very powerful at identifying exactly what they need to start healing. It saves time, is very specific, and brings about healing very quickly. I began using this in practice and soon began to see many wonderful results with patients.

Let me give you an example of how the structure of NRT works. One of the things done in NRT is to determine what the weakest part of the body is. We have three categories: organs, endocrine glands and body parts. Most of the time an organ or an endocrine gland is found to be the weakest. NRT doesn't use a statement to determine this but simply places a hand over that part of the body and performing AK. It is the intention that matters. Asking statements is quicker in my opinion, but it is fine to perform the test either way. Let's say you are testing to see if an endocrine gland is the weakest part of the body. You could either hold a hand over each gland or say the name of each one and perform the test.

- Pineal (test = strong)
- Pituitary (test = strong)
- Thyroid (test = weak)
- Thymus (test = strong)
- Pancreas (test = strong)
- Adrenals (test = strong)
- Testes/Ovaries (test = strong)

In this case, all tested strong except for the thyroid. Therefore, we know that we would need to support the thyroid with whole food supplements to be able to heal this part of the body. We can also test to see if a heavy metal, heavy chemical, food, pathogen or physical scar is affecting the thyroid. We would just have to use AK to test our way through each one of these. If it was a pathogen, for example, we would test for viruses, bacteria, parasites and fungi. Wherever we found a weak muscle response is where we know we would need to offer further support to the thyroid. A viral pathogen is a very common thing that shows up in testing the thyroid.

NRT is a great tool to deal with things on the physical level—and we all need healing on this level! Three things happened after I first learned how to use this for physical health issues. First, my skill with the tool improved over time. I refined it. Anyone can use the tool, but in using it repeatedly, you become a master and learn the power, subtleties, and finesse of it. Anyone can use a paintbrush to draw, but the tool in the hands of Michelangelo is a different story altogether. The tool is the same for all people, but the way an expert uses it can be much different. Applied kinesiology is much the same; it takes lots of practice to use it well.

Second, about 60%-70% of the people that I used NRT on had very positive results. However, on some level, some people were taking the best whole food supplements, exercising, getting chiropractic, and eating all the right things, and their problems still didn't seem to improve much. This is when I began exploring and found other levels in the body that NRT, as a construct, didn't readily detect. The energetic, mental/emotional, family emotional, and spiritual levels went beyond the physical level and were not being addressed using NRT. To help heal the whole person, one has to deal with the electrical system, mind, consciousness, and emotions that affect the body. What is held in the mind manifests in the physical body. The symptoms you experience physically are the way for you to know that something may be originating in the mind.

An ancient Ayurvedic saying tells us, "If you want to know the condition of your mind in the past, examine your body now. If you want to know what your body will look like in the future, examine your mind now." This was when I began to explore other energy modalities such as NAET, Psychokinesiology, The Emotion Code, and Body Talk. All of these modalities use AK as the tool to discover issues in these levels of the body and work to correct them. These constructs explore the contents of the subconscious and have a direct effect on the mind. Healing the mind is the most important aspect of helping someone heal.

Third, after pushing on people's arms innumerable times, I began to sense and feel the energy of responses a split second before applying the test. This was startling at first, and I didn't know that it was possible or even what I was really experiencing. However, it continued to happen to me and one day after months of being able to sense this intuitively, I decided to do all the testing this way and see what happened. What I discovered was that when our intention is focused on the substance, thought, emotion, statement, or question, the energy response that I would feel in the muscle test was something I started to sense intuitively within my own body. This took about six months for me to discover on my own. I had not discovered Dr. Hawkins' works yet, but he explains that this happens because, from a physics standpoint, the response is "happening" or "occurring" in the tester first.

After discovering this, I was reading a book by Dr. John Veltheim that discusses this phenomenon. You can tune into someone's innate wisdom and with more practice and a couple of week's time, the physical muscle test is no longer needed. Weeks?! It took me six months to realize this on my own, and I didn't know what was happening! I later discovered that other kinesiologists report having the same experience. You make a statement such as, "The weakest part of this person's body is their liver." and you feel the energetic response either "yes" or "not yes" from within. You begin to sense the energy, vibration, or truth of the answer to the question. This was key for me in further developing the use of my right brain, which has been called the intuitive brain.[185]

Donna Eden in her wonderful book, _Energy Medicine_, talks about this same experience, "Being energy tested (muscle tested) reinforces the link between your brain and subtle energies in your body, establishing new levels of internal communication. New areas of self-awareness begin to unfold. Many people find they intuitively know what the result of an energy test will be before they apply pressure to the other person's arm. It's not like guessing before the test, but rather launching a communication in which your awareness is working in tandem with subtle energies."[186]

Dr. Kam Yuen also mentions this about muscle testing in his book _Instant Pain Elimination_, that "As you practice these physical confirmation tests you are tuning into how it feels to be strong and weak. Essentially, there are only two distinct feelings. Practice trains you to differentiate between them. Once you become confident in knowing the difference between strong and weak mentally (intuitively), you no longer need to use the arm or finger-thumb confirmation. Your mind will quickly pinpoint what will weaken and what will stay strong."[187]

Dr. John Thie observed the same saying, "After some experience, we begin to get a deeper sense of whether or not energy is flowing. We may also be able to feel what's happening with our energy before we test the muscle. Some people will feel subtleties even if the muscle seems strong and locking in place..."[188]

Dr. Bradley Nelson, author of *The Emotion Code*, also mentions that same thing, "If you use *The Emotion Code* for very long, you may begin to notice an odd phenomenon. A split-second before you get an answer through muscle testing, the answer may suddenly appear in your mind, like a quiet little voice whispering to you. At first, it might be so quiet that you might overlook it...This intuitive knowledge flows into you from the universal database of consciousness, from the sea of intelligence and energy that surrounds us all...muscle testing is like training wheels for your intuition."[189]

We live in a left-brained dominated world, and none of us have been deliberately trained how to use our intuition or right brain like we have our left brain. In fact, when you look at people like Albert Einstein or Nikola Tesla, often the greatest discoveries they had came with the use of their intuition or access to more of their right brain. Information appeared in a flash that didn't make sense, but they had the guts to go with it. This intuition led to some of the greatest discoveries in the world. In practice, some of the craziest, most confounding and seemingly illogical things are discovered by asking questions about why people have the problems they have. Much of the time it doesn't seem to make logical left brain sense. But being able to feel the yes/not yes answer for any statement or question and being receptive to the answers, opens the door to the subconscious of each person. Using the left brain (NRT structure) together with our right brain (intuition) can bring understanding to health problems in amazing ways and helps people heal.

In spiritual terms, I once heard a charismatic pastor speak about the use of the miraculous Biblical gift of knowledge spoken about in 1 Corinthians 12 in the Bible. He said the gift of knowledge functions in one of two ways—like a radio tuner or a cell phone. Tuning in is when you are searching for information, and you have to go looking for it, much like turning the dial on a radio in order to tune into the station that you want. At other times, it is like picking up a cell phone, and information just drops into the brain directly. Using AK intuitively is the same as this gift of knowledge. We use the gift in the same way the Bible advocates; to help and love people so that they can grow and be healthy. As you begin to let go and allow divine love to flow through you, your intuitive ability rises exponentially.

"Your capacity to draw on your own, innate mental clarity, will determine the clarity of feedback you receive from the client's body. To put this in another way: The communication you receive from the innate wisdom of the body will be a direct reflection of your own innate, mental clarity. This mirroring dynamic always takes place, in some way or another, between client and practitioner." - Dr. John Veltheim

Knowing The Right Questions To Ask Is Half The Battle

For the average person, if they asked if the liver was the most damaged organ in the body and the response was "yes," what would they do with that information? This is where left-brained learning and knowing come into play. Having a map or energy construct that facilitates what to do with the information discovered is key in knowing what to do with the information you get. Each modality such as NRT, Body Talk or Psychokinesiology provides the left brain structure or map. Using AK intuitively to navigate through this information is using the right brain. For example, having a list of things that can affect the liver including foods, vitamins, liquids, toxins, anatomy, and physiological functions and much more would be helpful in pinpointing what is affecting the liver. You use a left brain knowledge based structure combined with intuitive right brain applied kinesiological and energetic sensitivity to navigate through someone's health issue. This is not used for diagnosing a health problem nor does it take the place of proper Western medical treatment, but is useful in addition to what Western medicine offers.

Intuitive abilities can be used by anyone. Intuition rises the more you let go of the negative emotions inside you. When you free yourself of them, you cut down on internal noise, giving you more internal peace, allowing you to be more intuitive. Using your right-brained intuition is amplified when you are able to access a rich left-brained knowledge that you have stored from studying and learning. Responses are clearer and deeper when you have a database of knowledge about liver function and tools to help the liver heal.

"Innate (intuition) is the mental clarity experienced when left brain, seemingly rational explanations, are infused by right brain, seemingly irrational, intuitive processes and vice versa. The concepts of left and right brain serve as imagery for describing two seemingly contradictory, mutually exclusive forms of mental function. Here the term seemingly is key, because rational and irrational or intuitive thinking processes never happen in exclusivity of one another. Unfortunately, this is rarely understood, particularly in societies where so-called left brain, logical/rational thought is considered superior to intuitive thinking." - Dr. John Veltheim, D.C., Body Talk

If you can feel/intuit the vibrational answers of truth when you tune into a body, substance, thought, emotion, question, or statement without the use of pushing on someone's arm, you quickly realize faster ways to extract information and help people. Someone's body (as energy) can be accessed anywhere in the world and is not limited to physical space or location. You can "tune in" to anyone's body from anywhere in the world, at any time. Someone does not need to be present to get the information you need to help them. Sessions can be done at a distance and are done this way by practitioners all over the world. Quantum mechanics has discovered that there are no barriers to energy and that energy can travel faster than the speed of light. While this concept may seem strange, because this is not common societal knowledge, that doesn't mean it isn't true. Arthur Clarke once said, "Any sufficiently advanced technology is indistinguishable from magic."[190] Cell phones, airplanes, and electricity would have been considered magic hundreds of years ago.

> "Intuition is a very powerful thing, more powerful than intellect, in my opinion. That's had a big impact on my work...I began to realize that an intuitive understanding and consciousness was more significant than abstract thinking and logical intellectual analysis." —Steve Jobs

I feel that energy medicine is the medicine of the future, especially when people discover how they can learn and grow by understanding why they are the way they are and have the problems they have. I affirm the words of Dr. Robert Jacobs, N.M.D., D.Hom. when he said, "The medicine of the future will be energy medicine, and chemical medicine will be a subset of medicine as a whole. Probably 80 percent of medicine will be energy medicine, and 20 percent chemical medicine." Dr. Mehmet Oz has also been quoted as saying that the future of medicine is energy medicine. Energy medicine is here, and AK may be its main tool.

When you realize the absolute power of the tool, our intuitive abilities as humans and putting them to good use to help facilitate healing in others, the results can be amazing. Being able to participate in this process is beyond humbling. You realize quickly that the body knows exactly how to heal itself, it just needs to be asked and reminded. The practitioner is not the healer; he/she is just a bridge that connects the unbalanced parts so that the body/mind can self-heal. We all have the ability to be able to tune into the wisdom of each person's body. This information is held within the database of human consciousness, which is an immense field of energy that encompasses everything. Since everything is energy, this information (energy) can be accessed to help people heal.

You can make any statement about anything and feel its energy either in a positive "yes" response or a negative "not yes" response. Nikola Tesla, the world's greatest inventor once said, "If you wish to understand the universe, think of energy, frequency, and vibration." Every question, substance, thought, emotion, and person has energy, frequency and vibration, and many people are starting to realize that AK is the doorway into feeling this energy within so that we can grow and help others do the same.

Dr. David Hawkins said, "Everything in the universe radiates a specific frequency or minute energy field that remains in the field of consciousness permanently. Thus, every person or being that ever lived and anything about them, including any event, thought, deed, feeling, or attitude, is recorded forever and can be retrieved at any time in the present or the future."[191] Bell's Theorem emphasizes that "No theory of reality compatible with quantum theory can require spatially separated events to be separate."[192] In other words, all distant events are constantly interconnected and interdependent. This implies that every electron must know exactly what every other electron in the universe is doing to know what it has to do itself at any given moment. This further implies that every atom in the universe is constantly "in touch" with "all that is." Few are born with the ability to intuit this information, but all can learn it.

AK is important to know because the use of this tool is astounding not only on a physical level but also on mental/emotional and spiritual levels. Every piece of information, all beliefs, and truths can be calibrated and discovered by all. In my personal experience, AK was used to discover the experiences and emotions that were contributing to why I was severely depressed. I never would have guessed that a memory I had when I was four years old was the root memory (and emotions in that memory) that was driving why I was depressed.

With the information I gathered with AK, I was also able to identify the exact emotions that were present in each memory that was contributing to the depression. With this information, I used tapping (discussed in the next chapter) to let go of all the negative emotions. Tapping has had such a profound impact on my healing mentally, emotionally, and spiritually.

11 TAPPING

"Enslavement by illusion is comfortable; it's the liberation by truth that people fear. People prefer their illusions rather than be confronted by truth. Taking a look at what emotions, perceptions, beliefs, and attitudes we hold onto deep inside is scary for most people." - Dr. David Hawkins

Thus far, I've covered three (AK, understanding emotion, and Chinese medicine) of the four tools I mentioned that have helped me change my thoughts, beliefs, attitudes, and emotions resulting in life-altering growth. Now, let's talk about the fourth: tapping.

Tapping is a modern addition to the ancient wisdom of Chinese medicine in the form of a tool to release unwanted emotions from the body. Many of my patients have made positive life-changing choices after realizing through tapping what was buried within and how impactful it really was on their present health. When we make the unconscious conscious, one of the most empowering things is knowing that we have a choice of what to do with what we have learned about ourselves. It is hard to change things we don't understand or even know exist as a part of a specific problem. Chinese medicine is a beautiful system of medicine that can help people heal on so many levels. Kinesiology helps to navigate the waters of our subconscious. Once we understand what the problem is, tapping answers the question, "What do we do about it?" and "How can we let go of the negative stuff that is within us?"

The very first time I was introduced to tapping was right as I was entering into Chinese medical school. I didn't even really know how acupuncture worked all that well. I remember watching a documentary called *The Tapping Solution* about ten ordinary people with a plethora of different problems including PTSD, low back pain, money and abundance issues, addiction, fibromyalgia, weight loss, and other issues. I saw all these people tapping on their faces, and I thought to myself, "This has to be one of the most peculiar things I have ever seen! And this is supposed to help people?!" This documentary showed that, by using tapping you see radical changes in the physical, mental, emotional, and spiritual state of each person involved. It was remarkable to see. One gentleman had chronic low back pain for 30 years that disappeared in days and healed permanently. Other stories shown in the documentary are just as amazing.

Now, after leading hundreds of people through tapping on many different issues and problems, I have seen just as remarkable things happen not only to patients but also to myself. The best thing about tapping is that it is super easy to learn and it is 100% free, if you choose to do it on your own. Even after reading this chapter or watching the documentary, you still may not feel comfortable doing it and may put off using it. This is where it is highly recommended to work with someone who can teach you how to use this extraordinary tool as it specifically applies to you. The learning curve is so much faster with someone who helps people tap through their issues for a living. With a skilled practitioner and this tool in hand, be prepared for substantial radical life change that will help you to change limiting thoughts, emotions, beliefs, and attitudes in your consciousness.

Tapping deals largely with emotions. Emotions create thoughts, and the thoughts and beliefs we hold then dictate behavior and the manifestation of problems in our lives and our bodies. This is why it doesn't matter what your health, relational, or financial problem is. The heart and center of most of our problems have a negative emotional base. This is why tapping has a powerful effect on just about any problem. Through intention, tapping helps your body to let go of the negative emotions and thoughts that are not helping you, and it allows you to start loving yourself more fully. This, in turn, will bring you more internal peace and healing.

Tapping is not a substitute for appropriate medical care. Tapping is not for diagnosing, treating or curing any disease or health problem. It is just a simple tool to release unwanted emotional energy from the body.

Who Created Tapping?

Tapping started with a brilliant gentleman by the name of Dr. Roger Callahan, a psychologist, who discovered by accident that tapping could alleviate problems that he had spent years trying to help people with. His book *Tapping the Healer Within* tells about this discovery and is a mixture of modern psychology and Chinese medicine.[193] Since his discovery other modalities arose that streamlined the process of tapping, and in my opinion, made it better. The most popular form of tapping is called Emotional Freedom Techniques (EFT), and I highly recommend books that explore EFT further. Gary Craig, a student of Callahan, is the one who started EFT. Other popular forms of tapping include Faster EFT and Mental Field Therapy. They all offer different aspects to tapping and are wonderful to learn about. The one I am going to teach you how to do is more along the lines of Mental Field Therapy (Dr. Dietrich Klinghart) because it makes a little more sense to me due to my training in Chinese medicine. I will point out the differences between these in just a moment. Most tapping practitioners haven't studied Chinese medicine formally, but knowledge of the medicine is not needed to do tapping. Anyone can learn it quickly and easily.

What Does Tapping Do?

We have already discussed the 12 major meridians or channels of electricity energy in the body. The Chinese would say that our emotions are "stored" energetically within the channels of energy and their corresponding organs. In fact, each organ in Chinese medicine has its own consciousness. Each organ has one particular negative emotion that affects it more than other emotions. Regarding emotional consciousness, for example, the main negative emotion that affects the liver is anger (or other emotions in the family of anger such as hate, frustration, or agitation). The main emotion affecting the kidney (adrenals) is fear (or other emotions of fear including anxiety, overwhelm, tension, stress, or dread).

Tapping involves using our hands to tap on various points on the body that correspond with the 12 major channels and the two extra channels (ren and du channels or conception and governing vessel). The 12 major channels correspond with all the major organs in the body and cover virtually every part of the body from head to toe. Think of them as power lines running through the body. The ren channel runs straight up the middle of the body starting in the genital area and ending in the mouth. The du channel starts in the genital area and runs up the spine over the middle of the head and ends in the mouth as well forming a full circuit with the ren channel. When we tap on these points combined with the intention of engaging the true reality of what we feel on the inside and our desire to let this negative emotion (thought, belief, etc.) go, the body lets go of this negative emotional energy. Your body will let go of negative energy and allow positive energy to shine forth. When this exchange happens, your body does remarkable things. This process allows love to heal us from deep within.

Tapping Starters

Let's first talk about a couple of critical things that highlight some differences in tapping, EFT and Mental Field Therapy (MFT). First, with EFT normally only two fingers are used to tap. The index and middle fingers are mostly used. Only two meridians of energy run through the index and middle fingers. However, with MFT, we use all five of the fingers to tap because then we access all six meridians that run through the tips of the fingers.

Second, with EFT, the tapping is done very rapidly. Tapping on a point can be done as much as 20-30 times in five seconds. Research done by Dr. Dietrich Klinghardt indicates that tapping this fast is a little too fast for the nervous system. His research indicates that tapping slowly at the pace of a waltz is the best speed in which to tap. I must stress though, that ultimately, your intention alone is the strongest thing that will make this process work.

Third, in EFT the first point that is tapped on is on the side of the hand, on what they have nicknamed the "karate chop" point. In MFT, the first point is on the top of the head. The reason this makes more sense from a Chinese standpoint is that the point on the top of the head is called "One Hundred Meetings" because five meridians intersect at this point. These five meridians combined with the six on the hand total 11 meridians out of the 14. Starting at this point accesses more of the other meridians than by starting on the karate chop point.

Fourth, the point sequence in MFT is a little different than EFT (essentially all the points are the same with a couple of exceptions in the sequence). Does it matter what points are used, in what sequence, and the speed at which they are tapped? Research done by Dr. Klinghardt indicates that it does make a difference, although it may not be a huge difference. I haven't observed it making a difference. These four differences make sense to me, but at the end of the day, I believe that any tapping is very effective. I highlight these differences because if you read anything about tapping, you are more than likely to see these differences and I wanted you to know why what you may be seeing is different. You are more than encouraged to explore the different options in the world of tapping. To learn more, one of the best resources on tapping is *The Tapping Solution* by Nick Ortner. Now that we have explored some of the differences let's get into how to actually do it.

Putting Tapping To Use

When tapping, you can use either hand in following the sequence below. First, put all your fingers together into a straight line and make sure they are all touching the body (see illustration). Then you're ready to begin tapping, in the following sequence:

1. **Top of the head**. This point is on the very top of the head, almost directly above the ears. Take your two hands and place one behind the other on an imaginary line that divides the head down the middle. Each finger should be aligned on the imaginary line running down the middle of the head.
2. **Eyebrow**. Put your pinky finger on the beginning inner edge of the eyebrow, closest to the bridge of the nose. Align all the other fingers over the rest of the eyebrow.
3. **Temple**. At the end of the eyebrow in the temple area, tap using all fingers together over the temple.
4. **Back of the head**. The back end of your skull bone is called your occiput. Find the edge of the occiput and right directly under the bone about 0.5 inches on either side of the spine is where this point is.
5. **Under the eyes**. This point is directly under the pupil of the eye on the bone below the eye.
6. **Under the nose**. Put one pinky into the philtrum (the groove directly under

the nose and above the upper lip), and put the other pinky slightly off to the side. Remember to continue using all of the fingers.

7. **Under the mouth**. Directly under your month, in the center, is a groove above the chin. Place one pinky directly in the center and the other pinky slightly off to the side touching the other pinky.

8. **Under the arms**. About 3-4 inches directly below the anterior portion of your armpit is where this point is. For women, this point is where the edge of the bra is. I called this the funky chicken point because instead of crossing your arms to hit this point, you want to open up the chest and bring the hands up as high as you can to hit this point.

9. **Under the collarbone/thymus**. You can do it in the middle of the chest or just under the collarbone, and 2-3 inches lateral to the sternum (the breast bone) is a depression. This is the last point in the sequence.

When tapping, start at the first point on the top of your head and work your way down until you are at the last point. You should tap at least nine times on each point at the pace of a slow waltz. After each tapping sequence and tapping through all the points, remember to take a deep diaphragmatic breath in and out. This is very important to remember when processing through emotional things. Breathing in is associated with our ability to breathe in new life and breathing out with our ability to let things go. Therefore, taking deep breaths is critical in this process.

On a humorous note, many people feel silly or even ridiculous tapping on their face and other places. This is a very common experience for many people. In fact, these emotions, while seemingly benign, are negative emotions, and when tapping with someone for the first time, I normally start with tapping on these very emotions. It is ok to feel silly when doing this for the first time.

The Set-up Statement

Now that we have learned the tapping points and sequence, we are going to go over what is called the "set up statement." Now that we know how to tap, we need to learn how to use tapping to work through our problems. The setup statement gives us a framework that we can use to guide us and to "tune" into what we are working on while also moving towards resolving the issue. The classic set up statement has two parts. The first part of the setup statement acknowledges what we feel and think and the state or condition we are in. The second part of the statement is the directive that we use which moves us towards the healing frequency of love. Here is a very simple example of a setup statement:

- "Even though I feel sad because my dog died, I deeply love and accept myself."
- Other variations exist because some people have a really hard time saying

that they deeply love themselves. If one of the following feels more congruent to you, use it.

- "Even though I feel sad because my dog died, I choose to love and accept myself."
- "Even though I feel sad because my dog died, I want to love and accept myself."

Wanting to love yourself is saying that even though I realize that I don't, I really do want to move in this direction. Choosing is a step above this because I may say that even though I don't deeply love myself, I think I can choose to do so at this moment. Deeply loving and accepting yourself may occur right away for some or it may require some time before you can honestly say this.

This first part of the statement is meant to give one the opportunity to acknowledge and take responsibility for the condition, state, thoughts, beliefs, or emotions we have. This is the part where we realize that we may be contributing or participating in the perpetuation of the problem we have. Our tendency as people is to want to blame things and people outside of ourselves for our problems. The setup statement gets us to agree about what the problem truly is. Below are some other examples that could be used to start working through things. Try to state everything in the present moment, because even things from the past are being experienced now. However, if it feels better to state something in the past tense, that is acceptable also.

- Even though I am angry about losing my job…
- Even though I feel cheated by what happened in the competition…
- Even though I feel embarrassed by my performance…
- Even though I don't feel good enough to date someone…
- Even though I hate this cancer…
- Even though my lower back hurts so bad…
- Even though I am devastated that my wife/husband left me…
- Even though I am so undisciplined…
- Even though I feel my thighs are enormous…
- Even though I'm so frustrated I live paycheck to paycheck…

Tapping Can Be Used On Just About Everything

Here are some different examples of things we can use tapping for as well.

- **State:** Even though my back is killing me…
- **Body Sensation:** Even though my stomach aches so bad…

- **Condition**: Even though I have a headache…
- **Emotion**: Even though I feel depressed…
- **Thought**: Even though she doesn't like me…
- **Belief System**: Even though having millions of dollars is wrong…
- **Attitude**: Even though I don't feel like cleaning…

When establishing a setup statement, it is very important at this point to ask ourselves how intense or strong it feels. Measuring the intensity of the statement will give us feedback in the future after tapping to determine if the intensity has gotten better, worse or stayed the same. Let's take the example of "Even though I have a pounding headache…" and rate the intensity at a 9/10. After a round of tapping, we can ask ourselves if the intensity feels the same, better or worse. Frequently after a round or two, the intensity of the feeling associated with our set up statement starts to lessen.

However, sometimes people are very unaware of how strong an emotion is within them until they fully access it, which is why we ask if something feels worse after a round of tapping. I was tapping with a woman about a house that she had built from scratch and had been in their family for many years. Due to economic factors, they now had to sell. When I asked her how intense the sadness was that she felt for having to sell it, she said it was a 4/10. So we tapped on this saying, "Even though I feel sad that I have to sell my house, I choose to love and accept myself." Intuitively, I felt it much stronger within her at a 10/10 but didn't comment on this hoping more of it would come out eventually on its own. After the first round of tapping was completed, I asked her if it was better, the same or worse in intensity. She began to cry, said it got worse and now rated it as at a 9/10. We continued to work through it until the sadness was gone. Always try to measure the intensity of what you are tapping on after each round of tapping.

The second part of the tapping statement involves what our true reality is and is a movement toward what we want to experience. If we hold true to the idea that "the Kingdom of Heaven is within us" and that what defines the core of who we are is divinity, then we are simply letting go of that which we are not to reveal what we already are—love, joy, and peace. Therefore, to reiterate, one of the common ways to finish the setup statement is by stating the following:

"…I deeply love and accept myself."

So if we combine that, we get: "Even though I have this pounding headache, I deeply love and accept myself."

If we have a lot of negative stuff inside concerning a problem we have, this is the primary indicator that we don't love ourselves. By acknowledging the feelings and thoughts we have, and with the intention that we are going to love ourselves, the body will start to let go of the negative energy that surrounds a problem we have.

I once had a patient who was anemic. The most prominent symptoms exhibited were fatigue, looking pale, feeling faint at times, and having low blood pressure. The general consciousness of anemia is having a "Yes but attitude. Lack of joy. Fear of life and not feeling good enough."[194] She was raised in a very affluent family that expected a lot from her growing up. Her mother was very demanding with everything she did and she never felt like she measured up. This squeezed all the joy of living from her, and since she never seemed to do anything right, she ended up fearing life and never did anything new because in the back of her mind was the thought that it would just be another reminder of how she didn't measure up. She was full of bitterness, anger, resentment, and hate towards her mother. She felt a tremendous amount of guilt for not being good enough and shame for being a disappointment to her parents.

Here are some of the things we tapped through as many times as needed until the emotions/thoughts left the body:

- Even though I'm afraid I will never be good enough for my parents, I want to love and accept myself.
- Even though I feel so exhausted every day carrying all this emotional baggage, I want to love and accept myself.
- Even though I look pale as a ghost and I feel insecure about my appearance, I want to love and accept myself.
- Even though I'm angry that they demand so much from me, I choose to love and accept myself.
- Even though I hate my mother for always demanding things from me, I choose to love and accept myself.
- Even though I feel guilty for never measuring up and have punished myself all these years, I deeply love and accept myself.
- Even though I feel so ashamed and hate myself for being a constant disappointment to my parents, I deeply love and accept myself.

Before we started tapping through each one of these phrases above, I asked how intense each one felt on a scale from 1 to 10. Normally, the answer was at least a 9/10. After every round of tapping, she was asked how intense it felt and whether it felt the same, better, or worse. Normally, it would take between 4–6 rounds of tapping on each phrase for the intensity to go down to a 1 or 0.

It is very common to blame one's mother or father (or someone else) for how things have turned out in life. During our formative years, being "programmed" to believe certain things by our personal experiences is very common. However, as someone grows up, one needs to take responsibility and confront the things that aren't true expressions of what they are on the inside. The truth is that she, like all of us, is powerful, loving, full of joy, and full of peace. The emotions she had felt all her life, had mostly drowned out the true essence of her Self or the Divinity that defined her within. When these emotions left her body, she began to feel the light inside of her by feeling "lighter," "calmer" and "more peaceful." This is very common after tapping through some heavy stuff and letting it go. Most of the time, someone has an instant knowing that they feel different.

One common question I get with patients at times is the following:

"Why do I have to say I love and accept myself when it is another person that I am angry at?"

But I think it's important to understand who the person is that is holding onto the anger? Who is the person that the anger is really affecting?

This reminds me of a well-known quote by the Buddha that says:

"Holding onto anger is like grasping a hot coal with the intent of throwing it at someone else; you are the one that gets burned."

Anger is not love, joy or peace. When you are holding onto anger, it is really only affecting you. When you are holding onto anger, you are the only one inhibited from more fully experiencing your true Self. This is why it is critical to intend to love and accept yourself because as you let go of anger, this will happen experientially.

Another common thing that happens with tapping is that people like to complicate it. Many times I get patients saying things to me like, "I wanted to tap but couldn't remember the words or what to say." Tapping is 99% about intention. If you intend to let something go and don't resist it, then it will release in due time. Your intention to let go is really all you need. When using tapping, it is good to remember to keep things simple. The setup statement is divided into three simple things:

- What are you feeling? Identify the feeling you are experiencing such as anger, fear, frustration, sadness, etc.
- Why do you feel what you feel? Come up with a short 6-10 word explanation as to why you feel what you feel. Like "I feel angry because Mike lied to me."
- Use the last part of the setup statement that feels congruent with you: "I deeply love and accept myself," "I choose to love and accept myself," or "I want to love and accept myself."

Add an "Even though…" at the beginning and you are all ready to tap: "Even though I feel angry that Mike lied to me, I choose to love and accept myself." Tap at least nine times on each point on the body. Once you are done with one point on the body, move to the next and repeat the same phrase while tapping at least nine times. After going through all nine tapping places on the body, stop tapping and take a deep breath.

Tap again through this as many times as you need until you feel the emotion release from your body.

Summary

Tapping has many other nuances and ways to delve deeper into your experience of your issue, but making simple set up statements as seen above can account for 60-80% of a great tapping experience. My knowledge of tapping was very limited when I started using the tool to release and experience profound healing and freedom. If you doubt that you are doing it right or are not saying the right thing, start with: "Even though I'm doubting that I am doing the tapping wrong, I choose to love and accept myself." Again, it is not so much the words you use or the things you say, but your intention to stop resisting your emotions, to welcome them and to watch them release from the body.

What follows next is my depression story. I describe why I got depressed and the memories that were associated with feeling so horrible for 11 years. After sharing these stories, in subsequent chapters I talk about how I processed through them with the tools that I have explained in this book. AK helped me to identify the memories and the emotions in each memory. Tapping provided me with what I needed to let these emotions go once and for all.

PART 4
THE PRACTICE OF HEALING

12 THE MINDFULNESS OF EMOTION

"Feelings, whether of compassion or irritation, should be welcomed, recognized, and treated on an absolutely equal basis; because both are ourselves. The tangerine I am eating is me. The mustard greens I am planting are me. I plant with all my heart and mind. I clean this teapot with the kind of attention I would have were I giving the baby Buddha or Jesus a bath. Nothing should be treated more carefully than anything else. In mindfulness, compassion, irritation, mustard green plant, and teapot are all sacred."
— Thich Nhat Hanh, The Miracle of Mindfulness: An Introduction to the Practice of Meditation

Dr. David Hawkins talks about the power of mindfulness in his book Healing and Recovery.[195] This information is important to know because many who have healed from a very difficult disease or health problem have ultimately discovered the deeper truths about whom and what they are. These truths, once realized, can drive healing into the physical body.

Our physical body cannot experience itself. A hand cannot experience itself. Something greater than the hand has to be able to recognize the movements, sensations, and experiences that one is having in the hand. This is the mind. The body is always experienced by the mind. The mind is composed of thoughts, emotions and belief systems. Through the mind we have a thought or feeling about the hand, "my hand is hurting, swollen or bruised." The mind is having an experience of the hand. Therefore, the mind governs the body.

On the level of mind, we begin to see that a thought or an emotion cannot experience itself. The mind cannot experience itself. A thought cannot have an awareness of itself. A part of you exists that knows it is having a thought or experiencing an emotion. This is consciousness, which is even greater than the mind. Consciousness governs the mind. Beyond consciousness is pure awareness.

The dictionary definition of identifying with something means to "make the same." Most people in the world are highly identified with their bodies and the mind. One of the most important things to learn in this life is to un-identify with the body and the mind. We think we are our bodies and minds, yet this is not true at all. We think we are our looks, abilities, talents, associations, jobs, money, relationships, thoughts, beliefs, opinions and emotions. But we are not. We must learn to stop identifying with those things. Many people look at me crazy when I suggest that healing needs to occur on a level far beyond the body in order to heal the physical body.

When we surrender the "I, Me and Mine" expression of the ego, we can then learn to identify with the Truth of ourselves. We say, "This is MY body!" No, it is just a body. "This is MY opinion!" No, it is just the ego-reinforcing itself through the mind. We can learn to identify with that which is aware of the mind within us. The more we learn to identify with this aspect of ourselves, the more we will see who we really are and then we can completely heal. Everything with the body and mind can change instantly. Why would we ever want to identify with something like the body or mind that can shift like sand in a moment's time?

All emotion, thought, and sensation is experienced in the physical body. The first step in healing is actually to create awareness and become intimate with how we genuinely are experiencing our bodies. Most people have never really paid any attention to their body on an intimate level. Have you ever just sat down and noticed, for example, the pain you have in your arm? How most of us experience pain, especially if the pain is intense, is to numb it by taking an over-the-counter medication hoping it will just go away. We try to run away from it, not embrace, welcome and notice it.

At this point, the temptation for people with depression or any health problem might say, "I know what I am experiencing in my body really well." I feel the pain and symptoms every day. And while this is true, layers of truth exist far beyond this, just as there are different layers of perception in the body (body $\rightarrow$ mind $\rightarrow$ consciousness $\rightarrow$ pure awareness). One may be aware of the pain, but may be completely missing the reason for the pain deep inside, what it means and the emotions that may be contributing to the problem. Many are in reality very unaware of why they have their health problem on a physical, emotional or mental level. They have no way to decipher its messages, so they ignore them or take medications to put a band-aid on them.

But when the question is asked, "Do you know why you have depression?", it is evident in many people that they really have no idea what is underlying the depression. A world of meaning is sitting behind it. I choose to see pain and health problems as God using something to draw you into your own story, so that you can grow, change and identify with inner Beingness. Nothing like human suffering forces us to grow and deal with what is on the inside of us. If you were to have asked me this question while I was at the height of my depression, I would have said I had no idea why I was really depressed.

Depression or any other health problem we experience may be 100% related to the trauma we went through when we were younger. This health problem is our body's way of getting our attention and truly being able to heal that part of us from the past. Your body always keeps the score. The good news is that when you delve into the depths of your being and become familiar with that which is inside of you then you will progressively begin to experience the ecstasy of love and joy.

Two steps exist on the road to emotional freedom. The first step is awareness.

Awareness is a term that can be used interchangeably with mindfulness. Mindfulness is being fully present and aware of how one is experiencing the present moment at all times. Mindfulness is being fully aware of all thoughts, emotions, judgments, perceptions, opinions, and beliefs one is having in the moment. Mindfulness is observation, being in a state of non-judgment towards anything one is experiencing. Included in being fully aware of the present is how the past is playing itself out in the present moment, including what we experience in the body as health problems. The mind is the ground on which our emotions, thoughts, belief systems, and programs can be seen and play themselves out. It is the movie screen that we are watching where the whole scene of our life is being acted out.

Scientist Dr. Bruce Lipton has mentioned that 5% of what we experience is only what we are consciously aware of at this moment.[196] It is the other 95% that is subconscious or unconscious, that which most of us are completely unaware of. Most people would like to think they are aware of why they react the way they do, why they have the health problems they have and what exactly to do to be the best and healthiest versions of themselves. But as the state of health in the USA exhibits, we see that mindfulness is something that we sorely lack today.

Mindfulness or awareness can take shape in many different ways. Physically, our bodies are in a constant dance of reacting to things that have built up inside of us for decades and also simultaneously things we experience acutely. Recently, I had some friends of mine tell me how they are so frustrated because their 3-year-old son was getting ear and sinus infections almost every month. It was getting so bad that they were considering having ear tubes put in (myringotomy). Through observation (mindfulness and awareness) clinically I have seen what the cause of this is in most cases. I asked the mother if he drinks cow's milk. Her response was, "He loves cow's milk!" I told her to stop giving him cow's milk immediately and replace it with organic almond milk. She did this immediately, and after six months had passed, I received a text stating that he hadn't had a single ear infection since they discontinued consumption of dairy.

Dairy (infant formula) is the culprit behind most infants and toddlers getting ear infections. It is a horrible food that no child should consume. However, she was not aware or mindful that this was the problem. Most people are not. Once someone becomes aware or more mindful, different choices can be made leading to a greater experience of health and vitality. We simply don't know what we don't know. However, we can constantly seek and search for answers so that we become more mindful.

Having said this, so many things happen in our world that we are unaware of. In this chapter the goal is simply to highlight things that are vitally important to how we learn, grow and change. Becoming more mindful is the first step towards real, sustained inner growth. Becoming intimately familiar with how we experience what is within us is the pathway towards the freedom and joy we all seek.

"One does not become enlightened by imagining figures of light, but by making the darkness conscious. The latter procedure, however, is disagreeable and therefore not popular." - C.G. Jung

What are the most common things to be mindful of that can help us to discover the pathway towards emotional freedom?

1. Become aware of the emotional states that you are in every moment of every day.

On a January morning in 2018, at the clinic, I was trying to get to the bottom of why a patient was depressed. So, I asked, "What do you think are the main emotions that are fueling why you feel the way you do?" After a few moments of silence, the patient's response was, "I don't really know." This response is fairly common. We don't pay attention to what we feel, so we don't spend much time contemplating the very emotions we find ourselves feeling from moment to moment.

We cannot expect to become intimately familiar with someone if we do not spend a significant amount of time being curious, questioning, listening, observing and noticing every little thing about them. In this same way, we will never become intimately familiar with how we experience the world if we do not do the same things with our emotions. Have you ever just allowed yourself to consciously and purposefully be with a singular emotion for more than 15 minutes? When people do this, the discovery that takes place opens us up to a whole new world. This is the fulfillment of the dictum, "know thyself."

2. Become aware of the cornerstone events or experiences where our emotions were planted in our subconscious for the first time.

In my own healing journey, one day I wrote a list of the most negative memories I could remember before the age of 18. This list has over 110 memories on it. When processing through them one by one, I would have so many "Aha!" moments realizing that with certain memories started the beginning of behaviors, beliefs, programming, and emotions that greatly affected me from those moments forward. All of these things are waiting to be explored by you as well.

3. Become aware of the emotions that drive us to behave the way we do.

So many people have sugar cravings these days. We tend to reach for sugar more when we are under times of stress. The other day I asked a patient when she tended to have more sugar cravings. She mentioned it was in the middle of the afternoon at work. When I asked her why she thought that was, she replied, "I just get stressed out!" I pressed a little further and asked, "What is (are) the exact emotion(s) that you commonly experience under stress that pushes you to do this?" After some moments of pensive thought, she answered, "I have no idea!"

For her, her workload often increases in the afternoon, and she is under a deadline to complete work. Therefore, she often feels overwhelmed. Overwhelm is an emotion within the family of fear. She is constantly afraid that the work will not get done and won't be done right because she has to rush to finish it. She is afraid because at times the work is very hard and difficult to understand and process. If she fails, she will feel like a failure. She will also feel guilty, ashamed of herself and angry that she won't be able to do her job the way she wants.

The sugar is a way to feel better instantly in moments when we don't feel good. Because she is in such an emotional state, she reaches for the sugar to feel better. We all have done this, many times very unconsciously. Sugar temporarily covers or blocks our experience of stress, pain, and negative emotions. We feel badly and since we are programmed to avoid pain and pursue pleasure, what better way to feel better than to fire up the feel-good hormones in the body through the consumption of sugar? But something within us doesn't want to feel like a slave to sugar or our emotions. We want to be free not to eat sugar. We want to be free to consume it when we are fully and consciously making a choice that isn't arising to cover up something negative we are experiencing at the moment. Behind our deepest cravings for things is usually deep and complex emotions and programs that are unconsciously running in the background, waiting for us to discover what they are and to surrender them so we can be free.

"In a true you-and-I relationship, we are present mindfully, non intrusively, the way we are present with things in nature. We do not tell a birch tree it should be more like an elm. We face it with no agenda, only an appreciation that becomes participation: 'I love looking at this birch' becomes 'I am this birch' and then 'I and this birch are opening to a mystery that transcends and holds us both.'"
— David Richo, When the Past Is Present: Healing the Emotional Wounds that Sabotage our Relationships

4. Become aware of why we say the things we say or do the things we do.

We all have said and done things that we regret. After we have said or done something regretful, we often ask ourselves why we did such a thing. It was as if what was said just escaped from us without any prior notice or notification. We acted without even realizing what we were doing until it was too late. We were in the "heat" of the moment. We were living that moment unconsciously, mindlessly unaware. Then we "come to our senses" later on and ask others for forgiveness for what we said or did that we truly didn't mean.

5. Become aware of how you are not your body.

You are NOT your body. In fact, one of the points of being here on this planet is learning to emotionally un-identify with the physical body. We suffer in countless ways depending upon how emotionally attached we are to our body. Most people in this world are highly over-identified with their physical bodies. They think they ARE their physicality. Their identity largely rests on how they look, what they have accomplished, how much money they have or who they know. But what we are is not something that can ever change. Love can never change, and that is what you are.

We see this obsession is every facet of life. Men and women are obsessed with physical beauty. We even make alterations to our noses, breasts, hair, face, abdomens, and buttocks. Plastic surgery exists for all kinds of things today. We see magazines of photoshopped women to whom other women can never measure up.

If you had a stunning face and then got into a car accident and were mangled, would you still be you? If you lost an athletic ability, would you still be you? If you had immense wealth and then lost it, would you still be you? Do you resist the process of growing older? Do you feel disgust towards the new lines, wrinkles, saggy parts or body parts that don't work like they used to? Think of all the ways we suffer because of how we experience our physical body or lose something we used to have.

Because of how obsessed we are with the physical body in our society today, sometimes I will suggest an exercise to people. When you get out of the shower, stand there and observe how you feel when you look at every part of you. Do you feel the need to change things? Could you let go of needing or wanting to change a part of you? If you see the extra weight you are carrying around, how do you actually feel about the weight? Do you see yourself as beautiful or as ugly? Do you spend time constantly comparing yourself physically to others? Look at your muscles, face, skin, hair, breasts, hips, legs, hands and feet. When you see each part, what emotions are stirred up inside you? Go to any gym and see people in front of the mirror puffed up with loads of pride because of the body or looks they have.

I was always super skinny growing up. I was made fun of for it. When I was in college, in an attempt to make up for my internal emotional deficiencies about how I felt lacking, I decided to lift weights and build muscle. People will surely like me more if I have bigger muscles, right? I put on about 30 pounds, but it never changed how I felt about myself on the inside. So eventually that fantasy ended, and I stopped lifting weights. About a year ago, a woman I dated asked me one day in a tone that implied she wanted me to change for her, "Why don't you lift weights and build muscle?" I responded, "Because I have made peace with my body. I love my body the way it is. My only goal now is simply to be healthy." The road to this being a reality was in letting go of many negative emotions about how I felt about myself and my body. It is still a work in progress and may always be as I continue to change and grow.

6. Become aware of how we are not the mind. We are not our emotions, thoughts, opinions or beliefs.

You are NOT your mind. Most of us have highly over-identified with the contents of our mind. You are not the thoughts, emotions, ideas, judgments, opinions, and positionalities you experience in the mind. Again, all of these things can change in an instant. Your true identity is not found in anything that can change in an instant. So we can stop identifying with such things and learn to identify progressively with that which we already are.

Have you ever shared an opinion with someone, only to have your opinion met by the other person with defensiveness and anger? We want the best for those we love, and if someone is doing something that we judge as being not as healthy or helpful as something else, we may wish to share something with them in an attempt to change that person. As crazy as it may sound, wanting to change someone, even though we try to disguise it as love, often is not love at all. We may feel afraid for someone making poor choices. We may feel grief or sadness over the choices another makes. We may feel guilty about someone making a choice that we know we contributed to. Our advice may actually be us simply projecting our own negative emotions onto someone else, and we may not even be aware of it. It is easy to say that we are being loving, but when we further examine our internal motives, the story might be more complex. I've been guilty of this many times.

No one wants to be judged. I find that people really don't understand what judgment is though. Judgment is when you share something and the energy driving what is being shared is negative. What is being said is one thing. The energy sitting behind what is being shared can be positive or negative. Let's say a friend is dating someone that I can clearly see is going to only bring them heartache. I can say in a tone of anger, "What are you thinking?! Why are you with this person?! You are only going to get hurt!" This may only spark anger and defensiveness. This is judgment.

On the other hand, I could pay very close attention to the internal emotional state I am in when I share. I release all my anger about the situation first and then in a loving state and tone of voice, I could say, "Why do you think this person is good for you? Do you see any red flags that would lead others to think that this person may not be the best for you? Whatever choice you make, I don't think this person is the best for you, but I will love you in whatever choice you make."

Such statements may also be met with anger and defensiveness, in spite of knowing that you communicated with love. Even if something is communicated in love, you may get the following responses: "Why are you always against me?! Why don't you want me to just be happy?! Why are you always so critical?!" You cannot control how others react. In fact, their reactions are reflections of what is inside of them, not you. If you truly shared something in love, what more can you do? The person they want to be with may crush their heart into a million pieces, and it may be the very best thing to help them grow emotionally and spiritually. So why rob them of their experience? But you can still share your thoughts with love, even in spite of others reacting negatively.

Love's highest expression can actually be for someone to go through unspeakable pain and for you to learn to be at peace with this occurring. Nothing is a catalyst for growth like pain. Nothing. We seek to hold our thoughts and opinions loosely because often, even in a state of love, we don't know what someone actually needs, even if that is more temporary suffering. Can we experience love even when someone we deeply care about is suffering deeply? Or does their suffering bring out your own suffering of fear, sadness, guilt or anger?

Have you ever met someone who has an opinion about everything? You bring up any subject, and they are quick to share what they know. If you disagree with them though, watch out! Whenever someone is very opinionated, another way to express this would be to say that they are very attached to their opinion. Remember, attachment is the root of suffering. It is also very difficult for such people to listen well to others or change their opinions about things. This attachment to their opinions can generate significant amounts of suffering. For such people, they think they are their opinions. When you disagree with them, it stirs up their internal suffering, and they can get very angry or defensive.

Opinions can change, and expressing opinions with rigidity is not the healthiest expression of being. You are not your opinions, so learn to hold them loosely and lovingly. The emotion that expresses itself very vibrantly with heavily opinionated people is pride. Pride is the emotion that asserts itself as, "I'm always right, or I need to be right!" Pride is a very fragile emotion and is always just a reactionary emotion to a deeper emotion. Behind all pride is insecurity (fear). Insecurity is the primary driving emotion behind very opinionated people. Prideful people are actually just very scared and fragile, although this is the last thing a prideful person would admit to!

It is hard to see beyond the pride in people at times, but much of the time a significant amount of fear can be found. From this fear, pride is generated. For example, someone could have grown up believing that they don't matter. So they are afraid of not mattering or not being good enough. To make up for this, they learn to have opinions about everything to compensate for feeling like they don't matter on the inside. But this doesn't resolve the internal fear. It simply is just a defensive or reactionary position. Learn to surrender pride and hold your opinions with love. If you find yourself trying very hard to convince someone of something, this rarely is love.

You are not the contents of your mind. Your hand cannot experience itself. Something greater than the hand has to experience the hand. This is the mind. The mind sputters off details about the hand because it is experiencing it. My hand is small, large, strong, broken, hurt, painful, etc. The mind cannot experience itself either. Something greater than the mind is aware that you think thoughts and feel emotion. This is consciousness itself. Learn to identify with this part of you. Learn to identify with the watcher or witness of the thoughts, feelings, and emotions. Learn to altogether transcend and surrender the contents of the mind through conscious awareness. As you do, suffering (emotionality) will progressively lessen as you fall into the essence of what you are, the essence of awareness (love, joy, and peace).

7. Become aware of others as we see beyond our own experiences and emotions.

Have you ever been having a conversation with someone and you are everywhere else but actually in your conversation with this person? You may be having a conversation, but are thinking about dinner, all the work you have to do at home, the fight you had with your husband/wife this morning, where to go on vacation next, or the growling in your stomach, etc. You may be physically present, but you are anything but present. How can you really be present, listening, attentive and tuned into the emotional state of the person sitting in front of you when you are only thinking about yourself?

The more you step into, become aware of and let go of the suffering inside of you, the more compassionate and aware you become of the suffering of others. You will learn to truly recognize suffering in others and be empathetic with it. As you continue to let go of what is inside of you, your mind will grow more and more silent and at ease. The incessant worrying, pondering and thinking will soften as you continue to surrender. When this happens, you will automatically be able to "see" others more fully and be more present with them.

At times, when you really want to tune into what others are truly feeling, you can actually develop this as an intuitive skill. Everyone has a "feel" to them, some more subtle than others. Everyone has met someone that has "given you the creeps" or "made you feel more alive." What is that energy that you sense? Often, people don't know what this is. They just simply sense it as something being "off" or "different."

What if you could learn to descriptively and specifically know exactly what this is in another? What if you could develop this skill? You can do this simply as a byproduct of paying attention to what emotions you feel and how you experience those emotions releasing from your body.

As you learn to identify and meditatively be with all of the different emotions inside of you and surrender how each one feels, you will develop a keen sense of recognizing when others are experiencing the same thing. Often in the clinic, I can sense, feel, recognize and name emotions in others long before they recognize it in themselves. This can be intimidating to others, especially if they want them to stay hidden or are not used to truly being seen by another. It can kick up fear within people. But yet, deep within, I think we all yearn truly to be seen by ourselves and others. We really do want to expose our heart and give from our heart into the world. What is there to be afraid of when one is truly open, vulnerable, loving and free?

"Mindfulness, also called wise attention, helps us see what we're adding to our experiences, not only during meditation sessions but also elsewhere." - Sharon Salzberg, Real Happiness: The Power of Meditation

8. Become aware of how to release unwanted feelings, sensations, memories and events from our body and our mind.

How do we release an emotion? How do we let go and know with certainty that we are free? The reality is that our emotions are just as much a mystery to us as some of the other deepest mysteries on this planet. They don't have to be. Emotional intelligence is something that should be taught to us in every single grade growing up in school. Harvard psychologist Daniel Goleman wrote a book called Emotional Intelligence outlining that emotional intelligence is a far more valuable thing to have than regular intelligence.[197]

People who are emotionally intelligent are more likely to get the jobs they desire, have more fulfilling relationships, be more secure spiritually, can adapt and respond to most situations with more peace, earn more money in life, and the list goes on and on. This is something that should be taught in schools from the moment we start attending. Think of the onslaught of emotions that children feel in school on a daily basis. In the back of Goleman's book, he discusses how they have implemented emotional intelligence activities in certain schools with some impressive results. How much more at peace would our world be if everyone were able to understand, be fully aware of and release negative emotions at will starting as children?

While I loved this book, the only critique that I would offer is that books such as The Tapping Solution[198] or The Sedona Method[199] are better when it comes to actually learning how to release emotions from our consciousness. I think the book was wonderful at pointing out how awareness of our emotional states is critical. These other tools take emotional intelligence full circle by teaching how to actually let go.

As you can see, we all experience the world in many mindless, unconscious ways. We don't know why we do or say certain things. We don't always know how to change those things. We don't know what is affecting our health when the answer is oftentimes very simple. We don't know why the same patterns repeat in our relationships over and over again. Reasons exist for almost everything we experience on many different levels. We simply don't know what we don't know. But, we can learn how to be mindful and to pay attention to things so that these insights arrive in our lives.

How do we bring the unconscious conscious? By being mindful. How can we begin to change something unless we are first aware or conscious of it? Being mindful includes knowing how and what to pay attention to.

The first step towards freedom is simply becoming more aware of how we experience our world emotionally and physically. The second step to bringing the unconscious conscious is actually releasing those emotions. What emotional states do we commonly find ourselves in? What is driving these states? What memories and experiences from the past are driving how we experience the present moment?

How do we experience these emotions in our physical bodies? Many health problems that we experience physically are simply just projections into the physical body that represent some emotional energy that we have been holding onto from the past.

Sense Experiences

Sights, sounds, smells, tastes, and touch are the sensory experiences we have in the physical body that are intricately linked together with our emotional experiences in life. Often certain senses get activated and stir emotion in us both negatively and positively. In every memory that we have from the past, our senses have made associations that are very powerful. For example, if I worked in a coffee shop and went through a horrible breakup or didn't like my job, I might begin to despise the taste and smell of coffee. On the other hand, if I have wonderful memories getting coffee with people I care for, I may love the taste and smell of it. It is warm, inviting, comforting and stimulating. As you heal emotionally, it is really important to become mindful of what senses are linked together with the emotion you felt in any particular memory.

Surrendering Emotions

The first step towards emotional freedom is awareness. The second step is surrender. Using tapping to surrender emotions is very simple. First, you identify how and what you feel. I feel cheated. Second, you ask why you feel an emotion. I feel cheated because I didn't get the promotion at work. Third, you make a setup phrase and tap through it. "Even though I feel cheated for not getting the promotion at work, I want/choose to love and accept myself." Tap through it as many rounds as you need in order to fully surrender it. Remember, it is not the words you use that are important, but instead your wordless intention to actually let the feeling go. Intention to let go and surrender is the very most important aspect of healing.

Besides tapping, two other resources have also been very inspirational in understanding and facilitating surrender and letting go. Those two books are The Sedona Method (Hale Dwoskin) and Letting Go: The Pathway of Surrender (David Hawkins). The quote below from Letting Go succinctly summarizes all that is needed to dissolve any feelings:

> "Letting go involves being aware of a feeling, letting it come up, staying with it, and letting it run its course without wanting to make it different or do anything about it. It means simply to let the feeling be there and to focus on letting out the energy behind it. The first step is to allow yourself to have the feeling

without resisting it, venting it, fearing it, condemning it, or moralizing about it (I shouldn't have this feeling). It means to drop judgment and to see that it is just a feeling. The technique is to be with the feeling and surrender all efforts to modify it in any way. Let go of wanting to resist the feeling. It is resistance that keeps the feeling going. When you give up trying to modify the feeling, it will shift to the next feeling and be accompanied by a light sensation. A feeling that is not resisted will disappear as the energy behind it dissipates."[200]

People have no idea how powerful this process can be. Dr. Hawkins used this process to let go of many incurable health conditions. Lester Levinson, the gentleman who originally came up with The Sedona Method, was given six weeks to live because of a massive coronary heart issue. Both of them surrendered the programs, memories, emotions, and sensations that were behind every one of the health problems they had. Both completely healed and ended up living another 30 years or more in good health.

Surrendering emotions is not a difficult thing. The mind likes to make it complicated. But it is very simple. The hardest part is not the process itself, but simply allowing yourself to fully feel (and then surrender) whatever it is that is coming up for you or what a health problem represents to you. Facing your pain may be the most difficult thing you ever do. For me, it has been the hardest thing I have ever done. But I would do it repeatedly because on the other side of the pain is freedom, love, joy, and peace. Nothing compares to being able to genuinely experience those things in your life.

13 THE STINGS OF THE PAST

"We repeat what we don't repair." —Christine Langley-Obaugh

The most exquisite sensation of pain ripped from the bottom of my foot through the rest of my small four-year-old body. There was so much pain. The pulsating, throbbing, and stabbing sensation on the bottom of the foot was almost unbearable. The waves of agony that followed were almost paralyzing. The world got so small and felt like it had collapsed in just a matter of seconds. Every piece of logic flew out the window due to the crippling feeling on the bottom of the foot. The only thing to do was to explode with buckets of tears and loud cries of whaling resembling a seriously wounded animal. This is the first memory I ever remember having that involved such great physical pain. How could the sting of a bee be this painful? How come no one had warned me about them?

It was a clear, beautiful, and sunny July day in the heart of a Michigan summer. My childhood best friend, Lizzy, and I were gleefully playing in her backyard in a small 6 foot round plastic "pool" that her mom had filled up with water for us. This entertained us for hours on end. She lived in a two story three bedroom white paneled house that was surrounded by a wooden fence about 5 feet high on one side and a chain link fence about 4 feet high on the other side. Opposite her house was a row of evergreen shrubs that almost perfectly closed off her backyard from the surrounding yards, including mine. Through a small gap in the shrubs was an opening that led caddy corner into my backyard. Both of our backyards were about 1/5 acre in size. We spent a lot of time playing in our backyards during the summer.

A common plant that grows in Michigan in the summertime in the grass is called white clover. It shoots up only a couple of inches from the ground and is found all over. Bumblebees and honeybees are commonly seen jumping from one to another pollinating as they go. I didn't claim to be the sharpest pencil in the box at the age of four. I honestly didn't know any better when Lizzy and I started jumping on top of the bees that were landing on the flowers of the white clovers covering her yard. Besides, how does a child know about the power of a bee sting unless it is experienced firsthand?

Lizzy and I squealed with laughter, giggled and ran from flower to flower stomping on any bee that we could find that day. Like all good parents, I am sure mine told me not to partake of this activity. But, Lizzy and I were playing in her backyard with sparse supervision as it was in those days. Even if I did know that bees "stung," whatever that meant, Lizzy and I were probably more caught up in our enjoyment of jumping through the grass together.

And then it happened. As soon as my foot landed on this creature and the fury of this fuzzy insect sunk itself deep into the soft fleshy part of the bottom of my foot, my world would never be the same. Literally. It took almost 30 years to realize the full significance of how this bee's sting would change me forever. I wailed, screamed and cried at the top of my lungs. My only instinct at this point was to run or should I say hobble/crawl home so that I could fall into the loving arms of my mother who would know what to do. Moms always know what to do. My mom was a critical care nurse, and at that age, I knew she helped people, so I knew she would love, care, and protect me and make me feel better.

I don't know how I made it those 90 yards home. The pain was so overwhelming that I remember almost passing out halfway to the house in the middle of my yard. I yelled and screamed, "Mommy, Mommy, help me!!!" Being a nurse, not much fazed my mom. She was trained to remain calm in the most brutal of circumstances. Upon opening the door to the screened patio attached to the back of our house, she had a look of bewilderment given the state that I was in. She quickly assessed my little body and didn't see anything "majorly" wrong and calmly asked me what had happened. Her presence made me feel better.

My mom inquisitively and concernedly asked, "What happened?"

After trying so hard to get the words out between the tears and convulsive crying, I said, "I got stung by a bee on the bottom of my foot!"

Knowing then that I didn't break a bone or wasn't suffering from a wound, she even more calmly asked, "What were you doing?"

I answered, "Lizzy and I were stepping on bees."

I know unequivocally that my mom's intent was not to harm me, make me feel bad, damage me, or cause me more pain. This is not who my mom is. And children can internalize things in the craziest of ways. My mom really did take care of me that day, I just interpreted it a certain way, which had almost nothing to do with her. A part of me now believes that even if what she gave me was unconditional love (which she may have fully done), I would not have been able to receive it because of the physical pain I was in. The physical pain was my filter in this moment and out of this filter only arose the potential for more pain. It was next to impossible to receive love and care in this state. We all like to blame, especially when we are in pain, and this is what I did, even when it was not her fault.

What came out of her mouth next is what really did the most damage. I had never consciously remembered feeling this amount of physical pain before. It was a time when I needed love, care, a tender touch and soothing words to make my pain go away. I needed help with my physical pain. What ensued was even more painful, but it was a different kind of pain. It was an emotional pain, and this pain was even worse than the physical pain. From this moment forward, I would carry it with me subconsciously for the next 29 years.

I don't know what my mom had been doing in the house in the moments leading up to my entry into the patio, nor do I know what state of mind she had been in. The only thing I remember was her response. From my point of view, it was a cold, crushing, brutal blow to my fragile four-year-old self.

In a very nonchalant, calm, and neutral way she said to me, "Well, you deserved it."

This was her response to my physical pain. Ouch. Ouch. Ouch. It was emotional pain on top of the physical pain.

I was crushed, leveled, pummeled on the inside. My innocent heart was thrown to the floor broken into a thousand pieces. I was broken and no one could fix me. Because I couldn't be whole, strong, and powerful, I became broken, hostile, powerless, and abandoned instead. This exact moment gave rise to how I would see myself and interact with the world from this point forward. She was right though. It is wise to leave bees alone, to mind my own business and be a lover of creation.

I felt ashamed of what I did to that bee. I felt rejection from the person I needed love from, even though she didn't reject me. My mom spoke the truth and sometimes the truth stings. I don't blame my mother because, after this moment, it became my story and choosing to hold onto its meaning was my choice. My mom is a wonderful, loving woman whom I love with all my heart. My distorted perception was that she wasn't present in this critical moment and that I needed something else in that moment.

My World Shifted After This

How did this moment change the way I perceived the world? How did her response alter the way I processed emotional information? In what ways did this emotion I took on affect me from this moment forward?

Trauma affects everyone differently. One does not have to suffer abuse or a deep trauma for it to be potentially as life-altering to someone mentally, emotionally or psychologically. What one considers to be minor can just as equally and radically change someone on the inside forever.

How we all personally experience trauma reminds me of a brilliant film made in 1957 called *The Three Faces of Eve*, which was based on a true story. Joanne Woodward won an Academy Award for portraying Eve White, who had three personalities. The trauma one would have to experience for a personality to fracture in three ways would be significant. What was discovered as the simple event or trauma that fractured her personality in three ways? Her beloved grandmother had died when she was six, and according to family custom, relatives were supposed to kiss the dead person at the viewing, making it easier for them to let go. Eve didn't want to do this. Eve's terror of having to kiss her dead grandmother led to her "splitting off" into two other distinctly different personalities to cope and deal with this trauma. Trauma is as deep, scarring and painful as it is perceived by the person who lives with the experience. Physical and sexual abuse are usually the only other things that trump all other trauma.

Let's fast forward 29 years from this momentous experience. One of the rooms in my home that was used as an office has a beautiful view of palm trees, a huge grassy area, and a long walking path. I was mesmerized watching a wasp crawl and fly up and down the window that was just four feet in front of me. While sitting there, I reminisced through the years about the different times, places and people I was with when confronted with bees. Whether it was at a picnic or playing baseball, bees would decide to grace me with their presence. The sight was always quite comical for others. As soon as I heard the very distinct buzzing of their wings, I literally would freeze in terror and at times, would run like a lunatic in whatever direction seemed to be the fastest escape route. As if one could outrun a bee?!

I sat there staring at this bee outside my window feeling uncomfortable just looking at the bee. My heart raced a little faster, with adrenaline beginning to pump through me in anticipation of a fight or flight response. I asked myself this one very reflective question. "When did I become so afraid of bees?" Having dealt now in practice with people knowing that every health problem has a context, my fear of bees most likely had a context too. So I waited for an answer to come into my awareness.

In the past whenever someone asked, "Why are you so afraid of bees?" my response was always the same: "I don't have the foggiest idea, I just don't like them." Saying I didn't like them was a very nice way of saying that I HATED bees. They terrified me. I would almost soil myself when they buzzed around me even as a grown man. I would shake, start sweating, and would freeze as if in a state of paralysis. My body continued to carry the trauma of getting stung at the age of four into the present moment even though I never would have linked the present moment to my past. When bees started flying around me, I was no longer an adult, but subconsciously was reliving the trauma of my 4-year-old self, even though I was completely unaware of doing this.

As I continued to sit there, ready to actually receive the answer to this lifelong question, the answer came very quickly. Four years old. Bee. Pain. Mom. Emotional pain. The memory flooded into my awareness and through my body. I can't remember the last time I had thought of this memory, but as soon as it came into my awareness, I knew there was a lot more significance to the memory than I had remembered. My fear of bees finally started to make sense to me. I found the original context to the fear. But besides being terrified of bees, what was the real underlying emotional significance to this memory and how did it relate to the depression I experienced for 11 years?

Most of us suppress, repress or escape from feeling our negative emotions. Who in their right mind wants to feel emotional pain over and over again? It doesn't matter what the emotional pain is that we have felt; most of us want to numb it away, stuff it deep inside or run for the hills. We just aren't taught to run directly into our emotions, welcoming them or knowing how to truly let them go.

The irony is that this pain, those emotions, and the memory are a part of us, whether we are acknowledging it consciously or not. They will fester in us unconsciously until we consciously deal with them. Life will eventually bring us to this realization in one way or another. If we are still carrying something around with us, every now and then something may trigger our pain, even though we are completely unaware of its original context or meaning. We aren't taught to understand or confront our pain and negative emotions. And this is the dilemma for the majority of us. How can we let go of something we don't know exists in the first place or that we are terrified of confronting because we might get lost in the pain and not be able to crawl out?

For the first time in 29 years, I allowed my body and mind to feel the full weight of this event, as I fully welcomed the entire experience into the present moment. I didn't expect what happened next. When the emotions and the physical sensations in my body were fully welcomed into the present moment, they were very overwhelming, all-consuming. I was soon buried under the weight of my tears, and the sobbing continued for hours. But this time it was different, I knew I would be able to truly release this emotional energy from my body and feel the relief and freedom from having done so. I had the tools to be able to help me come out the other side. I would not just crawl but would overcome this event like a victorious Spartan returning from war.

I had a plan and a map that helped me to navigate through the event. I used intuition to navigate through the memory and applied kinesiology to discover the emotions and negative beliefs in it. I discovered the underlying meaning I gave to the event. Then I had the tool of tapping to help me not only understand what was stored emotionally in this event but to help me let go and move beyond it victoriously. I would release these emotions from my body once and for all.

Using kinesiology, the emotions below were found as the "energy" that was fueling this event. This energy was still very much a part of my consciousness, which is the reason why there were so many tears when truly stepping into and opening myself up to the memory. Everything in the subconscious is actually in the present moment. I have heard many people say that they barely even remember what happened to them 20 or 30 years ago. Just because you don't consciously remember what happened to you, let alone how you felt, doesn't mean that your body doesn't still feel the full weight of that event every day since it happened.

For many people, as time moves forward, our memories from the past seem to fade more and more. As we become less and less conscious of our memories, some think that they just magically start to heal over time. The reality is that most of us just learn to repress, suppress or escape from the emotions that were caused by traumatic events in our past. When measuring the energy of an event and the emotions within those events through AK, it is discovered, most of the time, that it is just as powerfully active within us now as it was when it occurred many years prior.

Having said this, it is critical to identify what emotions are present for us in the memories we have. The emotions we experience give rise to everything else in our memory including our thoughts, actions, and behaviors.

Five very powerful emotions formed the basis of this memory for me. When analyzing these emotions and knowing that those emotions sunk deep within my subconscious from that moment forward, it was easy to see a context for why things continued to happen in my life as a result of going through this event. In physics, we learn that energy attracts like energy. What does this mean emotionally? It means that the energy of a negative emotion becomes a part of you and acts comparable to a transponder that sends out a broadcast signal to the world of whatever is on that frequency. What you get back are things resonating on that same frequency. If you hold onto anger, the world will manifest and show you angry people, situations, and events. The anger you are holding onto is reflected back to you in future events you may experience. You are subject only to what you hold in your mind. If you hold onto anger, the world will give you back anger. Until we let an emotion go, events "out there" will serve as reflections of what is "in here."

Processing Through The Emotions In Our Memories

Listed below are the emotions I experienced in this memory and the significance each one had not only in the memory but in my life from that point forward. All of these emotions were felt at a 10 out of 10 in terms of intensity.

1. Powerless

Consciously, for the first time in my 4-year-old awareness, I was heavily confronted with the limitations of my own power as compared to the power of that tiny flying insect. The world became much smaller for me. I became less powerful, less free. The world became a place of pain, where an unhealthy fear manifested in me for the first time that I can remember. I felt powerless against the pain, powerless to walk home, and powerless to deal with the emotional blow that I thought my mother gave to me.

From that moment on, I carried this powerlessness into my life as a child, adolescent, and adult. Many memories flooded into mind that were also reflections of the same emotions that I had chosen to hold onto from that day. Feeling powerless was something that I saw in my life over and over again through the years ahead. As a result of this memory, I had made an unconscious, silent agreement that I would live life feeling somewhat powerless. This silent, unconscious agreement I made was that I was powerless against pain, to changing things and doing what I wanted to do.

Powerlessness can manifest in many ways into our life. This may include not starting or engaging in things that seem too hard or giving up on things shortly after beginning them. The emotion can then degenerate into an apathy within that says, "Why bother? You don't have the power to do this or to change the circumstances, so why even try?" Obviously, this doesn't paralyze all of our life because life has a curious way of confronting the emotions that we hold within to give us opportunities to change. And for those who know me personally, I try to do almost everything I have ever wanted in spite of my fears or hesitations.

Doing tasks that have the potential to reinforce our powerlessness, but are overcome simply by the act of doing them and succeeding on some level, often diminishes the hold that emotion has on us. We can either reinforce our internal narrative or form a new more empowering one. Life gives us many opportunities to face ourselves in this way. But, we can also become even more powerless depending upon how we deal with the present circumstances. For some, instead of overcoming and feeling empowered, life becomes a continual paralysis due to how we face those moments.

2. Vanity

Vanity in this memory was experienced as futility. This vanity was related to pride or concern over my appearance from what had happened to me. I was broken that day, but I didn't want the world to see me that way. The whole neighborhood heard me wailing. Lizzy heard me wailing and saw how traumatic it was for me. The most important person that I showed vanity towards was my mother. I tried to muster whatever small piece of pride over what had occurred to not look like a complete weakling in front of the one person whose opinion counted most at that age. Vanity is a negative emotion that places too much emphasis on how we appear to the world and to those around us. The real question should be, not in a reactionary way, but in a loving way, "who really cares what others think?" For many of us, the opinion of others is largely all that matters. We live our lives to keep up with the Joneses. Our society is heavily influenced by vanity, the pride of life or others' opinion of us.

Pride is an emotion that is extremely prized in our society today because much significance is placed on skills, abilities, and the appearance of the body. It reminds me of the song that is sung by Matthew McConaughey and Kate Hudson in *How to Lose a Guy in 10 Days*. They were shouting "You're so vain!" at each other from the Carly Simon song. Interestingly, this word comes from a Latin word that means "empty." True unshakable value and worth never come from outside of ourselves, our physical appearance, abilities or skills. Relying on this to give us value and worth is true emptiness. I will admit that while growing up, much weight was put into this vanity because it was something I chose to make a part of me at the age of four. I cared what others thought, how people perceived me and saw me. When they approved, I felt great. When they didn't approve, I felt horrible. This isn't a healthy way to live in the world, especially since it is built on a foundation that is like shifting sand. Another silent agreement I made was: I care deeply about what others think of me to feel good about myself.

3. Hostility

The dictionary defines this as "unfriendly" and "antagonistic." Hostility is something I felt toward the bee and my mother. In this memory the identification is more with antagonism. This is the second most powerful emotion that affected me from this memory. I can hear my father's voice ring out very prominently throughout much of my childhood when he asked, "Scott, why do you antagonize others and push them away? They won't like you if you do those things." I never understood why I antagonized people as a child. I unconsciously pushed people away from me at the time. I never understood why I had this desire within me to push people away, to make sure I was unfriendly towards others, guaranteeing that they became unfriendly towards me. This part of me didn't start changing until about my junior year of high school.

The world was a lonely place for me growing up. I didn't connect well with others and digging into this memory explains in large part why this happened. Another secret agreement I made in this memory is that to protect myself from the pain within and from more pain, I could not trust those around me to safely help me or be present for me. In essence, this is like saying, I secretly and unconsciously am going to push people away just to make sure that they don't hurt me first. Therefore, to avoid people from getting close to me and feeling even more pain, I would instead be hostile and push others away in an effort to protect myself.

Why should I trust people who get close to me knowing that eventually, they would cause me great pain, much like my mother did? It took me 29 years to see this about myself. If we live to protect ourselves, life can be lived in a state of subtle hostility towards everyone and everything to avoid the true pain that we ourselves carry within. We all carry around these types of unconscious childhood wounds.

This was a very impactful emotion for me because it was hard for me to make friends at times growing up. I didn't consciously know why I pushed people away. I didn't want to do this consciously, but subconsciously a part of me was operating very strongly that had an immense impact on my life and my ability to connect with others. Sadly, a part of me became hostile towards my mother and others from this moment on. I just reacted, and this was the emotion that I held onto. I didn't know any better. You can't do better if you don't know better. It wasn't until much later that I reconnected more with my mother emotionally. In her defense, her childhood was not all roses, but she came out remarkably well given her circumstances, and she is a very loving, kind woman. It has been a wondrous relief to start becoming aware of, naming and letting go of this emotion.

4. Shame

This emotion hit me the moment my mom told me that I deserved what I had done. Guilty as charged. I had no defense. She was right. I did deserve what the bee did to me as it was just simply defending itself. The shame over what I had done sunk in deeper and my inner voice diminished. It was as if a muzzle was put over a part of me. Why should I speak up about anything in life? I deserve to be kept quiet. I am wrong for certain actions I take; therefore, I cannot speak up for myself because I am shameful. No one will stick up for me. My mother certainly didn't speak up for me. She was the judge, jury, and executioner, and I was guilty as charged. No words were available in my defense. My head hung low.

This doesn't mean I never spoke up about anything. Every once in a while this emotion would arise at various times in my life while I was growing up. It meant that I didn't have a voice or, when I did speak up, I wasn't listened to or felt like I was understood. I often felt like others didn't understand me.

From an Ayurvedic standpoint, part of the consciousness of the 5th chakra (which is associated with the thyroid and throat area) has to do with communication and self-expression. If you grow up feeling like you don't have a voice, like no one listens to you or you don't feel like you have the ability to express yourself freely, this can set up very fertile grounds for health-related issues in that area. For many, reclaiming one's voice in the world is a powerful part of healing. The body always keeps the score, and I started to take hypothyroid medication at the age of 17 due in part to not feeling like I had a voice.[201] This book is proof that I now have things to say, people listen, and I can freely express myself in the world, even if others disagree. But the subtle agreement I made from this emotion was that when it really matters, I couldn't express my voice and no one would listen to me.

5. Abandoned

Feeling abandoned was by far the heaviest and most damaging emotion that was embedded in me from this memory. The moment my mom told me that I deserved what had happened to me, my world shattered into a thousand pieces. My foot was throbbing. I barely made it home and it took every effort to tell her what had happened to me. And then she tells me that I deserved it.

A part of me died that day. I felt emotionally abandoned by her. If ever I needed an ally, someone to comfort and soothe my pain, it was then. I don't blame my mom at all because it was my choice to fiercely hold onto this emotion for so long. This emotion is closely linked to hostility because it affected all of my personal relationships moving forward. The full impact of this emotion is linked to some of the biggest struggles I have had in life.

Powerful Agreements

As we experience trauma in our childhood, we unconsciously make agreements about ourselves, others and the world. We are not aware in those moments that we are making these agreements, but our minds desperately try to make sense of what has happened. Our minds are programmed for survival. The mind of a child takes trauma and has no other choice but to make very concrete agreements so that we can be protected. These agreements we make are our defenses against life and the perceived threats to our survival.

The agreements that arose out of this experience that impacted me from that moment forward were:

- "Life is going to be very painful."
- "You don't deserve love from others."
- "Push others away so that you don't ever get hurt again."
- "In the end, everyone is going to abandon you on some level."
- "You can't freely express yourself because no one will listen."
- "You can't emotionally trust even those closest to you."

We live our lives wondering why we act and behave in certain ways. Much of the time the reasons for why we live the way we do can be traced back to agreements that we unconsciously made when we were children. Carrying around beliefs such as these will color your whole world and perception moving forward. I learned that the world is a very painful place and that people will abandon me in one way or another.

I made an agreement at the age of 4 that sooner or later everyone would abandon me. Little by little, over the years, this agreement grew stronger and solidified itself until reaching a crisis point. This crisis point happened 17 years later at the age of 21 while I was a senior in college. It was this crisis point that plunged me into 11 long years of heavy depression.

14 THE IMPACT OF OUR HURTS

"The purpose of the agonies, of the dark nights of the soul,
then became apparent - they're so intolerable that their
exquisite pain spurs one on to the extreme effort required to
surmount them. When vacillation between heaven and hell
becomes unendurable, the desire for existence itself has to be
surrendered. Only once this is done may one finally move
beyond allness or nothingness, beyond existence or
nonexistence. This culmination of the inner work is the most
difficult phase, the ultimate watershed, where one is starkly
aware that the illusion of existence one transcends here is
irrevocable."
- David Hawkins, M.D., Ph.D.

"Mom and dad, I don't want to live anymore! I want to die! I want to kill myself and end this misery!"

The desperation in my voice horrified and saddened my parents on the other end of the line. My phone calls to them progressively worsened over the months as all meaning in life seemed to be vanishing. No other option was seen and life was just not worth living. I was afraid for myself. My parents, who were very worried, said, "Scott, come home, and be with people who love you." So I moved from Virginia to Michigan to live with my parents. My parents were the lights in the darkness and comforted me during those very dark years.

How'd I get there? Why had things gotten so bad? Why had all hope almost vanished?

This phone call took place on a cold night in Lynchburg, VA in 2003; a couple of years after the depression had started. I was just finishing up seminary. At the time, I had some idea as to why I felt this way, but I wasn't completely sure, and I didn't know what to do about it. My parents, close friends or even the professional counselors couldn't really help me to understand why I was so depressed and what to do to overcome it. They were just as clueless and helpless as I was. It took another 11 years to be able to see what was going on and what the primary cause was that held this depression in place. As was alluded to in the last chapter, when I started seeing the theme of abandonment, I finally felt like things were starting to make sense.

My story starts out at the age of 4 with the sting of abandonment. I never fit in much as a child. I always felt like an outsider. I didn't make friends very well, even though I wanted to have friends more than anything growing up. After periods of time, people didn't want to be around me. I said and did things that purposefully pushed people away from me. This energy morphed and changed over the years, eventually coming to a head in 2001, when this emotion took on its most desperate meaning. I still couldn't see it though. I was so full of shame and blame to take any responsibility for it. I never understood why until 2011. It took 29 years to understand why, and 11 very rough years vehemently and tirelessly searching for meaning to feel better.

Abandonment sums up much of the energy, sadness, desperation, loneliness, and heartache I have felt through my past. A little fuzzy insect was a contributor to seeing darkness in me that didn't come to light until much later. I felt and internalized that my mother abandoned me emotionally. Or at least this is the way I perceived it then. No one makes us feel anything, as much as we want to blame others, our environment, our experiences, etc. No one can hurt you. Hurt is simply just your mind giving meaning to an event. The most powerful thing about our mind is that through surrender we can transform the meaning we gave something that happened to us long ago. We choose what we feel and how we interpret what happens to us whether we are conscious of it or not. A shift from blame to responsibility is an enormous leap in consciousness and awareness. It is perhaps one of the most important things in life and spiritual growth.

Until we transform the meaning of a major hurt in our life, the theme of our major hurt gets repeated and reinforced in the future. For me, four major events happened subsequent to getting stung that continued to shape how this emotion ran through my life like a plague.

Four Major Reinforcing Memories

From the moment I was stung, the world reflected itself to me as a place in which I would constantly be in pain and would be deserted. As I mentioned, I didn't make friends easily. No one wanted to be around someone who was constantly projecting out into the world subconsciously, "I need you to abandon me. I need you to desert me. I need to feel all alone!" I projected this energy out into the world because it was what I had chosen to hold onto and the world simply reflected it back to me throughout most of my life. I didn't know any better and as a result this emotion continued to manifest into a pattern of the same kind of events in the future. Four major events after the age of four repeated and reinforced this theme of abandonment.

Not Enough Time With My Father

I went to a Christian school until the 9th grade. My dad was the pastor of the church. It was a large church, a congregation of around 1000 people, and my father was the only pastor for a time. The school was very small, and of course, I thought I ran it. Throughout grade school, I was constantly getting into trouble. I would do anything for attention it seemed. When I wanted attention, I did stupid things, and when I was asked why I did those things, my response was always the same: "I don't know why." No one else knew either.

It wasn't until around the age of twenty one that, for the first time, I began to make sense of my story. I began to discover the issue that was behind the proverbial curtain. Things changed when I read a book called *The Family Crucible* by Augustus Y. Napier, Ph.D., and Carl Whitaker, M.D.[202] A crucible is a container that can withstand very high temperatures and is used to shape glass and metal. This book details one family's experience going through counseling together. It is a fascinating work. What better place to mold and shape us than within the crucible of our family?

I saw myself reflected in one of the characters, Don (the son). This is what I learned about myself from his character. From what I recall, Don was always getting in trouble and was a constant troublemaker in the family. The reason why he was always in trouble was that his father was never home and Don needed him in his life. The lights came on for me. I needed my father. I loved spending time with him and never got tired of throwing the baseball together, playing basketball one on one in the driveway or riding around on his moped looking for aluminum cans that we returned to the store for money. Spending time with my dad was precious…but limited. I craved and demanded more time from him than he gave me when I was younger. I craved his attention because I knew on some unconscious level that he would not abandon me no matter what and I didn't have that guarantee from anyone else in the world.

Dad seemed like he was always at church and never home. I craved and needed more time with him to feel loved and accepted because I didn't love or accept myself much growing up. Instead, he wasn't home much and I felt abandoned and that he didn't love me. This was my perception. This wasn't true, but it was my truth at the time. Therefore, in my mind any attention is better than no attention, so I misbehaved. I was convinced that this would get his attention. Negative attention is better than no attention I thought. His office was about 30 feet from my classroom, and if the offense was bad enough, my dad was consulted immediately. My dad got consulted a lot. I felt the pain at home because I constantly faced the consequences of my actions. My love language is quality time, something that I didn't get much of with dad while growing up.

Growing up, I never wanted to be at church, especially in high school, because it was a sore reminder of the thing that stole my dad away from me. I felt abandoned, deserted, and unloved by my dad; though these things weren't true. In truth, my dad has always been my champion and fiercest supporter. My internal lens of seeing the world through abandonment is what generated this for me. My dad is an incredibly loving man, who in many ways is my hero. But at the age of 21 for the first time, I began to realize why I always got into trouble. My dad and I sat down one day, and I poured my heart out about how this made sense to me. I forgave him and myself, and we have had an incredible relationship since, for which I am eternally grateful.

Dating Disaster

The second major memory, or should I say "memories," that continued to reflect back to me the emotional energy of desertion and abandonment happened during my junior and senior years of high school. I was so good at pushing people away throughout my adolescence, that I never had a girlfriend nor had many girls interested in me. This all changed with a girl that I met my junior year of high school. It was short lived though because I was awkward, very insecure and this, of course, led to me pushing her away. I really clung to the idea of someone liking me, and it devastated me when it never went anywhere. My proclivity towards pushing people away did start changing in significant ways when I turned sixteen, and by my junior year of high school I had a very wonderful group of great friends, people whom I am still very close friends with today. But that didn't mean it all instantly changed for me inside.

The same thing happened again my senior year with another girl I met. I fell hard for her as well, only to have things be very awkward again, leading to my eventually pushing her away also. While the specifics of these events would only embarrass me further and are not very important to tell in detail, you get the idea. I have since processed through and let go of all the emotions I experienced in these circumstances and am no longer awkward or insecure around women. Thank God. People and events simply reflected back to me the energy that I held onto. Life reflected my internal reality back to me. I just saw a projection of myself out into the world.

Deserted By God Himself

The event that broke the camel's back happened to me my senior year of college. This was the dagger to my heart, sending me into a tailspin for 11 years. When I was seventeen, I became a Christian. It was the most positive, transforming thing that I had perhaps ever experienced up to this point in my life, especially considering the way my life so radically changed from this point forward spiritually. I read through the Bible cover to cover that year and every day as I read it, the more I was changed.

Reading about Jesus in the New Testament was life-changing. I mean, what is not to like about Jesus?! And no I don't mean the version of Jesus that is mixed up with rules, and graceless religion. What I'm referring to is the divinity, love, forgiveness, sacrifice and deep grace he embodied for humanity. I enjoyed church now and was honored to hear two very gifted men speak at church every week (Ed Dobson and Rob Bell). It was fun watching Rob Bell grow and eventually leave Calvary Church to start Mars Hill Church.

Things were going great in my sophomore year of college. I got a scholarship and went with my best friends to Liberty University to study the Bible. I loved Liberty. It was a place where I grew leaps and bounds personally and spiritually. I felt the presence of God in my life all the time and many times in supernatural, miraculous ways. I fervently desired to take my relationship with God even deeper, and that's what I did. I spent an hour reading and studying the Bible and another hour in prayer almost every day. I led a traveling ministry team speaking, singing, and doing discipleship in churches all over the east coast.

I wanted more of God. I wanted a deeper relationship with Him. All of this was new territory for me and I didn't know what that looked like, but it became clear that deepening this relationship was the most important thing that life could ever offer. We were made to reconnect with our Source, the Creator of All That Is. This became clear to me while at school, and it was my innermost desire to continue to "progress" towards establishing and rooting myself in this mystical union. I now know there is nothing to progress towards as this mystical union is already a reality, but I didn't have this understanding at the time. I thought it was something I had to gain or achieve somehow.

So I continued to do the only thing that I knew how to do based on what I had learned until this point. I submerged myself in the reading and studying of the Bible and prayer. I loved what I was studying in school. We learned about theology, missional studies, Greek, Hebrew, exegesis, how to minister, methodology, etc. I soaked it all up.

The Final Blow

As my senior year of college progressed, I continued to learn, grow, minister, and above all to deepen my relationship with God. But one day arrived which was the final blow of abandonment in my life. Over the last couple years leading up to this moment, I felt a very palpable sense of presence from God in my life. It is hard to describe, but it was always there. Have you ever walked into a room and just intuitively felt like another person was in the room with you or was somehow watching you? Experientially, this was how I felt God's presence every day. I don't exactly know how, but I could sense, intuit and feel this presence with me every day.

Then one day, His presence deserted me. From one moment to the next, God was gone. It was the most unsettling, disturbing, and horrifying feeling. This rocked my inner world. It was like an inner panic attack. The foundations of my world began to crumble, and I didn't know why. I felt an increasing chill, a silence, and a lack of direction with regards to His presence and also the leading of His voice within that had previously guided and directed me. My world went from feeling free, open and rapidly expanding to being cold, alone, confined and small from one day to the next.

I can remember starting to feel shame that day. Something was wrong and it became internalized as something must be wrong with me. Something MUST be wrong with me? Why would God "abandon" me? The shame was heavy. The feeling of desertion was even worse. People who go from undergraduate Biblical studies into seminary are supposed to have their stuff together, right? Those becoming pastors are supposed to have the answers, especially for the people coming to them, right? The religious instruction one is given in seminary is supposed to be enough. Isn't someone who is becoming a pastor supposed to have all their beliefs figured out and to be so filled with hope so as to be able to communicate this hope heartily to others? This wasn't true for me. Instead, my life began to slip away.

After the initial shock, silence, and horror of this experience, I began the stages of grief.[203] At first came denial and isolation: "This can't be happening to me!" "I feel so alone." "Where did you go?" "What did I do wrong?" "I thought I was doing what you wanted me to do!" The fear of being deserted and abandoned got activated once again with the most devastating of blows, but this time by the One person or Being that promised to never do such a thing.[204] It was this abandonment that really broke me.

Rage After Abandonment

One night during this time as the ministry team I led gathered for practice, I decided to mention what was going on, what deeply troubled me. We divided into guys and girls and spoke about what was going on with each of us and how we could pray for each other. When it was my turn, I began to express what was going on inside of me, my struggle, the pain, the aloneness. My turmoil of what had happened to me was met with seemingly a lack of empathy and well-intentioned members literally said to me, "Scott, it is going to be ok; you just have to read your Bible more, pray more, and it will go away." I was dumbfounded and angered by this response.

The clear message was that I just needed to try harder and be more religious. This is when the second stage of grief started to set in, when you experience anger about what you have lost. The others didn't know what to say, feeling as desperate about telling me something, as I felt inside. I remembered feeling this rage boil within me that wanted to lash out yelling and screaming at them saying, "You have no idea what is going on inside of me! You have no idea about the level of pain I'm feeling! I feel lost, alone, cold and all you can tell me to do is read the Bible!"

So guess what I did? I read my Bible and prayed even harder. On my knees day after day, week after week, I wept profusely while crying out to God to feel the return of His presence. I questioned, "What did I do wrong?!", "Did I commit some horrible sin?!", and "Why have You left me?!"

Crickets. Silence. Nothing.

I continued to feel worse as the weeks went on. The more I told my friends, others, and my parents of what was happening to me, the more alone I felt as they had no clue how to respond to my desperation either. The anger, bitterness, resentment, and fear continued to grow within me. It didn't appear that God was going to show up. I felt abandoned by God, much like I did by my mother. As a result of being abandoned, I was angry. Anger is what drives most depression and I was very angry at God for abandoning me. How else is someone supposed to feel when everyone in their life abandons them? This experience is what began 11 years of dark, cold, lifeless, horrible depression.

The Hopeless Pursuit Of No Answers

Depression for many people is a loop of five primary emotions. The first is the activation of some kind of **fear.** For me, it was the fear of being abandoned. For others, it could be the fear of being rejected, unloved, or not being good enough. The second emotion is **desire** for something that we just can't seem to be able to get. The third emotion is the **anger** that arises in response to the fear. I was angry that I was abandoned. The fourth emotion is the **sadness** that ensues over having lost something. The fifth is the **hopelessness/apathy** that encompases it all because one feels like it will never change or be any different.

I was desperate for answers. This drove me to read, to try to find something from someone who had gone through something similar. The closest thing I found was in the books of Neil Anderson, Charles Solomon and St. John of the Cross's *Dark Night of the Soul.* I continued to read, listen and ask anyone about what I was experiencing. From 2001-2003, I probably read at least 75 books on Christian counseling, psychology and other materials which spoke about the deep levels of the heart/spirit. It was the beginning of an intense exploration of what was at the source of this pain. I was trying to answer the deepest and most profound question that anyone can ask in life – "Who am I?" I was asking this question, because who I thought I was had completely slipped away from me, driving me into depression.

It wasn't difficult to intellectually understand my identity about who I am in Christ, but how it applied directly to me was a different matter altogether. I read all the identity-confirming passages of the Bible about who I am in Christ, and tried to tell myself these affirmations day after day. But this did absolutely nothing for me. Understanding identity intellectually and trying to tell myself these things never really touched my being. I have found that you can try to tell yourself any kind of affirmation until you are blue in the face, but getting these affirmations to firmly root within takes something more. The concepts of "giving it all to God" and "laying it all on the altar" are a part of and are heard in the Christian world. When I pressed pastors, counselors and theologians about how to actually do this, I found they all were just as clueless as I was.

As a result, the ultimate answers I found were not found in the Bible or books by Christian authors. This is not to say that I didn't find my answer with God's help. I did find my answers from God, just not through traditional Christian channels and resources. The answers that finally helped me not only understand the struggle I had for so long and how to alter this reality came into my world through Chinese medicine, non-duality, the works of Dr. David Hawkins, and understanding consciousness and emotional release.

Two years passed with things only getting worse, and in 2003 I found myself on the telephone with my parents telling them I wanted to end this struggle. The one thought that drove this whole conflict was this: "God, if you are not going to be 'present' in my life, what is the point of living?" It was like being permanently separated with the one person that you loved, needed, and wanted more than any other in life. And when that person abandons you and never appears in your life ever again, the separation is unbearable.

The Reason God Abandoned Me

A very well known quote by the Buddha says, "Attachment is the root of suffering." This same concept is expounded upon identically by Jesus too, but in a different way, using different language and words. When we attach to something or someone in unhealthy negative emotional ways, and then that person leaves us or we lose something, the loss can reveal the attachment we have. If we are attached, we suffer and experience many negative emotions. I "lost" my connection with God. I "lost" this close personal palpable feeling experience. As a result of losing this connection, the depth of my attachment came out as the true nature of what I was holding onto internally. My attachment to my relationship with God being a certain way eventually revealed very deep emotional suffering.

Love is the ultimate definition of non-attachment (not detachment), whereas attachment is the root of suffering. Attachment is finding emotional meaning or significance in the exterior world-- in things, people, objects, abilities, etc. What drives attachment is the sinful nature, or in more modern terms, the ego. Attachment in this sense is not love.

True, divine, unconditional Love is free and is attached to nothing. When one realizes and fully steps into Love itself, one is free from needing to attach to anything. One is free, unbound, and therefore loves and gives freely to all without reservation, specialness or judgment. Love is expansive; attachment is restrictive. Therefore, if one truly and unconditionally loves, when you lose something, no suffering arises. At the heart of it, suffering comes only at the hands of drawing from our internal negative emotional reservoirs.

For those who have experienced a huge loss in a personal relationship, I am sure you can relate to how this feels. Grief and sadness are not love; quite the opposite. Grief, sadness, and loss reveal the depth of our emotional attachment and how much we projected getting love from what we lost. Grief and loss are the result of needing to find love in something "out there," rather than discovering that the Source of all unconditional love has always been "in here." The Kingdom of Heaven is found within.

Grief and loss are excruciatingly painful emotions. When you place your happiness in things and people outside of yourself, and they leave, you suffer because of what this situation reflects to you. Loss will bring out our true attachment. Redemption comes when these things are set free, knowing that they don't have to be experienced. We can release them at any time.

I didn't know how to let go, to ease my internal pain of being abandoned, being angry and grieving what I had lost. Life seemed better ended than continued. The root of suffering is attachment. I was attached to God. As healthy as this may sound, it was not. I was not experiencing the fullness of the mystical union with God because all I experienced was separation. My attachment only revealed my true separation internally from God. Jesus prayed for us to be One, as he and the Father are One. In reality, I was more attached to hearing God's voice and the "specialness" of the relationship we had than I was to becoming more like Him and merging into this mystical union. My attachment to God wasn't Love, but a house of cards which had fallen over.

Therefore, God in His wisdom knew that this was my attachment and by taking it away, the suffering would come up from within me. This sort of attachment is seen in the parable in the Bible of the man that had great wealth. Money is not bad, but when you are attached to it, God knows exactly what buttons to push to address your deepest attachments. When Jesus told the man to sell his possessions and follow Him, the text reads that he left feeling very sad or sorrowful. He was very attached to his wealth, and Jesus knew this. He knew that in losing it, the man would feel great suffering – sadness. In the same way, the degree of my suffering showed me the extent of my attachment. My attachment was rooted in feeling deserted. God cared so much about dealing with this in me that He used this event to help me to see it and grow. It just took 11 years to finally see it.

I spent the next 11 years in what clinically would be considered a deep depression as I went through a process of discovery about these truths. I learned to keep most of my struggles from everyone. This was not done to be hypocritical, but who wants to be around someone who constantly talks about their struggles without knowing how to help? Those who were closest to me knew, and I was never afraid of telling anyone who got to know me well in those 11 years. But mostly I kept it to myself and continued to suffer.

8 Years Of Abandonment

I mentioned that four major events reinforced this theme of abandonment for me. The last major one had to do with one of my best friends. My college experience was amazing. I loved every minute of college in spite of having this experience my senior year. During the year in which this depression started, I experienced even further insult to already existing injury. In my life I have had the most amazing friends anyone could ever ask for. Most of my college friends are still the people I am closest to.

One of my best friends was someone to whom I had grown very close. Life has a way of testing relationships to see if they really are solid or not. In the year this depression started, I stood up as the best man at my best friend's wedding. We had a close friendship for many years or so I thought. Throughout my life this theme of abandonment didn't just affect me in the experiences I have described in this book. Many other less emotionally damaging things occurred as well. In the theme of being deserted and abandoned, I never got called to do things when I was growing up. Given the context of what has been written about in the last two chapters, it is easy to see why this occurred. Most of the time, I proactively called people to hang out and do things, but people rarely called me.

Having to initiate things first has always bothered me, and at various times throughout the decades, I would stop calling people. When I stopped calling, I would never hear from certain people ever again. This actually showed me how these relationships weren't all that solid to begin with. My best friend got married and moved back home to Michigan after graduating from Liberty. I remained in Lynchburg, VA. We spoke on the phone often, and to his defense, I was no fun to talk to because my world was so deeply clouded with depression. Also, in his defense, he didn't know how to help me either. One day, I stopped calling him. When I did this, we didn't speak for eight years.

This, yet again, was the broadcasting and solidification of the abandonment that I held onto. I wasn't completely to blame, but I do take responsibility for my part in creating this distance. As a result of being abandoned by him too, I was very angry. After eight years of silence, I finally called him. I apologized for the anger and resentment that I had towards him. He apologized as well. We reconciled and made peace with each other.

We all have these emotional themes in our life, whether you are depressed or are experiencing something else in your life. In what ways can you perhaps identify with this theme? Can you think of a theme that has been present in your life and has driven you subconsciously for many years?

Everyone I have worked with in the clinic has at least one, if not many, negative emotional "themes" that have driven their lives in some powerful way. I find that most people don't fully understand the things that really drive them. Or, if they do understand them, they are not sure how to change them or what to do about them. I voraciously tried to understand this in my life, and it took 11 years looking vehemently for answers to find what I was looking for and what the problem was.

15 FREEDOM FROM OUR HURTS

"I am the prodigal son every time I search for unconditional
love where it cannot be found."
- Henri Nouwen

"Catastrophic experiences (negative events) are the seeds, the
very essence of the ultimate spiritual experience. Within it and
following it to its very center core, totally walking off the cliff
in complete abandonment, the full surrender (to God) of the
experience is the very seed and core of that which the
spiritual seeker has been searching for all along." - Dr. David
Hawkins, M.D., Recovery and Healing[205]

So after 11 years, what finally broke? How did things change? How was I able to resolve the abandonment?

It was a regular day just like any other, but an awareness finally came that it was really time to sit down and process through what really happened to me when I was a child and then later in college. I didn't know exactly what I was going to find or how difficult it was going to be. But, with courage, I wanted to face myself and take full responsibility for what had occurred. I sat down, and I decided to identify all of the emotions and thoughts that were wrapped up for me in these memories. This was very painful and difficult, but I felt ready.

Just the simple act of sitting down and being honest with myself about all the things I felt was refreshing in and of itself. Many people find it difficult to be really honest with themselves and even more difficult being honest with God. If we are angry with God, most don't feel the inner freedom to be able to voice this. Additionally, many may feel guilt about being angry at God. In the Bible, we have an awesome example of someone who was brutally honest with God - David. God wants us to be honest. We can be just as resentful, bitter, and unforgiving with God as we can be with anyone else. What we must realize is that this is a projection of ourselves wanting to assign blame rather than taking responsibility for our internal state. I was livid with God. So in my attempt to be honest about my memories and emotions, here is what I did during this time frame.

First, I decided to write down the emotions which captured and summarized what was felt and experienced in each of these two memories. Eventually, I did this for all the negative memories I had from my past as well. Second, using AK, the charge or impact behind each sentence was measured on a scale from 1-10. Third, all of the emotions were given meaning by me. Once the emotion was identified, the question "why did you feel this emotion?" was consciously identified. I was able to give real meaning to the things I felt and why I felt them. This would also provide the information needed that was used to tap out all these emotions from my body.

Identifying each emotion and why I experienced them took about 10-20 minutes for each memory. Once they were identified and fully explored, each one was processed through using tapping. I wasn't afraid any longer to face this darkness within me. With intention, my spirit was opened up and allowed to feel the full weight of each emotion. Tears flowed heavily and only by the grace of God was I able to give my body full permission to consciously feel every bit of these emotions to finally let them go. Some of the phrases below took many rounds to process through due to how heavily they were felt. It took about three hours to process through each memory.

Tapping Through The Bee Sting Memory

The first memory that I tapped through was the one of getting stung by a bee at the age of four. Below are the phrases that I used to tap through every emotion, thought and agreement I had made in this memory. I gave each emotion or thought a number in terms of how intensely I felt each one. I continued tapping through each one until I no longer felt the emotional energy sitting behind each one. All together, it took me about three hours to process through this memory. I honestly didn't know if this was going to work or not when I first attempted it. All I did was have faith and trust that it was going to work. Some of the emotions were so heavy and I felt like I was going to drown in them forever, but with continued intention and courage, they all began to subside and disappear. I tenaciously tapped at least nine times on each point while I repeated the whole phrase. After tapping through all nine points, I would stop and take a deep breath. At the end of each round, I would check internally to see if it was the same, worse or better.

1. Even though the stinging pain in my foot is excruciating, I deeply love and accept myself. 10/10
2. Even though bees are terrifying and inflict pain, I deeply love and accept myself. 10/10
3. Even though I feel so powerless to do anything about the physical or emotional pain, I deeply love and accept myself. 10/10
4. Even though I am trying so hard not to be weak (vain) right now, I deeply love and accept myself. 10/10

5. Even though I feel so ashamed and silenced by my mother, I deeply love and accept myself. 10/10
6. Even though I feel so hostile towards my mom and want to push her away, I deeply love and accept myself. 10/10
7. Even though my mom abandoned me, I deeply love and accept myself. 10/10
8. Even though I don't deserve my mom's love, I deeply love and accept myself. 10/10
9. Even though I am worthless, I deeply love and accept myself. 10/10
10. Even though I am so stupid (guilty) for having stepped on that bee, I deeply love and accept myself. 10/10
11. Even though life is painful, I deeply love and accept myself. 10/10
12. Even though I deserve bad things, I deeply love and accept myself. 10/10
13. Even though it's not safe to freely express myself, I deeply love and accept myself. 10/10
14. Even though I can't trust those closest to me, I deeply love and accept myself. 10/10

Tapping Through Feeling Abandoned By God

Below are the thoughts and emotions that I felt about the memory I had in college. I worked through this memory a little differently. It just felt appropriate to list all of the thoughts I had about what happened in the memory first and then work through the emotions. I just let myself go and thought/felt through things as long as was necessary. This memory also took about 3 hours or more to work through. Even after 11 years, I could still intensely and consciously feel these things because the memory had occurred for me as an adult. In all of the things listed below, each thought or emotion had an intensity of at least a 9 out of 10 in intensity.

My thoughts about God abandoning me in college:

1. I feel like God didn't listen to me.
2. God is distant and far away.
3. God is a liar. He says He will never leave us and forsake us, that is total bull.
4. I feel forsaken, forgotten.
5. My voice isn't important to God because He's not listening to my pleas for help.
6. I am not important to God.
7. He left me to drown spiritually.
8. He stopped talking to me.
9. He abandoned me.
10. He hurt me by not responding.
11. God is mean and cruel.

12. He must be punishing me for my sins.

Here are the emotions I felt towards God in order of importance in this memory:

1. Abandoned. I am four years old all over again. Almost everyone else has abandoned me, including You.
2. Hard-hearted. My heart turned to stone and grew cold because of You. My feelings were callous, and all the tenderness that I had toward You left me.
3. Unmerciful. You are unmerciful because You didn't take pity on me and help me when I begged You to for 11 years.
4. Uncaring. How can Your silence be caring for me?! How can You expect to have a relationship when You don't care about me?! How can a Father care for His children without communicating with them?!
5. Contempt. You are worthless, despicable and not even worth consideration anymore, so I will forget You as You have forgotten me and have left me to die.
6. Rage. Anger doesn't even describe what I feel towards You for leaving me all alone.
7. Pain. Nothing has been more painful than not having You in my life. The pain in my soul is beyond excruciating. I am numb, just existing.

Here are some ultimate negative thoughts (The things we tell ourselves about what we go through):

1. God is a liar, can't be trusted and is never going to be there for me ever again.
2. Everyone is always going to abandon me and I will forever be alone.
3. I will never open my heart up to anyone ever again.
4. I am terrible and shameful, something must obviously be wrong with me.
5. I am not good enough.
6. I deserve only bad things.

If it seems as bad reading through this as it really was, then you are starting to see why the depression was so intense. This is a glimpse into the darkest recesses of my soul and the baggage that I had carried around for 11 years and beyond. Letting this all go was the most freeing thing I had ever done.

In exactly the same way as the first memory, I followed the same format and started tapping. To give an example of how the above was processed through, the first statement "I feel like God didn't listen to me" will be used.

Set-up statement: "Even though I feel like God didn't listen to me, I deeply love and forgive myself."

I tapped on each point at least nine times. After tapping through all nine points,

I took a deep breath. After every round of tapping the thought or feeling was assessed to determine if it felt like it was the same, better or worse. I simply asked myself at the end of every round, "Do you feel this is better, worse or the same?" Much of the time in both of these memories, even after tapping on something for a long time, the emotion seemed to remain the same. I was letting go, but each emotion was so intense that I didn't seem to make much progress at times. Eventually, even emotion and thought would begin to diminish and disappear.

At times, a person can identify an emotion at 7/10, but once they give their body permission to welcome, work through and feel it completely, it may get temporarily "worse." Negative emotions are finite things, so if we maintain the commitment to surrender the emotion for as long as it takes, eventually it will release. When it gets worse, what this really means is that one was able to identify with it more strongly. Nothing can actually get worse, but we can open ourselves up to feeling more of something we are holding onto. We simply are just allowing ourselves to feel something more fully.

Each one of the thoughts and emotions listed above was tapped out until the energy of them was no longer felt or intuited. Let me give an example of how the emotion of "hard-hearted" was processed through. This was done more freely, and I didn't follow the setup statement as I did in the last chapter. Again, it is not what you say, but it is allowing yourself to welcome the emotional energy of something. When you welcome something, combined with the heart intention to let go, releasing happens. Tapping is a very free process, so you can use it very freely. With the emotion of being hard-hearted, a round of tapping was done in the following manner. On each one of the nine tapping points, a different statement was made. When we simply name what this means to us in many ways, it can also help to release the energy of the emotion. Here is what was tapped upon:

- Top of Head: My heart is hard because of You
- Eyebrows: You took all the warmth away from my heart
- Temples: When You left me, my heart turned to stone
- Back of the Head: Why did You have to do this to me?
- Under Eyes: My heart is so hard towards You
- Under Nose: Just so hard-hearted…
- Under Mouth: Every part of me is callous towards You
- Under Arms: I release and let go of my hard-heartedness.
- Under Collarbone: I release and let go of all hard-heartedness. (Deep Breath)

After several rounds of this, I still felt the emotion, but it lowered to an 8/10. It still felt very strong. It is very important to take a deep breath at the end of every round. Sometimes it is helpful to take two deep breaths. Breath in Chinese and other ancient traditions is very powerful. After doing an intense round of tapping, it is important to breathe so that you feel more grounded and centered. Taking a deep diaphragmatic breath facilitates movement and is also a way of releasing and letting go as we let go of our breath.

On the next round, the following was repeated on all nine tapping points:

"Even though I feel so hard-hearted toward You because You left me, I deeply love and *forgive myself and forgive You.*"

After a couple of rounds of tapping on this, it released much more down to a 4/10. What is interesting about this round is the idea or concept of forgiving God. We may think to ourselves that God cannot do anything wrong, but in my view, God had done me serious wrong. Therefore, I literally needed to forgive God. This may seem like a strange concept, but for many it is very helpful. I needed to let God off the hook. I told Him I forgave Him and understood it wasn't His fault.

All along it was just my emotional expression projected outwards that caused me to think that God had offended or hurt me. The ego/flesh loves to blame everything and everyone for hurts, pains, and offenses. In reality, we end up seeing that, on the highest level, we are responsible for our reactions to things and that no one really can hurt us. When we forgive, what we are also doing is taking responsibility for our emotions. We realize that it is not about blame if we want to heal. It is about taking personal responsibility to forgive and let go. This is something that many people have a very hard time with. Our society loves to blame, but we have a very hard time taking responsibility. When we forgive, the person we are really freeing is ourself.

After tapping on all these things, the emotions were no longer felt and they were completely gone. The beautiful thing about memories is that once you let go of the emotions and energy from past events, they never come back. You cannot change the events of the past, but you can alter your emotional perception of them. You have control over the emotional energy that you choose to hold onto as a result of what happened to you. This is what you can let go of and be free from.

When people begin to use tapping as a tool, they frequently ask about what to say when tapping. They get concerned that if they don't say the right thing that it will not work for them. What is said is not important at all as compared to allowing yourself to truly feel what is inside of you. Welcome and befriend the negative emotions inside of you. Fully allow them to surface and let go of your resistance to feeling them. In reality, nothing needs to be said at all to let something go (as is the case with The Sedona Method). It can just be done by allowing the emotions or thoughts to surface while holding the steadfast intention of releasing or letting them go. Now, in practice, I use The Sedona Method more frequently, and in using this tool, nothing at all is said while releasing.

After processing through both of these memories, the feeling I had was astonishing. I realized that this was a very heavy burden that I had carried for a long time. When I decided to finally let go of the burden, my body instantly felt it. I felt lighter, freer, and ultimately more loving. I can't begin to describe what this felt like in the days and weeks after. **The cloud had lifted and the 11 years of depression**

was gone. I can't even begin to describe how amazing this FELT. The "sun" started shining again and color returned to my world. Vast relief was felt after 11 long years of choosing to carry this junk around.

Letting these memories go didn't mean that all my internal problems were solved that day, but it did mean that a lot of negative thoughts and emotions were released from me. My heart warmed toward God. That warmth had been absent for 11 years. A tenderness was beginning to rekindle within me. Prayer, which had been mostly avoided the last 11 years, began anew. Conversations with God began to happen again spontaneously. My consciousness was altered. More awareness of my internal world was revealed. I felt different. I felt alive. I felt so much better. This made the essence of my being more able to subjectively experience Truth as a result of letting go. When you release and let go, the way you see yourself, God, and the world changes. I felt more love, joy and peace.

The most important lesson that was learned as a result of processing through all this was what it really meant to me. I was more attached to God showing me things and speaking to me rather than actually experiencing Him with unconditional love or actually being love. The Buddha said, "Attachment is the root of suffering." I was attached to God because of what he was "giving" to me. I idolized or lusted after this part of the relationship I had with God. But, as you have seen, because I was so attached, when the "giving" stopped, the problem got much worse, and the suffering began (or was revealed). It wasn't really love that I had or displayed towards God, it was a projection of what I thought He could give to me to fulfill what my ego craved. While I know there was some good inside of me at the time, only by His Grace, was I able to let this attachment go.

A person filled internally with unconditional love does not need to attach to anything because nothing is "needed" in the world. Love needs nothing because it is whole and complete in and of itself. If one fully experiences the internal Presence of God, what else could one really need?! This is the essence of Oneness in God and the realization of Love within. This Love is all one really needs in the world. Worth and value are found completely within, because love is really all there is as an objective reality.

If something is lost and one is truly experiencing a full state of divine Love from within, no negative emotions can arise because there is no room for attachment to objects, people or experiences. This is not normal in the world today, but those with this deep, loving level of consciousness experience this in every moment. Divinity does fully express itself this way in people that are living on this planet currently. It is not very common though. In such a state, little to no suffering is subjectively possible. Suffering is emotionality. The full expression of Unconditional Love is not experienced as emotion, but Being or Beingness.

Unconditional Love doesn't need or want anything, it is fulfilling in and of itself, which is why it is one of the primary qualities of God. God doesn't need or want anything; He is Completeness. Dr. David Hawkins states, "The more evolved the person's level of consciousness, the less the pressure of needs. With major evolution, wants and needs disappear because the satisfaction arises not from what one has but from the realization of the Source of one's existence, which is therefore not dependent on any externals or artificially altered brain physiology."[206]

The culmination of life led me to see myself loud and clear, in bright colors, in this brutal event. This experience in college served as the perfect way for God to communicate and speak, I just didn't know how to listen for a long time. It was in Him not speaking to me that the most was spoken. God knew exactly how I needed to be loved for me to discover this Divine Love for myself. These memories were a reflection of me to me. Letting it all go was God's gift to me so that I could grow and realize the Oneness of the mystical union. This experience was now looked upon with gratitude. The best part is I rarely if ever feel abandoned or deserted now; it is simply not a part of me anymore. I feel more complete because I experience Him more as the completeness that has always been me. I'm not perfect and have many more things to work through, but so far letting go has been amazing and life-changing.

16 THE BEGINNING OF FREEDOM: YOUR PERSONAL MEMORY LIST

"We can never obtain peace in the outer world until we make peace with ourselves."
- Tenzin Gyatso, the 14th Dalai Lama

"The greatest disease in the West today is not TB or leprosy; it is being unwanted, unloved, and uncared for. We can cure physical diseases with medicine, but the only cure for loneliness, despair, and hopelessness is love. There are many in the world who are dying for a piece of bread, but there are many more dying for a little love. The poverty in the West is a different kind of poverty—it is not only a poverty of loneliness but also of spirituality. There's a hunger for love, as there is a hunger for God."
- Mother Teresa

So far we have discussed how emotions affect our lives in so many powerful ways. We have looked at applied kinesiology, Chinese medicine, and tapping as tools for helping us to understand our inner landscape. And we just have finished talking about the two primary memories and some auxiliary memories that were the full context of what drove why I was depressed for 11 years. Lastly, I revealed the process of how I let these emotions, thoughts, sensations, and feelings go from my body to be free of the depression that plagued me for 11 years. This chapter was written to help you take the first step towards feeling better. And that begins with making a memory list.

You may not be depressed. You may not even have a health problem that you want to work on. You may have resonated with things that you saw in my story that helped shed some light on things to work on in your own story. Your story is different from every story that has ever existed. It is unique. You are unique. No one in the world has the memories and experiences that you have had. But one thing is for certain; we all have things that are affecting us emotionally.

How do you dig into your own story? How do you know when and where your emotions took solid root in you for the first time? How do you begin to explore the richness and depth of your own story?

Honestly, I never in a million years would have guessed that the memory of getting stung by a bee at the age of four held such massive significance for me. It wasn't until I began to dig deep into my own story that I stumbled upon this memory and the significance it held for me. I can't remember where I read about this next fascinating exercise. But, upon hearing it, it resonated with me instantly.

It was suggested to me that I make a memory list. The instructions were to write out a list of all the most negative memories that I have ever had that I can remember. This especially included the memories that happened before the age of 18 back into childhood.

After really digging into the memory of getting stung by a bee, seeing the powerful emotions that were locked up in that story and how it felt to be liberated from those emotions, it dawned on me that every other negative memory I have ever had could potentially have significance and meaning much as this memory did. Eventually, this theory proved to be very true. Nothing in my life has had more value in helping me grow spiritually than processing through all my negative memories. Letting go of what was in each memory and feeling massive, instant relief each time was euphoric. If you don't have a map or plan for spiritual growth and resonate with this, I highly encourage you to do it.

I wrote out my list of negative memories and came up with 110 that I could remember before the age of 18. It took me about 2 hours to make this memory list. In the days, weeks and months after sitting down to do it, more memories surfaced that I didn't remember when formally writing out this list for the first time. When I remembered other memories, I simply just went back and added them to my list. I was surprised that I had so many memories, mostly of things that I had almost forgotten that I experienced.

We generally only remember two kinds of memories from our past – positive and negative memories. If you ask me what I had for breakfast 30 years ago on this date, I would have no clue, because nothing emotionally significant is a part of that experience for me. If you remember something from the past and it has a negative connotation about it, it is significant. The adult mind likes to diminish the significance of things. You may think that something as insignificant as Johnny stealing your popsicle in the 3rd grade couldn't possibly be worth noting on a list of negative memories. If you remember it, and it is negative, it is significant.

You may be thinking that I had a horrible childhood if I have 110 memories on my list, but I actually had a wonderful childhood. I was never physically or sexually abused and always had my basic needs provided for. If we really put our heart into this exercise, we will quickly realize how many things we actually remember from our past.

This chapter's aim is really to try to fulfill the dictum in life to "know thyself."

Even among the most intelligent and successful people that I see in the clinic, a relatively high degree of not knowing oneself is present. This is true for all of us. What I have observed is that we really don't know ourselves all that well. The ultimate goal of knowing yourself is letting go of that which you are not and allowing that which you already are to shine forth. Our "Self" (capital S) is the divinity within every one of us.

This chapter is about exploring the content of your problems which inevitably will lead you back to the context of the problem. The context is the meaning behind the events that happen to us. It is the emotional energy that is trapped in the body that continues to cause problems. We may not consciously remember, but subconsciously, the body/mind always remembers. Exploring these memories for me has given me so many clues into why I am the way that I am and how I show up in the world. Often, the exploration of our memories can answer many questions. These questions could be "why do I have the problems that I have?", "why do similar things continue to happen to me?", and "why am I the way that I am?" Your past is the context that has formed, shaped and molded every aspect of your consciousness both good and bad. Exploring the past in full and intricate detail and letting it go is what begins to bring life to the ancient phrase to "know thyself." This is because when you let go of what you think you are, what you truly are begins to shine through.

Once the negative energy of what lies within you, as a result of your past, surfaces consciously, then the process of surrendering it to God can truly begin. Letting go of your negative emotions as they arise from within you, in your ego, is the path to growth, true spiritual change and realizing what your ultimate destiny is. The more you let go of the negative, the more the love, joy, and peace of God can radiate from within. Heaven then is allowed to burst forth from within you. This process is not your doing though. Therefore you (your ego) cannot lay claim to making this change. It is activated only by Divine Grace. When one surrenders, one doesn't do anything, one simply surrenders. Surrender is to stop resisting God by letting go of what has stood in the way – negative emotions, thoughts, and the ego. Experientially, peace is about removing the obstacles that stand in the way of its realization.

So how do we do this? What are the next steps?

> "Peace comes from within. Do not seek it without."
> —Siddhārtha Gautama (commonly known as "The Buddha")

Steps To Knowing Yourself And Realizing Peace Within

Step 1

Make a list of every negative memory you can remember having at any time in your past, starting with your earliest memories then working your way up to the present moment. If you don't find at least 50, you are either going at this half-heartedly, or you have been living on some other planet. Many people will find *hundreds* of events, memories or circumstances that were negative. Write them all down. What has been discovered is that most of the events that have the most meaning and significance for most people are the memories that happened when you were young; in between the ages of three to eighteen. Even more specifically, the memories from age three to eight seem to be particularly impactful. Once you make your list you can work with an applied kinesiologist, if you wish, and a top ten list can be made of the memories that had the most impact on you. Or you can simply just start to process through them one by one by yourself or with a trained practitioner. I would highly suggest working with someone trained who can hold sacred, loving space for you as you work through your past.

Step 2

While making your list, you may find that some events don't seem to cause you any current discomfort in the present moment. That's ok. List them anyway. The mere fact that you remember them suggests a possible need for resolution. Without really opening yourself to a memory and what it meant to you, you may not feel anything in the present moment about it. Did I get stung by a bee? So what? This is what my adult mind said about this particular event. People go to extensive lengths to suppress and repress memories and their true impact in life. We do this because this is our subconscious way of protecting ourselves. If we don't have tools or the structure to be able to let something fully come up and deal with it appropriately, we simply just stuff it down.

Step 3

Give each specific memory a short title as though it was a mini-movie and rate the intensity of the memory from 0-10. Also, write down the approximate age when the memory happened if you can remember. Once you get done making your list, in the coming days and weeks, more memories may surface that you had not previously thought of. This is very common. Simply add those memories to your list upon remembering them. Here are some examples:

- Dad cursed at me in the kitchen. Age 4. 9/10
- I stole Mike's transformer toy. Age 5. 10/10
- I almost slipped and fell into a deep well. Age 6. 8/10
- My teacher ridiculed me when I spelled a word wrong. Age 6. 9/10
- Mom hit me in the arm. Age 7. 10/10
- Mrs. Williams told me I was stupid. Age 8. 10/10

Step 4

Another idea that is helpful for remembering memories is to work backward from an emotion. Take the following emotions and ask yourself how you experience them currently or in past events. For example, take FEAR. List all of the ways you experience fear and the related emotions to the fear family. You may say, "I fear _____," and it may be 20 things. With each fear (or emotion related to fear), give it a number of intensity. Think of any memories related to this specific fear. Do this for every emotion listed below. It could be the fear of being worthless, being rejected, of failing, of not being lovable, etc.

For example, I am afraid I am not good enough. Memories:

- Not ever doing my chores to mom's expectations. Age 8, 8/10.
- Not getting good grades, especially 5th grade. Age 10, 7/10.
- Failing to win the 3rd-grade long jump competition. Age 8, 8.5/10.
- Not feeling good enough for Jenny, so she dumped me. Age 13, 8/10.

Here are some other major categories of emotions that may evoke different memories you had growing up:

- **Shame**: Self-hatred, close to death, head hung low, banished, cruelty, abuse. List all the related memories you have where you felt ashamed or shameful in life.
- **Guilt**: Punishment, remorse, self-incrimination, masochism, preoccupation with sin, self-condemnation, cruelty, unworthy, worthless, suicidal. List all the things you have done to make you feel guilty in life.
- **Apathy**: Discouraged, defeat, impossible, given up, isolated, estranged, withdrawn, desolate, depressed, depleted, pointless, careless, humorless, doomed, useless, negative.
- **Grief**: Loneliness, abandonment, nostalgia, melancholy, longing, irretrievable loss, heartbroken, anguish, disappointment, pessimism
- **Fear**: Scared, afraid, panic, stress, anxious, frightened, shy, tense, overcautious, threatened, trapped, timid, insecure, dread, suspicious, distrustful, fear of loving, fear of dying, fear of rejection, fear of failure, fear of criticism, fear of inadequacy, fear of disapproval, fear of boredom, fear of responsibility, fear of change, fear of losing control, fear of fear, fear of heights, fear of sex, fear of being naked, fear of loss of security, fear of public speaking.
- **Desire**: Greed, obsession, hunger, envy, jealousy, exaggeration, selfishness, lust, possessiveness, control, glamorization, insatiability, never satisfied, never enough.

- **Anger**: Resentment, unforgiveness, spite, vindictiveness, contempt, wrath, argumentativeness, negativity, aggression, annoyed, agitated, impatience, frustration, rebellion, abusiveness, abrasiveness, smoldering, sullenness, pouting, stubborn, explosive behavior, meanness, revulsion, hatred, revenge, fury, indignation.
- **Pride**: Over-evaluation, denial, playing the martyr, being opinionated, arrogant, boastful, inflated, one-up, haughty, holier-than-thou, vain, self-centered, complacent, aloof, smug, snobbish, prejudiced, bigoted, pious, contemptuous, selfish, unforgiving, spoiled, rigid, patronizing, judgmental.

Use this list of different negative emotions to stir your mind to remember and situations from the past that still contain suffering for you.

Another way to bring out negative emotions from within is by thinking about the emotions we currently feel or have felt about specific people. Make a list of the most negative memories you have involving mom, dad, brothers, sisters, grandparents, other relatives, spouses, children, coworkers, etc. Write down any negative emotions that you feel for these people and why you feel those emotions. Many things tend to come out this way.

One day, I was testing a patient to see how many negative emotions she felt towards her abusive father, and the number was 63. She was holding onto 63 negative emotions towards her father that spanned many memories throughout many years. Just simply by thinking of her father, at that moment, she rattled off 30 emotions in a matter of minutes. Each of these emotions had a context in various memories from the past that surfaced more easily when thinking about it in this way. Thinking of these emotions helped to bring out much of the pain that she felt towards her father over the years. We were able to process through many of these emotions, and she was able to forgive him and herself for having held onto them.

In a similar way, I once tested myself for all the emotions I felt towards a woman I had dated. Using AK, I identified 37 negative emotions I felt for her. One day, I sat down and processed through each of these emotions. This took about 4 hours, and was exhausting.

But, I felt totally and completely "free" of this relationship from this moment forward. It felt wonderful.

"Each one has to find his peace from within. And peace to be real must be unaffected by outside circumstances." —Mohandas Gandhi

Step 6

Another way to think about possible memories is by progressing through each year of your life and remembering things at specific times. Did anything negative happen to you in 3rd grade, 4th grade, junior year of high school, etc.?

Step 7

When you decide to process through a memory for the first time, think of all the emotions that you can remember feeling as a part of that event. Walk through the memory in your mind from start to finish. Think of a memory like watching a movie. Start in the beginning of the memory and stop anywhere in the memory that you remember feeling something. Give each emotion a rating of intensity. When you are watching a movie, you can pause it at any time. When going through your memory, pause and ask yourself if you are feeling something different than what you felt a second or a minute ago in the memory.

Perhaps you felt multiple emotions at the same time, or at least it could be perceived that way. When you have identified the way you felt and have released the emotion, continue on. Hit the "play" button of your memory and pause it again when you arrive at another time in the memory when you think you may be feeling something else. It is also constructive to notice if you felt or feel any unpleasant physical sensations when doing this because those are very important as well. The body literally holds onto emotions in various parts of the body. People routinely report things like feeling a pressure in the head, pitting in the stomach, shortness of breath in the chest, ringing ears, etc.

Let's process through another memory as an example, when I got blamed for sticking out my tongue at the teacher at age 4. The intensity of the event was 9.7/10. Here were the negative emotions:

- Forced – 10/10
- Shameful – 10/10
- Frightened – 10/10
- Simmering anger (resentful) – 10/10

If you need to get a list of emotions, consult a dictionary or thesaurus for better understanding the meaning of an emotion. If you cannot label an emotion, this is not a problem. You know what the feeling felt like and this is what is most important. When tapping on a feeling that you don't know how to label, you just tap saying something like "this feeling." For example, "Even though I feel this feeling, I deeply love and accept myself." You can identify with it and let it go because even though you may not know how to describe it, you definitely remember what it felt like, and that is the most important thing. Giving the feeling a name or labeling it is ultimately not important, just as long as you know what the emotion meant for you and what it taught you in the memory.

Step 8

Give each emotion meaning. Why did you feel the way you did? List all of the reasons or ways you felt a particular emotion. For example again, when I got blamed for sticking out my tongue at the teacher.

- **Forced**: 9/10 – I was forced into admitting that I did something I didn't do. I was forced to admit to her side of the story. I was forced to admit this to my parents. I was forced to apologize to her. I was forced into betraying myself.
- **Shameful**: 10/10 – She made me feel like something was wrong with me. This made me feel ashamed in front of my parents because they were disappointed in me and I didn't want to disappoint them.
- **Frightened**: 10/10 – I was scared about how my dad was going to punish me. I was also afraid of how my teacher may hold this against me.
- **Anger**: (resentful) – 10/10 – I was so angry that she blamed this on me. I was so angry because my parents didn't believe me. I resented her for doing this to me.

Step 9

Ask yourself what you learned about life, yourself, others, and the world as a result of your experience. What did this teach you about you? What did this teach you about life/world? What did this teach you about others? What did this teach you about God (if applicable)? What kind of agreements did you make in your mind about how life was going to be from this moment forward, even if those agreements were made unconsciously? Every child is constantly formulating what something means to them. Once you identify the agreements, put(them) into setup statements and process through them one by one.

Here are some agreements or things that were learned from this memory:

- I can't trust authority figures. 8/10 (Process example: "Even though I can't trust authority figures, I choose to love and accept myself.")
- I can't trust my parents to believe me when I tell them things. 9/10
- I will get punished for doing things I didn't do. 8/10
- People are out to get me. 9/10
- I have to be cautious and careful with what I say and do. 9/10
- There must be something wrong with me for "deserving" this. 8/10
- My parents or others may not stick up for me. 10/10
- My voice in the world doesn't go far or count because people don't believe me when I say things. 9/10

Step 10

Notice any particular smells, thoughts, visual images or anything else that is significant to this memory.

I once had a patient who told me about a painful breakup she had that devastated her. The one phrase that stuck like a record in her head was when she was told by her ex-boyfriend, "You're gonna be ok, kiddo." This phrase was charged with so much anger for her that whenever she heard the word kiddo, she got super fired up. We tapped on this phrase many times before she let go of the energy behind it. She was able to heal and move beyond the sadness and grief of losing her boyfriend.

I heard of another person who had terrible memories of his mother yelling at him when he was a child, while she baked in the kitchen. Every time he was disciplined, he was forced to sit in a chair next to the oven. This person had a terrible allergy to bread from that point forward. When he smelled bread in the future, he always felt bad and never knew why. Going into a pastry shop was never pleasant for him due to the emotional associations with this smell. Tapping on something as simple as "Even though I detest the smell of bread, I deeply love and forgive myself" helped to remove his aversion to the smell of bread and reduced his allergic reaction. Allergies can form with physical substances because of the emotions we experience when we are around certain things or are eating certain substances. Arguably, the three most common food allergies are to milk products, wheat products, and refined white sugar. These just happen to be the most common things people consume in the USA. If they are in your system and you go through an emotionally charged event, an allergic association can form.

Another patient abhorred geckos. She was from the north and one summer when she was a child they went to visit family in Florida for the first time. Her cousins played a trick on her and threw a gecko on her. It terrified her because she didn't know what it was and it stuck to her shirt. She remembers yelling in terror, "Get it off me", as they stood around and laughed at her. Even as an adult, she was terrified of geckos. We processed through this memory and her fear of them disappeared. She was shown a picture of geckos, and we tapped through the emotions that came up for her and within minutes her fear of geckos went from a 10/10 to a 1/10. She had never even been able to look at one before without cringing in fear. Now she actually was curious to hold one.

Particular aspects and details of your memory can hold emotional charges and are important to note when remembering what happened to you.

Step 11

Try not to be dismissive of any memory that may not appear to hold much meaning or significance for you. People are often very surprised how powerful a memory is when they actually step into it and discover its meaning and significance. The adult mind loves to think that events that happened to us couldn't possibly be that significant. We need to keep in mind how we experienced it and when it happened to us as a child, rather than interpreting the memory through the adult mind/lens. Even I thought, at one time, "You got stung by a bee, so what?"

Step 12

If you wish to set a goal, try to process through at least one memory per week using tapping (or *The Sedona Method*). I made a goal to tap through all 110 memories within two years. I processed through one memory per week and had processed through my whole list in two years time. Tap on everything in the memory that has an emotional charge for you until you feel like the emotional charge of the event is down around a 1/10 or below. At times, you may sense that there are still some remaining aspects of the memory that are holding a charge for you, but you are not sure what they are. This is where a trained tapping practitioner can help you explore these aspects further. Again, there is no one better than someone else who has been professionally trained to reflect back things to you and help you discover things in yourself.

In the case of the woman who abhorred geckos, there were four or five reasons why she was terrified. We had to explore all aspects of her emotions and used the following phrases as we started tapping. She didn't like the way they looked ("Even though I also can't stand the way they look, I choose to love and accept myself"). She said they were very fast and sneaky ("Even though they are fast and sneaky…"). She said they are always hiding and watching you ("Even though they are always spying on me…"). Each one of the ways in which she described geckos was an aspect that had energy in it and was tapped on so she could let go of all the negative energy she had towards them. Consciously she knew that they could never harm her. However, when she saw them, her body was subconsciously replaying the memory she had when she was younger. Momentarily, she became a child again, and she was struck with fear and panic.

Step 13

Once you identify a memory and are immersed in it, begin to process through the memory from start to finish, stopping anywhere where you feel something negative. From the example memory in this chapter, here is how that memory was processed. A slight variation was made in this memory as my understanding of tapping had continued to progress. "Even though I was forced into admitting that I did something I didn't do, I deeply love and accept myself."

On the 5th point on the body, underneath the eye, instead of repeating the entire phrase, I simply said the word "forced," tapped nine times and repeated this until I was done with the nine tapping points on the body. Just using a one-word reminder is the only thing that is needed once you have tapped on this phrase four times. It is like the ball is rolling and instead of needing a big push to keep it going, it just needs a little nudge to maintain momentum.

- Top of Head: "Even though I was forced into admitting that I did something I didn't do, I deeply love and accept myself."
- Eyebrows: "Even though I was forced into admitting that I did something I didn't do, I deeply love and accept myself."
- Temples or sides of eyes: "Even though I was forced into admitting that I did something I didn't do, I deeply love and accept myself."
- Back of the head: "Even though I was forced into admitting that I did something I didn't do, I deeply love and accept myself."
- Under the eyes: "Forced."
- Under the nose: "Forced."
- Under the mouth: "Forced."
- Under the armpits: "Forced."
- Under the collarbone or Thymus point: "Forced."

I continued to tap through the rest of the things that were negative using the following phrases:

- "Even though I felt ashamed of disappointing my parents, I deeply love and accept myself." On the 5th tapping point - "Ashamed."
- "Even though I was very afraid of how my dad was going to punish me, I deeply love and accept myself." "Very Afraid."
- "Even though I was so angry that she blamed this on me and that my parents didn't believe me, I deeply love and accept myself." "So angry."
- "Even though I can't trust authority figures, I deeply love and accept myself." "Can't trust authority figures."
- "Even though I can't trust my parents to believe me when I tell them things, I deeply love and accept myself." "Can't trust my parents."
- "Even though I will get punished for doing things I didn't do, I deeply love and accept myself." "Punished."
- "Even though people are out to get me, I deeply love and accept myself." "Out to get me."
- "Even though I have to be cautious and careful with what I say and do, I deeply love and accept myself." "Cautious."
- "Even though there must be something wrong with me for "deserving" this, I deeply love and accept myself." "Shame."
- "Even though my parents or others may not stick up for me, I deeply love and accept myself." "Didn't stick up for me."
- "Even though my voice in the world doesn't go far or count because people don't believe me when I say things, I deeply love and accept myself." "No

voice."

- "Even though I am worthless, I deeply love and accept myself." "Worthless."
- "Even though I am unimportant, I deeply love and accept myself." "Unimportant."
- "Even though I cannot trust anyone, I deeply love and accept myself." "Distrust."

It is my recommendation that you process through your first couple memories with a trained professional. This is especially true for those of you who have very painful memories such as rape, abuse or something severe of this nature. Don't work through these things alone. Many people have expressed a severe aversion to stepping into their most painful memories. They are hesitant because they remember how painful, devastating and awful their memories are. They think that if they allow themselves to go there, they might not be able to get out of that space safely again. This is a very real fear for many people.

Having a trained professional by your side will ensure that you don't get stuck or feel like you can't get out of the memory you are processing through. Once you go through your toughest memories with a trained professional and come out on the other side free of the negative energy, which has encumbered you for so long, it will make processing through other memories much easier.

Another way to get started is first by ignoring the most devastating memories that you have gone through. Instead, start with more recent and fresh memories that are painful, but not devastating. It is difficult for most people to be able to jump into the worst of their memories without being super familiar with the process or even knowing first what letting go or surrender feels like. By starting out this way, you will become more and more familiar with the process and how it is going to work. This can bring a certain level of confidence and trust to the process. You will also get very used to how to bring things up, face them and know exactly what it feels like when emotions release from the body. The more repetition of the process, the more familiar you will become with releasing.

With that said, I'd like to add a disclaimer: tapping is not a substitute for appropriate medical care. Tapping is not for diagnosing, treating, or curing any disease or health problem. It is just a simple tool to release unwanted emotional energy from the body.

"Inner peace can be reached only when we practice forgiveness.
Forgiveness is letting go of the past, and is, therefore, the means for
correcting our misperceptions." —Gerald Jampolsky

17 QUESTIONS AND BUMPS ALONG THE ROAD

"The moment of surrender is not when life is over, it's when it begins."
– Marianne Williamson

When someone begins the process of looking within, facing the darkness and releasing on what comes into awareness, some questions, hurdles and bumps can occur along the way. This chapter addresses some of the most common things related to this.

What if I can't remember my childhood or anything that happened to me when I was younger?

This is a question I get in the clinic with about 1-2 in 10 people. Recently, I encouraged someone to make a memory list, and his response was two-fold. First, he didn't make a list or even really attempt to do it (he was making excuses because this inner work brings up painful stuff). Second, he said that he couldn't remember much that was negative from his childhood. I have heard this many times in the clinic before, so I asked him to talk to me about things he remembers his mother doing when he was younger. He didn't have a good relationship with his mother growing up. Within 5 minutes, he rattled off 10-15 negative memories. Many more memories existed, and I simply said to him, "You just spoke of at least ten negative memories that you remember in 3-5 minutes. Imagine how many you would remember if you sat down and did this exercise for an hour or two?"

I've learned that two general groups exist from the 1-2 out of 10 people that say they can't remember things from their childhood. One group is people that just don't see value in this exercise and are making excuses about not wanting to do it. This is what is occurring in the majority of these cases. They either want to avoid doing this soul searching or don't think that it is all that important. This is a sign to me that they just aren't ready to do this kind of work. It also reveals inner resistance.

Not wanting to do the exercise is totally and completely ok. It's not for everyone. This exercise really resonates with people when they see the tremendous value it can have in helping them to heal and realize their fullness and wholeness. In these cases, I drop it right away, and we don't normally discuss it anymore and just focus on acupuncture or physical healing. It doesn't make sense to insist on something that someone isn't ready for.

The second group of people is those that genuinely and honestly don't remember much of their childhood. This could be for one of three reasons. One reason is that long-term memory just doesn't serve them very well anymore. We could focus on a heavy metal and chemical detox, brain-nourishing supplements, and foods that will heal brain chemistry. This may help to jog the memory over time or it may not. A second reason is that some patients have had such traumatic childhood experiences that they have subconsciously blocked these memories completely out of their awareness. This appears to happen as a way for them to protect themselves. The pain of their memories is so intense that the mind literally blocks them from remembering at all. A third reason is that people simply don't remember. Their brain is fine and they didn't have a particularly traumatic childhood. This third reason is a possibility, but would be extremely rare.

Many years ago, when I was first getting into helping people release emotions, I remember working with a woman who had been violated sexually when younger. She honestly didn't know if it was her imagination or if it really did happen to her. We began to gently explore the memory. What happened next was astounding. While we were tapping on the possibility of this being a memory for her, from one moment to the next, the whole memory with vivid details came flooding back into her mind. Instantly, she felt all the shame, helplessness, fear and anger come flooding back. She did an amazing job of processing through it, but it took her a few days to recover and to fully let this go. I had the suspicion intuitively that other memories for her were blocked out as well to protect her. Some people have had very traumatic memories, and so much healing is needed for them to start feeling better. It is a process that consciously and with strong dedication can take a good amount of time. The mind can get very creative when the need to be protected is invoked.

Even if you don't remember your childhood or anything in it, your body (and mind) keeps the score.[207] In reality, no such thing as time exists. Everything is always present. Everything can only occur now because now is all we ever have or will have. Therefore, every problem that happened in the past can be surrendered in the now because it is happening to you now. The woman with fibromyalgia at the beginning of the book is a perfect example of this. Even though she was violated 40 years ago, she was still being violated in the now. This was not consciously being done, but her body had kept the score over "time." Every sensation, emotion or feeling can be surrendered in this moment because now is when we are always experiencing it.

If we feel fear frequently and are still holding onto fearful things from our past, the fear will manifest in many ways as we experience life now. We don't have to label a feeling, remember a memory, or even give an experience a name or an emotion. We can just simply surrender what is being experienced now either acutely or chronically. This is not in any way an excuse not to pursue appropriate medical treatment and is not a substitute for medical care. One must use every available resource to heal, especially appropriate medical care.

"Lord, make me an instrument of thy peace." - St. Francis of Assisi

When I am releasing on an emotion or a memory, will it ever come back?

The answer to this question is twofold. First, it has been my observation that when working on a specific memory and after having truly released emotions from a memory, they never return or the intensity is lowered significantly. Once it has been processed through, surrendered to God or let go of, it is gone forever. Out of curiosity once, I wanted to test this theory. I asked a woman, with whom I had processed through a rape, to do an exercise with me. When I asked her to think back on when she was being raped, she felt nothing negative at all. In fact, she mentioned to me how she felt sorry for the person who did that to her and actually held this person in a state of genuine forgiveness. This is how we know that healing has truly occurred. Forgiveness and compassion are what is felt towards someone who has done us unspeakable harm.

Secondly, I had encouraged another friend to pick up a copy of *The Sedona Method* and begin his inner journey of healing and surrender. He texted me after about two weeks with great excitement about his new experiences. He said, "Scott, I have been releasing on all kinds of things, and I really can feel the negative emotions and sensations leaving my body. I feel so much lighter and at peace when I do the releasing."

About four weeks after this, I got another phone call, and he was a little distraught. He mentioned that a significant memory surfaced that held a lot of anger for him. He released on it for about 45 minutes, and the anger just wouldn't seem to budge. He called and asked me why. I told him that some things could and do release very quickly from the body. However, certain memories and experiences are so deep and so profound that they take considerable time and diligence to surrender. It is entirely possible to be free of something very harmful that happened to us in a very short period of time. However, at times, surrender to God must happen on a whole different level.

Personally, I have released for days or on one singular emotion or experience. Certain emotions and memories that may be driving the expression of a very chronic health problem may take a significant amount of time to release from the body. Many memories and emotions spanning decades may be fueling something very chronic. Make it your steadfast intention to surrender it all. With this encouragement, he had an intuitive awareness that this anger he was holding onto was going to require tremendous courage and considerable time to face.

Negative emotions are finite things. They are not infinite, and an inexhaustible supply does not exist within us. With the complete and total willingness to surrender a feeling or emotion, in due time, the energy behind it will run out. If you do not have the courage or even the will to dive into what you know to be a mountain of negative emotions and memories, just take it one step at a time. If you have resistance about a memory or other feelings, surrender the resistance to the memory first. For example, if you feel overwhelmed about where to start, simply start with how overwhelmed you feel.

It is very frequent for me that when I think about sitting down to surrender something that has been bothering me, a certain amount of resistance arises about even getting into the process. I know that on the other side of my negative emotions will be peace and freedom. However, frequently, I experience the resistance about how hard it may be to get into the act of surrender in the first place. Some days I succumb to the resistance, on other days, the Grace is given to me to have the courage to face it. Ask God for the courage and the will to face what is inside of you and Grace will show up when it is needed most.

In the case of Lester Levenson, the gentleman who created *The Sedona Method*, he committed to surrender every negative feeling, sensation, emotion, and judgment that arose for him in every instant of the day.[208] He was faced with a prognosis of only living for six more weeks and decided to totally surrender. Through complete and total surrender, his body completely healed, and he lived for almost four decades longer than expected. Out of this experience arose *The Sedona Method*. I suspect that when faced with certain death, our willingness to surrender greatly increases. It normally takes something of this magnitude for us to get to the level of commitment to totally surrender. Rare would it be without a catalyst in life for a person to just wake up one day and decide to totally surrender. Dire and grave health problems are normally the wakeup call that people need to pursue this level of surrender.

This was also the case for Dr. David Hawkins, author of *Letting Go: The Pathway of Surrender*.[209] He had more than 20 incurable health conditions, many of which brought him to the brink of death multiple times. He arrived at a point of complete and total surrender and over the course of three years was healed of every one of these health conditions. Both of these men began to experience advanced spiritual states of consciousness that most of the world doesn't think is even possible for human beings. The mind literally goes silent, because it has been totally transcended and a peace that passes mental understanding is experienced. Very few humans experience this, but it is entirely possible with total and complete surrender of all of life to God.

Why is it that I seem to release emotions much easier when you guide me through them?

At one point in time, people thought it was impossible to run a mile in under four minutes. When this record was broken and people knew with certainty that it was possible, in a short period, many other people were inspired to accomplish this feat for themselves. If you are someone who has gone into the depths of your own darkness and are now relatively free of something, it is much easier to inspire others to do the same or to help others through their emotional pain. Many people that want to look like Arnold Schwarzenegger in his prime, have found tremendous inspiration just seeing him and hearing about his story of what was possible. We can find tremendous inspiration in others that have achieved what we seek to achieve.

People are capable of doing this on their own, but having a guide, mentor or teacher to help lead the way can make surrender easier to do, especially at the beginning of this inner journey. Additionally, the inner strength and love of a guide may be what is needed to hold space for someone or to direct them out of their own inner emotional hell. We, as people, need each other, especially during the most distressing times. Therefore, a simultaneous truth exists about needing someone and not needing them; both can be true. At times we may need someone to help guide us. Releasing can be easier with someone present, but with the help of God, people are capable of surrendering all on their own.

What if I have fully released something and yet still have a health problem?

On the highest level, the ultimate goal or expression of divinity fully experienced within is complete and total peace. The goal is not to be healed of anything. Emotional releasing doesn't guarantee that someone will be healed of anything. It is not a cure for any health problem. Emotional releasing is done for the sake of emotional releasing, for your inner freedom. As emotions are continually released and surrendered to God, the mind grows increasingly still and silent. Emotions and thoughts progressively diminish and their hold on the mind and the body lessens. However, it has been my experience and observation that if someone has totally and completely surrendered something, the majority of the time it will be released from the body. It has been extremely rare for someone to be truly released on something, and the body doesn't heal. At times, people can convince themselves they are totally released on something, but this could be just a form of denial. I have had patients where I can feel their inner emotional turmoil, yet on the outside they deny that they are holding onto things. Self-delusion is a negative emotion and some are experts of this emotion.

This state of consciousness of total experiential peace is exceedingly rare among human beings. But, if one has truly surrendered something and is at peace, one will not care if they have a health condition or not. When the mind is at peace, one literally could care less about what is being experienced in the body. Pain is one thing, but suffering is entirely different. They are not the same thing. The body can be in pain, yet one is so completely surrendered and in peace, that no suffering is actually occurring for them. If they are not suffering, pain will be experienced completely differently than how humans normally experience it. Dr. David Hawkins went through multiple major surgeries without anesthesia due to this fact. Anesthesia is a consciousness blocking agent. But if one is fully surrendered within consciousness, one's experiences within all of consciousness are handled, including what is happening in the body. It is entirely possible to be free of suffering (emotionality) but be in significant pain.

One last factor that must be considered is that over time the body, cells, and protoplasm naturally age and decline. In the later stages of life, it may be nearly impossible to physically heal a part of us, because having an aged body is part of being human. Therefore, the process of growing older must be surrendered too. The body may not be able to recover or be like it was when we were younger, but we can surrender and be at peace with growing older as well. Resisting the aging process will undoubtedly make things worse. Growing older with grace, peace, and understanding is the ideal way.

How do I know that I have really surrendered?

When you have completely surrendered, you will be totally at peace with whatever it is that the mind focuses on. I still have days occasionally when I feel a little down, discouraged, depressed, unmotivated or any other negative feeling. Previous to embarking on the inner journey of surrender these feelings were very intense. I would rate them at like 9/10 or 10/10 constantly. Now, they are qualitatively different in feeling, duration, and intensity. Certain emotions are experienced less often, and when they do crop up, they are only experienced at perhaps a 3/10 or 4/10 or less.

In fact, the pathway of surrender can lead one down one of two roads. One road is the increasing progression of just feeling progressively better as you surrender more and more. When I feel a little down, I have the know-how and the tools to be able to sit with, notice, and welcome what I am feeling in the moment. I generally don't fear it, push it away, escape from it or feel helpless to do anything about it. With the intention to welcome any emotion, feeling or sensation that arises, surrender usually is soon to follow.

Another road may be followed in which things that were impossible to handle before will now arise because you have the inner resources to deal with them. In other words, because you have been surrendering things in your life, even deeper things may now arise that need handling. With constant surrender you gain completely new inner resources, not because of what you have done, but because of the expression of divinity that emanates from within you. Another way of saying this is that life may continue to throw problems your way, but since you have a totally different way of seeing them and experiencing them, they may appear to be even more complex and difficult because they will require a much deeper level of surrender than you experienced before. Even then, it may not be perceived as a problem due to where you are within your conscious experience. Saying that something is a problem is a judgment. A judgment is a duality. On the highest levels of consciousness, duality and judgments drop away, and the mind is only left with total peace and love, which are states of non-duality and non-judgment.

A difficulty may present itself in your life simply to aid you and deepen your level of surrender. Instead of asking, "Why me, God?" or "Why do I have this problem now?" a deeper level of intuitive awareness arises. On this deeper level you can see more clearly how something is being used to continue the process of your inner transformation, so that you may be mature and complete, not lacking anything.[210] Reality is that you don't lack anything. You are whole, perfect and complete as you are. But, if you feel you do lack, it is just one more thing to surrender. Lack is judgment and duality. Wholeness is non-judgment and non-duality.

How do you really welcome an emotion, feeling or sensation in the body?

It is our conscious or unconscious resistance to our experiences that continues to cause problems for us. For example, if you are totally at peace with having a particular health problem, it will not be perceived as a problem for you, even if you continue to have it. When total peace is experienced from within, the world could be falling down around you, and you will be totally at peace with it. Peace is an unshakeable and immovable inner experience. What is "out there" will not be able to influence what you feel "in here."

Peace is not equated with inaction though. People may tend to think that peace, love, and joy are states in which you check out of the world and don't "do" anything. This couldn't be further from the truth. These states of being have driven the most profound moments of consciousness in all of human history. The individuals that truly embodied them have been the catalysts for the most profound changes the world has ever known. Modern examples of people that embodied this peace were Mother Teresa and Gandhi.

When most people feel pain or discomfort of any kind, it is resisted, either consciously or unconsciously. Pain brings up various inner programs, emotions, judgments and belief systems related to our experience of pain. When you place your hand up against mine, and together we push against each other (much like arm wrestling), this resistance to each other's pressure over time will cause physical discomfort in both of our arms. We may begin to feel weakness, soreness, and even pain if the pressure is resisted long enough. However, if from one moment to the next you or I decided to welcome the pressure, all of the symptoms in the arm that arose from the resistance would disappear. When we stop resisting our emotions, with grace, we permit them to go.

Another more crude analogy would be what happens when people resist being arrested. Even if you didn't do anything wrong and it was "unjust" for you to be arrested, resisting arrest never fairs well for people. When people resist being arrested, the consequences can be mild to quite severe. They get cuts, scrapes, bruises, dislocated body parts and in certain cases even broken bones. Things of this nature rarely if ever occur when people are not resisting arrest.

Alternatively, I only get to see my best friend 1-2 times per year. When I see him, I fully and completely welcome him in every way. My arms are completely open, my countenance is positive, and I am smiling. When we go to hug each other, we give each other a strong embrace. We are excited to see each other. We are in a full state of welcoming each other. This is what it means to fully welcome what you are experiencing in the moment. Do this with your negative emotions. Embrace, open, and smile into them.

Things can have little power over us if we are fully welcoming them in the moment. Try to welcome your problems like you welcome seeing your best friend or someone that really cares for you. Notice all the various ways that you are resisting whatever problem it is that you are having in the present moment. The experience of any negative emotion, thought or sensation that is being judged as bad, wrong or painful is resistance. Always try to bring awareness into what the driving motive within you is and the underlying resistance you have for the problem.

What are the main drivers behind why we experience our problems?

The philosophy of The Sedona Method explains the main drivers behind why we hold onto and resist life. The underlying motives of our negative sensations in the body, memories or experiences are normally because of four main things.

- Wanting approval (or disapproval or rejection)
- Wanting control (or no control or letting something control us)
- Wanting security (or no security or wanting to die or give up)
- Wanting separation (or oneness or connection)

Let's say that you are a struggling, broke college student and your car just happened to break down…again. You check your underlying emotion, and it is mostly fear. You are afraid. Where will you get the money? How will you pay your bills? How will others perceive you knowing that you're having financial struggles again? You're going to have to ask my parents for money yet again, and you don't want to do that! When you ask yourself if the fear is coming from wanting approval, control, security or separation, you may notice just one of them, or you may notice all four are driving the fear and keeping it in place. Wanting something means we lack it. Wanting (lust) is the feeling driving all of it. So all we have to do is let go of the feeling of wanting that we notice.

A first question to ask yourself simply could be: "Could you let go of wanting to change this situation?" The mind likes to think that if you let go of wanting to change something that nothing will get done. This couldn't be further from the truth. Wanting to change something means that you lack. If you want something, it means you don't have it. The reality is that your true core lacks nothing. You are whole, perfect and complete already. When you let go of wanting to change something, you allow openness and spaciousness to be experienced, which often opens up the very means for something to change effortlessly.

Let's say wanting approval is driving this fear. You want to be independent, make your parents proud and be able to take care of yourself. But you are broke and need their help. You want your parent's approval. The car breaking down generates fear that you will somehow lose their approval or they will disapprove/reject you because you were the one that bought this old junky car in the first place. Could (implies ability) you let go of wanting their approval? Would (implies volition) you? When (an invitation to do it now)? Continue to ask yourself this question until you feel the release of it. Or you could also tap on this with the following statement: "Even though I'm afraid my parents will reject me, I choose to love and accept myself."

Let's say wanting control is driving the fear. You try and try to get ahead, but something always continues to happen that is out of your control. You want to control what is happening to you. You want to make this situation be exactly the way that you see it in your mind. So you struggle and struggle to try to get ahead, secretly controlling everything. If you feel like you cannot control things in your life, it brings out a very real sense of fear. People who control things are normally just afraid. Could you let go of wanting to control? Would you? When? Continue to ask yourself this question until you feel released on it. Or you could also tap on this with the following statement: "Even though I'm afraid, struggling and wanting to control this situation, I choose to love and accept myself."

Let's say wanting security is driving the fear. You don't feel safe and secure in the world because of this added expense of $700 dollars. You are afraid of not being able to pay your car insurance, heating bill, and water bill this next month. The car breaking down and not having enough money does not make you feel very safe or secure in the world right now. Could you let go of wanting safety and security? Would you? When? Continue to ask yourself this question until you feel released from it. Or you could also tap on this with the following statement: "Even though I have no idea how I'm going to pay my bills next month, I choose to love and accept myself."

Let's say wanting separation is driving the fear. By constantly having issues with your car, you feel separated, disconnected and different than other people. Secretly, you think that no one else has the same problems you have and these problems seem to separate you and make you feel different than other people. It doesn't bring a sense of connection and unity to your life; it brings about separation. Could you let go of wanting separation? Would you? When? Continue to ask yourself this question until you feel released on it. Or you could also tap on this with the following statement: "Even though I feel like these problems don't happen to anyone else and I can't catch a break, I choose to love and accept myself."

With any problem that we have, health or otherwise, one or more of these primary drivers can be sitting behind the reason they stay in place for us. Whatever we resist, either consciously or unconsciously, persists. From the highest levels of consciousness, true reality is that we are already fully approved, in control, safe and connected to everything and everyone. When we let go of what we want, we realize that we already had it by nature of the divinity that defines us from within. The

Power within us embodies all these things. God fully loves and approves of you, is in control, is safe and is connected to everything. When you release the "wants" in your life, the revelation is that these things were true the entire time. You simply couldn't experience them because you were choosing to hold on to them and the emotional experience behind it.

When you want approval, for example, it points a spotlight on how we are not approving of and experiencing love towards ourselves, our bodies and others. Love is what you already are. Surrender the <u>want</u> of approval, and you will step back into the reality that you are already fully loved and approved. You don't have to want or desire something you already fully have. If you surrender the wants you have, the fullness of reality comes more into view.

How often should I release on my emotions?

Any sensation, negative emotions, or judgment can be released and let go of. I find that if we don't make a plan, we can plan to fail. Having a written plan to deal with our inner world can take us a long way. Let's make an analogy that hopefully will drive this point home.

Let's say one day you decide that you want to start working out, lose 50 pounds and build lean muscle. To do so, you must have a plan. Currently, you don't exercise or monitor what you eat. Therefore, embarking on such a journey would require a major change for you. To achieve this, you need to have a plan for eating and working out. Having a goal usually requires a plan that we need to implement and steps to take to achieve the goal. You cannot accomplish such a goal if you plan on frequencing the gym two times a month or sporadically working out. A plan requires discipline and consistency.

Likewise, if you only spend time releasing things in your inner world once per month or only when you are forced to deal with a problem, you will not be able to reap the full richness of embarking on a consistent journey into your inner world. When we make a practice out of something, we give ourselves the ability to experience the fullness of what making such a choice can mean for us. Just as we set aside an hour to go to the gym 3 or 4 times per week to have the body we want, the same case can be made for letting go and experiencing the fullness of our Being.

After we have made our memory list, make a concrete plan on how to process through each memory. If you set aside 1-2 hours each week to process through one memory per week, you will be able to process through 52 memories in a year. Next, you could divide things by topics such as money, relationships, work, sports, etc. You might spend a couple of months only dealing with the emotions, belief systems, and thoughts surrounding money. A great tapping book that explores this very theme is called _Tapping Into Wealth_ by Margaret Lynch.[211]

Another exercise that you could do once per week is to remember all of the activities that occurred throughout the week, paying particular attention to the times and places when you felt negative things. Write down what comes to mind and then release on all that comes up for you. Throughout the course of a week, so many things can happen that we dismiss or don't pay much attention to. But if we place our attention on them, we can easily enter into a space where seeing these things and processing through them can bring a profound depth and richness to our world.

We can also release on positive emotions. Releasing on positive emotions is not talked about very much because in the releasing process we focus mostly on the "bad" that has happened or is happening to us. But, we can even surrender positive emotions to God. For example, happiness carries with it a certain good feeling and experience. Being happy is wonderful when it is truly experienced, but joy is an entirely different level of experience. Happiness is a much richer experience emotionally than any negative emotions. However, happiness is not love, joy or peace. Happiness still lacks, whereas love lacks nothing. We can consciously surrender the happiness and progressively experience even more joy. Continue to notice the resistance you have to even feeling positive things.

Many times I see people that don't make time for themselves to process through their emotions outside of the clinic. They are at the mercy of everything and everyone else, thinking that the most loving way to be is by constantly making sacrifices for everyone else. The ultimate price for this is that their own health is sacrificed. It can come to our attention when a health problem arises that we are paying more attention to everything and everyone but ourselves. Or many minimize taking care of themselves until a problem has progressed to a stage where it might be impossible to ignore and will be more difficult to heal from. Many people feel badly for even thinking about taking time out for themselves for self-care. They feel a tremendous sense of guilt about doing even simple things for themselves. I wouldn't have believed this until it came up as a constant theme in the clinic. Making time for yourself is a radical act of self-love. Set a goal, make time for yourself, and give yourself the care that you need and deserve.

How do you get started processing through things?

Simply setting aside 15 minutes of time every day to engage your emotions is well worth it. I suggest you set this as a goal at first to get into the habit of doing it. This is so hard to do for so many people. When I set aside time to process through things, I usually start by doing two things. First, I start by taking deep slow diaphragmatic breaths. Diaphragmatic breaths are done with the stomach, not with the chest. For some, learning to breathe from the stomach is something that needs to be practiced because most of life has been spent breathing very shallowly and from the chest.

Focusing on your breath is the first thing that is done in most meditation practices. One of the reasons for this is because breathing is something you are always doing in the present moment. When you are focused solely on the breath, you are not in the past or the future; you are right here and now. Now is the only reality you will ever have. The reason we are able to let go of our past now is because the past is only experienced now. We can feel the sting of the past now. We spend so much time ruminating over the past or fearing the future. Both are actually happening now. Bringing the attention to the breath, here in the now, is very centering and grounding and is a wonderful way of bringing our attention inward.

Secondly, I usually spend time noticing and focusing on the resistance I feel in the present moment about not wanting to turn inward and face my emotions. To be honest, 97 percent of the time when I focus inward, my attention is brought to negative things that are waiting to be released. Seeing my reflection of these things and taking responsibility for them is rarely pleasant. Therefore, a small part of me resists digging into this process every single time. Once attention and intention are brought to the resistance, it usually releases very quickly. Walking into the storm isn't always pleasant, but the peace, clarity, and calm that come after the storm is the best part about facing yourself. Peace, love, and joy are always waiting for you on the other side of surrender.

Reviewing The Last 24 Hours

A practice I encourage people to do is simply taking a review of the past 24 hours. 15 minutes can be spent remembering all the negative things that were felt throughout the last day. If people say they can't remember anything or don't remember feeling anything negative, they are either in serious self-denial or are unconscious. They may not be aware of what is streaming through the mind. The last 24 hours usually holds plenty of things to discover that can be held in awareness and released. If you can't find anything negative, then find something positive and release on that.

Most negative things that happen during an average day are manageable. Someone cut you off in traffic, you spilled your coffee on your work shirt, the dog peed on the carpet, your husband/wife made a snarky comment, and your kids were sassy and disrespectful to you at dinner. These are many of the "little" things that happen throughout an average day. We experience negative emotions in every one of these situations. During the 15 minutes we have set aside each day, we can bring these emotions up, welcome them, and let them go. Doing this for 15 minutes every day can have a profound effect on our mental state and the way we experience the world.

If you set aside a longer period for yourself once per week, you can dig into one of your memories on your memory list. If you are unsure of which one to go through, just start with any memory on the list. Simply try as best as you can to remember every thought and emotion in the memory, welcome all the feelings and sensation and let it all go. Discover the meaning of the memory and what agreements were made about yourself, others and the world. With anything that needs releasing, sit with it as long as needed and set it free as best as you can.

If we want to change the physical body, we have to go to the gym and work at it.

You cannot expect to look like Dwayne "The Rock" Johnson if you are going to the gym once a month. Likewise, if you only spend one hour every month going inward and discovering the world of your perceptions, then growth will be very slow. The more we go inward to be with ourselves, we will continue to see, experience and partake of the Source of life itself. This is what is meant by the verse "Be still and know..."[212]

The Consciousness Of Depression

Every disease, health problem and body part has consciousness. In this case, consciousness means that specific emotions, thought patterns and belief systems are a part of every disease, health problem or body part. Depression has a very specific consciousness. Clinically, I have read the consciousness aspects of people's health problems to them over the last five years, and what I hear almost 95% of the time in response is this: "That describes me exactly" or "That is very accurate" or "Many of those things apply to me."

The best book in the world that is a brilliant tool for understanding the consciousness aspects of health problems and body parts is Inna Segal's *The Secret Language of Your Body*. With the definitions you find in this book, you can hone in and make tapping and releasing more specific. Below is the description of depression and anxiety found in her book:

> "**Depression**—Pressure to survive. Feeling overwhelmed, hopeless, disappointed, and disillusioned. Wanting someone to save you. Suppressed anger and resentment. Feeling and acting like a victim. Blaming others for what is not working in your life. Feeling unmotivated and uninspired. Can't be bothered to do anything. Stuck in an old story that's only getting gloomier."
>
> "**Anxiety**—Thinking about the past and the future, and not trusting the flow of life. Feeling insecure, unsupported, and helpless to change your situation. Focusing on negativity and limitation, and allowing yourself to wallow in fear."[213]

If you struggle with depression and anxiety, some or all of the things mentioned above may apply to you. If the depression/anxiety you are experiencing started at a very particular time in your life, I would invite you to curiously investigate and contemplate in more detail about the life circumstances that were occurring around the time you started feeling depressed or anxious. If you resonate with any of the above emotions and thoughts consider exploring the following questions:

- Do you feel a pressure to survive? What things in your life feel like they put the most pressure on you? Is it a relationship, work, family, certain responsibilities? In what way does life feel like it is just a pressure to survive? When did this start for you?

- Do you frequently feel overwhelmed? If so, what things commonly make you feel this way?

- Do you feel hopeless? If so, what things have occurred in your life that have felt hopeless? When did the hopeless feeling start?

- What are the most disappointing things that have occurred in your life? Describe in detail how this disappointment has affected you.

- When did you become disillusioned in your life? Who or what was involved in this?

- Have you always wanted someone to "save" you? For example, one woman was very depressed because all she wanted in life was to get married. She had put so much of her power into this idea that when, by the age of 35, she hadn't married and became very depressed. She was convinced that getting married would solve all her problems. Some think having a child will save them or their marriage. The word "save" simply implies that you think something outside of yourself will make your circumstances better or more complete.

- Are you carrying around a lot of anger and resentment towards someone surrounding a certain circumstance that occurred? This tends to be a very central theme behind depression for many people. I would highly encourage you to make a list of the people towards whom you are most angry.

- If you are honest, do you feel and act like a victim? Being a victim is a state of mind. Our circumstances can be tremendous catalysts for growth, or they can become a narrative that keeps us stuck in the role of victim. I was a victim for 11 years. I felt there was nothing that could be done to change what happened to me in college. The opposite of being a victim is taking full responsibility for everything that happens to you. Even if something very harmful or negative happens in your life, you ultimately have the choice as to how you want to react to it. One of the most beautiful stories that exemplifies this is the story of *Man's Search For Meaning* by Viktor Frankl. Frankl lived in a concentration camp during the Holocaust and realized that although he couldn't control the horrible atrocities and things that were happening around him and to him, he could choose how he wanted to react to them. He chose to do so not as a victim, but as someone who wanted to express love no matter what.

- Do you blame others for what isn't working in your life? This is very similar to being a victim. Do you find yourself complaining about the same things over and over again (for example: traffic, parents, significant other, kids, the government, the disease you have, etc.)? When we blame others the emotion that usually is sitting behind the blame is anger. Who or what are you blaming?

- Do you feel unmotivated or uninspired? When did it first occur that the winds of inspiration were swept from you?

- Do you feel like you can't be bothered to do anything? Most of the time a very specific reason or theme exists that serves as the fuel for why you might not feel like doing anything. What is this theme or reason for you? When did someone or something crush the inspiration in you?

- What is the old story of your life that continues to get gloomier over time? What is the story in your mind that has been replaying over and over?

- Do you constantly find yourself thinking about or secretly ruminating over something that happened in the past? Did a particular event occur in which you felt very afraid that you knew had a major effect on you?

- Are you constantly thinking about the future, and projecting fear into what may or may not happen? Fear usually projects itself into the future. Do you find yourself constantly worrying about things?

- Do you feel insecure about yourself, your body, your abilities, etc...? What are the memories in your life that have been a source of a significant insecurity for you?

- Do you feel unsupported in life? If so, why?

- Do you feel helpless to change your situation in life? When was a time in your life where you felt the most helpless?

- Do you find yourself constantly focused on the negative things or limitations in life, or things that can go wrong instead of what is going well in life? I had one mom contact me because her kids were always getting sick. After getting to know her, it became very apparent that she was constantly projecting fear into their lives. She wanted to control everything because she was always afraid they were going to get sick. Anything the kids did, she was afraid they would get hurt, sick or that something bad would happen. When she let go of her fears, the children got sick much less. Instead of being afraid around them, she was able to love them better. Our emotions can directly affect those around us, especially children, who are sponges and absorb everything until a certain age, including the emotions of those around them. Fear is that powerful.

If you are like me, the temptation at this point is just to read over the above questions, but not really sit with them and engage them. Instead, I encourage you to really engage each question. Grab a pen and paper. Write down the memories, thoughts, and emotions that come into your mind as a result of answering the above questions. The essential root of the problem as to why you are depressed or anxious could be "hiding" in plain sight in one or more of your memories. Answering the above questions may take you hours. This is completely normal. Take all the time you need. These are crucial things we are talking about here. Once you have really delved into the above questions and things begin to reveal and unravel themselves, you can then use the Tapping process to let go of those emotions and memories.

For some people, simply talking about what has happened to them or becoming more aware of things can be very helpful. This can be a mild form of letting go, which is why counseling and therapy can be very helpful. However, this was not the case with me. I knew I was angry at God, felt abandoned, and I constantly talked about how angry and abandoned I felt. But talking about something and actually letting it go are two very different things. Sometimes we get a lot of juice by rehashing our story repeatedly to the next person who will hear it. We are getting attention, sympathy, pity or whatever. Sometimes we continue to hold onto our destructive narrative simply because we are not willing to let go of the payoff or the juice that the narrative is giving us. Would you rather be free of the problem by letting it go or would you rather continue to have the problem and the payoff that you are getting from it?

Exploring what is inside of us with no judgment or condemnation, but with curiosity and wonder, can be the start of really understanding why you have been depressed or anxious. Most of us over-identify with our bodies and our emotions. Our emotions and physical body are not who we are. Many people think they are their bodies, thoughts or emotions. We claim possession of them. The body will one day fade away, and our attachment to it is something that we can let go of with love and understanding.

PART 5
LIVING IN SURRENDER

18 PEACE

"The day the power of love overrules the love of power, the world will know peace." - Mohandas Gandhi

What begins to happen when you start to surrender the negative emotional energy that has dominated your life for so long?

When surrender occurs at very deep levels in your life, everything will begin to change. Ironically, everything will appear as though it is changing, yet, not much of anything may have changed. You are simply becoming aware of the substrate of all life, the divinity that pervades all of life and is permeating you in greater ways. You simply are now more aware of Reality than ever before. Reality is the pervasive expression of divinity that can be seen in every aspect of life. You begin to identify more and more with the truest part of you.

Life can become quite magical when we surrender into divinity. Even when life is perceived as being tough, or we have "bad" things happen to us, we handle them differently than before. We look at life through a very different lens, a lens that can help us see love, joy, and peace even in the midst of what the world might consider tragedy, pain or suffering. We will finally start to fulfill what every person truly wants in life. The reason for this is because we are all innately programmed for this as our eventual destiny.

The Answer To Life's Most Essential Question

Whenever I ask anyone in the clinic what they ultimately want from life, the answer is almost universally the same.

"I just want to be happy."

Happiness (and beyond happiness – joy) is an inside job, which is why so many people that are chasing things in the physical world are constantly disappointed once they acquire what they thought would bring them the happiness they desire.[214] As you go progressively inward, you will find the Source of life, the Source of joy, love, and peace. This is what true "happiness" is because we all carry this ultimate desire within us. In fact, it is what drives all of life, whether we are aware of it or not.

Therefore, this chapter is dedicated to talking about what can be experienced when we go inward and how we will see this change our lives. If you want happiness (and joy beyond that), all you have to do is let go of and surrender that which is not love, joy and peace inside of you. It is THE eternal paradox. You are already what you seek. You just haven't stepped into the full reality or knowledge of this truth yet.

So many times, we need convincing that something is the pathway towards what we ultimately want. People work out hard in the gym because much of the time doing so will ensure the outcome they desire, which is a chiseled or toned body. People work hard because they desire to have "success" in whatever way they envision that to be. People date and get married because of how they think this other person will fulfill them and make them happy.

Benefits Of Letting Go And Surrendering

Humans behave in agreement with what they think will meet their needs and wants. For many, these needs are being projected out into the world. We mistakenly think that something outside of ourselves will make us happy. Letting go of your inner emotions gets to the root of everything. Rather than chasing after the projected happiness we think we desire, we simply realize that we already are it and then dedicate ourselves to surrendering into it. It truly is an inside job. Below are some of the things that we benefit the most from as a result of continually engaging and surrendering to what is inside of us.

Your consciousness changes.

Consciousness is a measure of how aware or awake you are in the world. The more you surrender, the more you wake up and see life as it really is. You begin to see more and more clearly how life is pervading and influencing everything you see and experience. You are less confused about things and have more clarity about yourself, others, and what is happening in the world. Rather than just seeing the appearance of things, you begin to perceive the essence of things instead.

"Real health has to happen somewhere inside you, in your subjectivity, in your consciousness, because consciousness knows no birth, no death. It is eternal. To be healthy in consciousness means: first, to be awake; second, to be harmonious; third, to be ecstatic; and fourth, to be compassionate."

- Rajneesh

You become more loving.

How many times a day do you judge what you are feeling or doing in the world?

How aware are you that you are even judging yourself in the first place? No one wants to be judged. All judgment of others is just self judgment. Judgment is just anger that is being projected onto people or the world. The more you surrender anger, the less you judge and the more loving you become. Greater self-love automatically means more love for others and for the Source of Life or God, which is your very life. You cannot love someone more than you love yourself. "Be the change you wish to see in the world," Gandhi once said. By loving yourself in this way, you will become the love that you have always wanted. You become the object of your deepest desires.

Love begets more love. If you want to be loved, love more. Yet, you are not loving so that you get more love. This would not be love. This would just be cravingness and behaving so that you can selfishly get something from others. Love doesn't need anything from others because it is whole and complete as it is. The more you love it just automatically floods your world simply as a byproduct of what you have become. The more you love, the more it constantly surrounds you. We are all projecting our emotional frequencies out into the world. As you experience more love, you will attract more love from everyone and everything naturally in your world through situations, people, and experiences.

Your filter of the world changes.

We don't see the world as it is; we see the world only as we are. If we are angry, we are going to see a world of anger. If we are afraid, we see the world as a place that only generates and perpetuates our fears. The same goes for any negative emotion that dominates our consciousness. If you are filled with pride, all you might see in the world is competition, opinions, being better than others and seeing others as a threat to you. As you become more loving, love becomes your filter in the world. You start seeing the world through the lens of love, even in the toughest and most brutal of circumstances. So no matter what happens to you, instead of reacting with anger, fear or guilt, you don't experience these things as you once did because of the love radiating through you into every circumstance of life.

You are no longer a victim of events, circumstances, people or bad things.

You choose how you want to experience life by way of what you have become. Much of our world is driven by a victim mentality. A victim mentality is one that people feel when life gets out of control. Victimhood in the emotional world is driven by fear and anger. When we feel oppressed, we get angry and lash out. This anger is simply just a smokescreen to the fear that we feel. Life isn't really out of control or unfair. It simply is the perception we have based on the fears we are carrying around. Being at peace though does not mean that you continue to allow someone to take advantage of you. It is not loving to yourself to allow things to happen to you that you can change. The changes in your life are made from love rather than reactivity and anger.

Many of the movements worldwide defending those who are marginalized today arise because of fear and anger. While desiring a better world for everyone is good, healthy and noble, movements that are driven by fear and anger will never change the world. Even in the face of being marginalized, people can still choose love. But this is not what happens many times. Instead, a movement or organization forms that is perpetuated by force (anger) and not true power (love). We can advocate for anything, but we must be aware of the emotions driving us to advocate. Love is the unstoppable force in this world. Love also doesn't mean inaction. Mother Teresa was a woman who embodied love, yet she did not sit around all day doing nothing. Love drove her to even more intense action in the world. She brought dignity to those who didn't experience much internal dignity.

> "When you complain you make yourself a victim. Leave the situation, change the situation or accept it, all else is madness." – Eckhart Tolle

You feel more urgency or a calling to help others surrender their lives to being, love, and peace.

Upon deep inner transformation, you may find yourself wanting to participate in more activities which help others experience the same thing. Often, people may feel a deep desire to change jobs, explore the world and help others in some way. Something wakes up and stirs in you that helps you realize that nothing else in life is as important as waking up, growing spiritually, and surrendering into Being.

While the image of someone fervently trying to proselytize another may come to mind, this is not what happens in states of love. Being at peace means that if someone talks to you, wonderful. If they do not, that is wonderful too. No attachment to needing or having to share anything with anyone arises. Things just naturally and lovingly take place. Nothing is forced. Nothing is pushed. No such agenda exists with love. When someone's ears are open to hearing, truth has a special way of finding its way to souls that crave it.

Life may drastically change.

The people, jobs, and experiences you have vibrate on a certain frequency. As you change and wake up, expect change. You may lose a job, friends, relationships, positions or other things. Don't worry when the fears that you have held for so long have mostly gone. You will face the new changes with courage, fortitude, and more peace. You will gain new friends, relationships, jobs or other things that are more supportive of the person that you have become on the inside. This may be very unsettling at first. In fact, it can cause some very significant disruption in your life. Those around you will fiercely want to keep you the way that you have always been and may outcast you when you don't fall in line. You may not resonate with them like you used to. This is not a reason to reject them or push them away, but instead to realize that they may not be what is best for you anymore.

When you change and love more, those around you may be inspired by the love bursting out of you and desire to experience this change too. Or they will resist, and it will result in phasing them out of our life. This can bring up even more things for you to process through as well. This can be perceived as loss in life. Loss is usually experienced with sadness or grief. If you experience sadness, you will have an awareness that the change and shift that is happening is also helping you to see the sadness you have been holding onto deep inside.

Change will ultimately not stop you though. It will be the catalyst for an even more rich experience of life. You want to continue growing and evolving as the driving force in your life. You may disappoint others, but you will feel compelled to continue to follow the road less traveled because it will make all the difference.

Your desire to serve increases.

You may find that you feel an urgency to contribute more to the service of God and mankind in some way. I became a physician because I knew that I wanted to help others heal after seeing profound healing for myself. What better way to help others to heal than to help them have the tools, understanding, and resources to reclaim health where disease, pain, and sickness may abound? You don't have to become a doctor to serve God and mankind in some way. It will develop naturally and whatever you do will be perfectly suited for you in whatever circumstance you find yourself.

New temptations will be easier to handle.

Temptations will arise that constantly try to suck you back into where you were. However, since you are more awake, the energy to surrender temptations will be much stronger. Most people try to "fight" the temptations they feel. Fighting something is only resistance. The war on drugs will never work because it is based upon force, not power (love). When we desire to fight something, counter-resistance will always be found. The best way to deal with a temptation is not to fight it but to surrender it. When surrendered, the temptation will disappear on its own, and no "fight" need occur.

Food cravings are some of the most difficult temptations to deal with in the health world. A craving can be handled by seeing it for what it is. A craving is just a feeling that the body is experiencing. Most cravings can be summarized by the emotion of lust. If we pay attention to and are mindful of what is sitting behind the craving, we can create awareness around it so that it can be surrendered. Cravings can occur for many different emotional reasons. But with more and more practice of learning how to let go and surrender, an inner source of power will be accessed that can make a temptation easier to handle. They can still be quite tenacious and persistent. If we fail, we also create more awareness around the guilt, self-loathing or anger we feel for having given into the craving or temptation. We can then choose to surrender that as well.

You begin to trust the process of life like never before.

In higher states of consciousness, you are more in tune, and in touch with The Source of Life. Therefore, you begin to trust life more and more, even in spite of rough and difficult circumstances. Life does want to support you in every way. You may not think that "support" is the hard times that you are going through. But, the hard times you are going through will ensure that whatever negative emotions are inside of you come out through these circumstances so they can be faced and surrendered. With this understanding, whether you are in what we judge as good times or bad, life is working for you not against you. Your understanding of this very idea deepens, strengthens and grows. You can trust that it is going to work out for good no matter what. All things work together for our good.[215] We can surrender our judgments of things we label as "bad" or "difficult" and trust life more deeply.

You will deal with hurt and wrong more lovingly.

When people do wrong to or even hurt you, you have a more compassionate response. You have an understanding that what they do is all they know how to do. If people knew how to do better they would, but they don't, so you have more compassion. You have more compassion for the suffering of others that they project onto you or into your life because you realize that you too, at one time, largely projected your own suffering and negative emotions in the world. Forgive them (and yourself), for they know not what they do.

You have more compassion for others because you have more compassion for yourself. The mind likes to judge when people do bad things to us, and we say things like "They should have known better!" What people do is one thing, your response to them is always and forever a reflection of you. Instead of focusing so much on what others do or don't do and judging them, you tenaciously notice how you are experiencing them and are more committed to surrendering your reactions than needing to change them.

The need to change people lessens.

Needing to change someone often is more a reflection of us than it can be for the person you wish to change. We want people to be the way we want them to be, or we judge our life as better. It is such a frequent experience in our relationships when problems arise to blame your friend, boss or partner. We see them as the problem. "If so and so would just change, things would be so different or better." How many times have you thought this or even said it out loud to yourself or someone else? On one level, one of the most futile things in a relationship to do is to expect someone else to change and meet your expectations. This is one of the ways to ensure that problems will continue to occur. The only person you can ever really change is you and your reactions.

As we continue to see and take responsibility for how we are reacting to life, we focus less on others and more on ourselves. We progressively find ourselves less and less concerned with changing others and much more concerned with changing and dealing with what is arising out of us. Love can be curious. Sharing occurs when necessary. And holding the tongue until our opinion is truly desired may be the best response. Love always knows how to respond, even when met with anger in another. The more we focus on how we are experiencing things and surrendering what is occurring to us, we increase our capacity to be genuinely more loving to others in the present moment.

You're more willing to forgive others.

Your willingness to forgive others is made stronger because you have committed to forgiving yourself of all the negative emotions that arise within you as you experience life. What you forgive in others is also what you choose to forgive in yourself. Forgiving others is all about how forgiving we are towards ourselves. If we are all one and oneness is the heart and center of beingness, then forgiving oneself is also forgiving things in others. They are inseparable. So many people live holding onto bitterness, resentment, and anger about things that have been done to them in the past. As you forgive yourself more, you are so much more willing to forgive others. Forgiveness is the literal and full expression of unconditional love and joy in this world. When you are unforgiving towards others, you realize that you are only allowing yourself to continue to suffer.

Relationships are deeper, richer and more fulfilling.

Relationally, you begin taking responsibility for every negative emotion you experience as you relate to others. Doing this brings more peace to the relationships you have, at least in the way that you experience them. Relationships become more loving and are so much more rich and healthy when each person takes full responsibility for how they project their own emotions into each relational experience. They even get better even if you are the only one taking responsibility for your emotions.

You stop blaming others because you are taking full responsibility for your anger and the fears sitting behind the anger. You also begin to see how often relationships serve as a way to secretly meet our selfish desires. You stop projecting your happiness into what a relationship can give you and you begin to be more giving. You start owning the source of power within yourself, rather than needing to get it from another. You are more giving not because you expect something in return and get resentful when someone doesn't reciprocate or give back to you. You aren't trying to get someone's approval or trying to control as frequently. You simply give because you love to give with no expectation of anything in return.

As a consequence, relationships are built on love, trust, care, genuine concern and seeking another's well being as much as your own well being. Power struggles, control, selfishness, and abuses fade away. These friendships and relationships are so life-giving that they often bring you to tears. The gratitude that wells up from within you and overflows out of you is quite surprising.

Sex becomes more and more amazing.

Sex is a sacred gift that reflects the deepest part of our divine programming for oneness and connection. On the deepest levels, we find ourselves connecting to and loving someone rather than simply meeting a need. Oneness and connection are the supreme focus. It is an act that ultimately expresses the oneness you have come to experience within and wish to share with another. It is less about just wanting to feel good and is no longer localized to the physicality of the body. Orgasms become more intense and change as you grow. Orgasms are experienced beyond the physical body and can feel as though they fully encompass both of you. Both people more fully trust and open their vulnerable hearts to one another.

Being one with and molding into the presence of the one you are with becomes possible. Sex can morph into it being a physical expression of the oneness, connection and love you feel with someone. Separation from others, which is just an illusion maintained by the ego, diminishes. The oneness you feel with another is heightened to new levels. Sex draws us into the narrative that our separation from God doesn't exist either and is an illusion supported only by the ego.

The more loving you are towards yourself, the more you are free to love another. A sense of enjoying the naked presence of another becomes quite intoxicating. You are free to explore, try and do anything in harmony with one another. You find yourself naturally wanting to ensure the pleasure of the one you are with. Sex becomes an experience of mutually giving and receiving and meeting your partner's needs physically, emotionally, and spiritually. You not only are vulnerable physically, but you become more vulnerable emotionally, not just giving your body to another, but your soul and spirit as well. The real magic of sex is not being physically vulnerable, which seems more common than ever in society today, but being vulnerable and open emotionally (which is quite rare).

Everything in the world becomes more beautiful.

In reality, everything is not more beautiful, but since our inward beauty is shining more brightly, our eyes are increasingly opened to see the beauty of all things. Our perception of everything changes because we have changed deeply from within. We begin to see beauty in the world in ways we never have before. Before deeply letting go of my emotions, I had many painful nights filled with tears and often fell asleep crying. Now, I may cry myself to sleep, but the tears are ones of joy. Thinking about certain things, people and circumstances have brought such joy into the present moment that I am just moved to tears. I no longer hesitate to cry, because I don't have much resistance to tears or crying. It just flows freely if this is what presents itself at the moment.

Additionally, upon hearing a beautiful song, viewing a touching scene from a movie, seeing an act of kindness or when someone thinks of you, tears of joy bubble up freely from within. This is not just oversensitive emotionality either. Many people cry because they are feeding off of negative emotions, yet this is an entirely different experience. When one encounters beauty, it is seen in all of its stunning radiance, and you can't help but cry by the sheer magnificence of what you are witnessing.

Boredom lessens and needing to be entertained diminishes.

Boredom is a negative emotion within the family of resentment, a gallbladder emotion. Boredom is a form of resentment that life is not entertaining us the way we want. As we let this go, we become more happy and content wherever we may find ourselves. We can shut our eyes and go deep within to a meditative state at any time. We can be content doing nothing or doing anything.

Many people may watch television for hours at night, watch sports all day long on the weekend or binge watch Netflix without realizing that it is a subtle form of escape. What are we escaping from? Perhaps it is the constant, continual chatter of our minds? Or the pain we hold deep within or the suffering that we are unwilling to really take a look at within? For some, being quiet and sitting in silence is brutal and very difficult. I have heard people say the silence drives them crazy.

Stillness and silence are the substrates of life itself because they are synonymous with peace. When peace is the prevailing experience within, the mind literally goes silent. This is what the Buddhists refer to as No Mind. This is what Christians refer to as experiencing The Mind of Christ. This is another reason why so many people struggle with meditation. The mind just simply won't shut off and frustration ensues. Try to sit for even 2 minutes and you will find your mind wandering to some or many thoughts. But like doing anything well, meditation requires constant dedication and perseverance.

I can attest that I used to analyze, overthink, and worry about anything and everything. Now, after having released so many emotions, my mind is more silent. I still struggle like everyone else to still my mind, but it has gotten easier over time. I do escape from time to time and enjoy entertainment just like anyone else. But, needing to escape from life is not the primary motive now. I have rough days, but more consciously choose to engage how I feel and face my feelings head-on rather than having to escape from them or numb out. Life is filled with more wonder rather than boredom and this can be seen anywhere we look.

Our opinions about things soften.

Opinions are completely natural for the mind to have. But an opinion plus negative emotions are an entirely different experience. Have you ever met someone who is constantly arguing with others about everything and defending or needing to prove what they think? They need to let everyone know that they are right and have all the answers. On the surface pride is the constant need to be right or superior to others. As mentioned before, pride comes from our inner insecurities. This fear is what most truly react to in pride.

People can sense the difference between when one is defending their point of view, rather than just lovingly sharing it. When it is being defended, it is being done out of a deep fear or insecurity. As we let go of our negative emotions, we also let go of being so attached to our opinions of everything and needing to be right. When you begin to embody the truth from within, love softens our perspectives, and an inner stability shines forth. When you embody the truth as a reality from within, you find that you no longer need to defend anything. Truth doesn't need a defense. If you disagree with others, you can make your point of view known, but find no need to defend it. You also are more open to hearing about the experiences of others, always wanting to learn and grow, even if you disagree. You ask a lot more questions and remain curious even if you don't agree.

When you have a conversation with someone, if they are interested in what you have to say, you will find a curiosity develops between the two of you. You find yourself asking questions and questions being asked of you. You are more interested in learning, expanding and growing. You can only grow if you are curious, open and constantly asking questions in order to learn. We all have found ourselves in situations sharing something that has impacted and changed us, and our words fall on deaf ears or, even worse, people reactively argue and negate what you say. People may take no interest whatsoever in what you are sharing and this is completely ok. You simply become aware of this and either continue to ask them questions or realize that they are not all that interested in learning or getting to know you and stop sharing. Amidst all this is just a softening to life and the attachments you have as you see the world.

We are constantly pulled more into the present moment.

Often our lives are lived either in the past or in the future. We may live every day in regret, sadness, shame, guilt or anger of the past. Or we live in fear over the future. Have you ever been with someone who was physically present with you, but emotionally they were on a different planet? They are not here and now. They are in the past or the future. Technology has made this seemingly worse. We are tethered to our phones and many have difficulty disconnecting from technology.

I have been at a restaurant seeing everyone on their phone rather than being fully and completely present to the company in front of them. Have you ever been listening to someone but are not present and are only thinking of the next thing to say or to defend your opinion? Being present is being with someone and not trying to change them or having an agenda but being fully engaged with them and with what they are saying. It is exploring with curiosity, love, and non-judgment as to what is being said and communicated. I have struggled with this and continue to struggle with it. It can be difficult to be present and to hold space for another. But it gets better the more clear you become on the inside.

When present, we can focus on another rather than just ourselves. We can see other needs and desires more clearly in the moment. We can anticipate things in the moment. Clarity is much more a part of our interactions with others. We can see the emotions we are having in each moment rather than being completely engulfed by them. We can take increasingly more responsibility as to how we are interacting and reacting to every single moment. Being present is being in tune with life as it is, and we begin to see the magic and marvel of what is truly in front of us.

We become more aware of our bodies.

When we feel pain we are less resistant to it. Instead, we become more inquisitive, non-judgmental, and out of curiosity and meditative awareness, we ask our bodies to tell us if this pain is a messenger of something that needs attention in our lives or if it is something we have been holding onto that yearns to be surrendered. Much of the physical pain that is experienced in the world today is emotional. It is not often seen this way, but when you see hundreds of people let go of the emotions sitting behind pain, and it disappears, it becomes very convincing. We become one with and stop resisting the pain we experience, rather than wanting to escape from it or take a drug at the first sign of it in our body.

Our diets and eating habits also become much better because our physical body experience is largely a reflection of what we are carrying emotionally. We become so aware of our body that we can almost intuitively tell whether something we eat is good for us or not instead of it just satisfying an emotional craving. Emotional love for self automatically translates into better eating habits. We consume more vegetables and fruits and are more concerned about what is in our food and whether something is really healthy or not. Is our pain a way of telling us we need more water, certain nutrients, rest or something else? We pay more attention.

If we take the time to be present and tune in, normally the message is there waiting to be received as long as we are ready to listen. Or if we don't have the answer because of our intention to want to heal (which is a form of prayer), we find the resources or people who can supply the answers for us. They appear serendipitously in our life. Support and healing are always available.

The more conscious we become, the more we use our right brain.

Our intuitive sense of the world develops at an alarming pace. We experience more of an inner knowingness, trust, and peace about things rather than worrying about them. Seemingly supernatural things may start to happen that are associated with intuition and the awakening of the right brain. These have been historically known as spiritual gifts. We may resist it at first or things may seem strange because they are new to us or don't appear to be logical. Over time, if we surrender to them and let go of the fear and confusion that may arise, we begin to see the gift that is offered to us in tapping into this side of our consciousness.

The right brain is more creative, intuitive (we don't know how we know, we just do), fluid, emotionally intelligent with feeling and sensing, sees the big picture and is imaginative. Clinically, when I used to do acupuncture, I followed exact point prescriptions because this is what I was taught. I thought that finding the exact right point or following the perfect protocol would be what made people heal. Needling the right point is important. However over time, I learned to take the left brain book knowledge I have and am aware of and combine with an intuitive sense about how to treat a patient. It is less about getting things right or wrong but learning that if I needle someone with love, care, and intention, the treatments are always more "powerful." I still use my left brain knowledge combined with a right brain intuitive sense of how to help someone. It makes practice more lighthearted, fun and creative and treatments more healing.

We begin to sense and intuit the thoughts and feelings of others more clearly.

We are more sensitive to how the world feels around us. Our own noise (negative emotions) diminishes as we let go, enough so that we can be more sensitive and aware of what others are feeling. You can more easily perceive and sense exactly what others are feeling. When you spend hundreds, if not thousands of hours learning to recognize and feel the emotions within yourself, you intimately become more aware of these same emotions in others. Often in practice, I find myself being very aware of exactly what someone is feeling because I literally can sense and feel it within them.

Intuition is a learned skill that anyone can learn to have and which all have on some level. But it needs practice and attention to be sharpened as a skill. It is the heightened, subtle levels that take much time and practice to master. This is called true empathy because you have learned to have increased empathy and forgiveness for your own negative emotions. We don't take on other people's emotions or let them affect us. This is not healthy. We simply learn to sense, name and know emotions when they are present in another.

This may make some people feel very insecure because nothing can truly be hidden. Emotional energy cannot be hidden even if someone is projecting an appearance outward yet feels the opposite on the inside. Emotions can be tuned into within anyone at any time. I only tune in to people that I have permission from or in situations where tuning in can help to keep me safe in unsafe circumstances. My favorite questions to ask in the clinic are, "What was the emotion you just felt as you expressed that thought?" or "What was the emotion driving such and such behavior in that memory?" or "What emotion is driving the pain or sensation that you are experiencing in your body now?" We can be curious together. As we do, we experience the right brain in all of its creative, imaginative brilliance.

Life appears to slow down or intentionally slows down.

A desire to move out of such a fast-paced life may begin to kindle within. We care less about achievement, approval, money, success and having to have the latest gadgets and toys. We care more about living and loving well, and helping others to do the same. We begin to long more and more for silence and retreat, because complete silence (peace) is the end of the road on the spiritual journey. However, when we come out of daily moments of silence and retreat, we bring the silence with us into our world, even into a life that can be fast-paced.

We increasingly crave growth and knowledge.

We may begin to read more, have more desires to grow and may engage in activities such as meditation, prayer, and contemplation. We humbly realize that many other people that have lived before us were much further along on the path than we are. So we learn from them and their life experiences to grow and become. Harry Truman once said something to the effect of, "Not all readers are leaders, but all leaders are readers." I recently heard a statistic that most CEOs read an average of one book per week. People who are thirsty to grow will usually engage in activities that help them to continue growing. Reading is one of the best ways to grow and learn.

The source of all real knowledge is within, yet we learn more outside of ourselves first to learn how we can foster true inner knowledge. The heart behind "Know thyself," the famous quote attributed to many people throughout time, is the driver of this endeavor. It is the simultaneous paradox of being the knowledge we seek, yet also seeking it at the same time. We move between the paradox of this idea until we may reach the point of being fully what we already are and realizing there was nothing to seek all along. This is true knowledge, true knowingness.

Our listening preferences for music may change.

We may find ourselves being drawn to music that reflects higher levels of consciousness and the beauty of such music. In other words, we feel more drawn to music that reflects or embodies love, joy, and peace. Music that speaks of drugs, betrayal, hurting others, sex and lust, selfishness, anger, fear and other such qualities are left behind. The worst of such music would be gangster rap and heavy metal/death music. People who embody the love that they are have no need to listen to such music.

Often, I will put on a relaxation station after a difficult day of work and can feel how such music revives me from within. If I have spent the day being stressed out and haven't been living in the love that I am, a song that reflects this can pull me into a loving space almost instantly. Mozart, Beethoven, Pachelbel, Debussy or other classical music can bring us back into serenity and peace. Chinese flute music is something that I play in the clinic at times during acupuncture, which can help people relax and fall asleep rather quickly. You may also find yourself drawn to something like Gregorian chants. You may have another form of music which has the same effect on you.

19 FREEDOM

"The food you eat can either be the safest and most powerful form of medicine or the slowest form of poison." —Ann Wigmore

We have covered so much ground in this book and now it is time to put it all together. If you are wondering where you should start and what you should do in order to get started on being depression free, what follows will be a short guide that brings together what we have discussed thus far. Whether you are depressed or have another health condition, what follows doesn't just apply to depression, but can be beneficial to many other health conditions.

The Pareto principle, which is also known as the 80/20 rule, says that roughly 80% of the effects come from 20% of the causes.[216] A few critical health practices will be covered which, in my estimation, make 80% of the difference. In other words, we can do a few select things that will have a huge impact on our health.

Action Steps To Heal From Depression

1. Cut out all inflammatory foods from your diet.

As we discussed, people simply do not realize how inflammatory and disease promoting the following foods below are. We are caught up in the moderation idea of things. If you want to be healthy, depression and disease free, moderation is not the answer with regards to the foods listed below. Start at first by cutting down on your consumption of these foods and over time, it will get much easier to not have them, especially when you start seeing how awful they can make you feel.

Foods to avoid

Wheat – breads, pasta, pastries, donuts, muffins, cakes, and cereals. Organic sprouted bread might be the only exception that I might make to this list. However, when muscle tested, even the organic sprouted forms of wheat found in bread generally don't test well. Therefore, I would even suggest not having wheat at all for a few months in order to really heal your digestive system.

Dairy – Cow's milk (even organic lactaid), cheese, yogurt, sour cream, cottage cheese, and kefir. In the natural health world some practitioners advocate for some of the fermented forms of dairy. I do not. When a muscle test is performed, even the fermented forms do not test well for most people. Additionally, even though you can find dairy products organically, I have seen repeatedly how much they contribute to poor health.

Sugar – Refined white sugar is an additive that is found in so many things these days. Even organic sugar that is added to organic products should be avoided. It is so critical to read food labels and avoid sugar as best as possible.

Fried foods – Oils/Fats are the hardest thing for the body to digest. Excess fat puts tremendous stress on the liver to produce bile in order to emulsify and digest it. The liver is the organ that gets the most stagnant in people who are depressed. Fat contributes to even more stagnation due to how hard it is to digest. Fried foods should be completely avoided and other fats should be kept to a minimum. Organic chips and crackers also have oils in them even though they are organic. These oils have normally been heated, are polyunsaturated (sunflower, safflower, soy, corn) and are not healthy. It can be easy to justify eating such things because it is from an organic product. However, just because something is organic does not make it healthy.

Eggs – I usually get flack for suggesting that eggs are inflammatory, especially as they contribute to increased bacterial issues. Eggs have been used in Chinese medicine for a very long time in food therapy and tonify or strengthen yin in the body. I love the taste of eggs. However, when I started to muscle test people, most did not test well for them. I even started testing the organic, pasture raised eggs that are the most expensive ones. Those didn't test well for most people either. Based upon this, I suggest for people to avoid them, at least until you are symptom free.

Corn - Over 90% of the corn in the US is genetically modified. Corn crops use the same carcinogenic herbicide glyphosate.

Soy - Over 90% of soy in the US is genetically modified. Crops of soy use the same carcinogenic herbicide glyphosate as well.

Pork - Pork is one of the top transmitters of Hepatitis E virus (HEV), has been linked to cirrhosis of the liver and liver cancer, and raises your risk of getting a parasitic roundworm called trichinella.

Alcohol - Regular alcohol consumption is linked with depression. This makes sense because alcohol is very inflammatory and depression is inflammation of the brain.

I know avoiding these foods can at first seem very restrictive and difficult.

Believe me, I know. I personally have successfully avoided consuming these foods for very long periods of time. You can do it too. Considering the amount of rampant disease and health problems we have in the world today, if we keep doing what we have done for the past few decades, we will continue to get what we have gotten (increase disease and health problems).

2. Start consuming large amounts of vegetables and fruits.

Start a 10 day (or longer) detoxification

Consuming large amounts of fresh vegetables and fruits is perhaps the most powerful way to alleviate physical depression. Physical depression is inflammation of the brain. Vegetables and fruits put out this inflammation. Therefore, the challenge is simple - consume nothing but vegetables and fruits for 10 days straight. As we mentioned in chapter three, the average American eats only 1–2 servings of vegetables and fruits per day. To have optimal health, we should be getting about 4-6 servings of vegetables and 2-4 servings of fruits per day. People with chronic disease or health problems may need the nutritional equivalent of 8–30 servings of veggies per day to help restore health! A good rule of thumb is to eat twice as many organic vegetables as fruits. Fruits have many life-giving nutrients that vegetables do not and vice versa, and both are wonderful for detoxifying and cleansing the body.

The immune system needs a whole range of nutrients to remain strong and have the ability to rebuild and defend itself on a daily basis. Vegetables are the most nutrient-dense foods on the planet, which is why we need so many of them. Without them, you can count on being sick more often and will be more susceptible to disease later in life. You may already be asking yourself how you might consume that many servings of vegetables in one day. The answer to this is simple. Instead of eating vegetables, the key to getting the servings you need per day is through juicing.

This 10 day detoxification will cleanse the body of toxins and will also supply you with the nutrients you need in order to be healthy. It's that simple. When people take this on, after the end of 10 days people usually report a whole wide range of benefits including:

- More energy
- Better sleep
- More brain clarity, less brain fog
- Less pain and inflammation
- Less anxiety
- More calm
- Weight loss
- Skin clears
- Feeling more empowered

If you wish to take on this challenge, below is a suggested plan and some tips for helping you have the best experience possible. First things first - be sure to check with your physician to ensure that this would be best for you, knowing that you do so at your own risk.

If your goal is to lose a little more weight, it would be advisable to cut back on fruits and have more vegetables. If you eat more fruit, it is totally ok, but most people would like to see a little more weight loss. If you are already relatively thin and don't wish to lose much weight, eating a good amount of fruit (for calories) would be recommended. Remember, the goal is to detoxify, not lose weight, although losing weight is usually a big benefit for everyone that does this challenge. Some lose more than 10 pounds in 10 days.

It is highly recommended to drink 5 vegetable juices per day and then eat any other raw fruits or steamed vegetables you want throughout the day. If you don't have a juicer, I recommend a Breville. If you don't have a juicer and would still like to have juice, you can use your blender. Cut all the produce into small enough pieces to fit into your blender. Blend produce and dump the contents into a cheesecloth or a nut milk bag and strain. We are after the nutrients, not the insoluble fiber. The vegetable juices contain soluble fiber, so you still will be getting plenty of fiber. **All produce should be organic.**

Sample menu for a day:

1. Breakfast upon waking. Make 16 ounces of raw celery juice (to reboot digestive system). Drink juice immediately after making it. Don't add anything else to it. If you cannot do 16 ounces, try a lesser amount and try to work up to 16 ounces.
2. Make 12 ounces of grapefruit juice about ½ hour after drinking celery juice before you go to work in the morning. Grapefruits are a relatively clean fruit and don't have to be organic. Use a citrus juicer to make this juice.
3. Lunch: Make a juice of celery/cucumber/1 apple. Make 12 ounces. If you can't make this at lunch, make it in the morning and store it in a container in the fridge to keep it cool. Juices are best consumed fresh when possible because enzymes, which are very critical, die quickly after making juice.
4. Dinner: Make a juice of carrot/1 apple, enough for 12 ounces.
5. Dinner (2 hours later – 7-8pm): Make a juice of romaine lettuce/1 apple, enough for 12 ounces.
6. Great vegetables to steam throughout the day are broccoli, asparagus, cauliflower, okra, Brussels sprouts, and green beans. Steam vegetables using a steamer basket for no more than 5 minutes, just enough to warm them up. Use Himalayan salt or organic spices to add flavor.

In between you can eat unlimited amounts of raw or steamed vegetables and fruits. Good health is about balance, so we want to make sure that we include a few important pieces of information. Raw food, especially vegetables and fruits are generally on the thermally cold side of things. So if you feel like you are swinging to the cold side of things, measures can be taken to have more balance. Some of the most warming spices are ginger, garlic, cinnamon, black pepper, nutmeg, and cayenne pepper. Other common warming foods include onion, sweet peppers, raspberry, cherry, blackberry, dates, asparagus, peach, apricot, fennel seed, and basil. Consume thermally warm foods for breakfast or lunch only, not late in the day. Keep in mind that most people in the USA today have some kind of inflammation, which normally presents itself as heat in the body. Adding ginger to celery, cucumber or other juices can balance the thermal quality. Below is a soup recipe which is ingested warm (heated up) and can feel good in the middle of the day.

Hippocrates Soup (www.gerson.org)

Equipment:
Use 4-quart stainless steel pot
Assemble the following vegetables
Cover with pure filtered water

Ingredients:
1 medium celery knob or 3-4 stalks of celery
1 medium parsley root – if available
Garlic as desired
2 small leeks (if not available, replace with 1 medium onion)
1 ½ pounds tomatoes or more
1 medium onion
1 pound of potatoes
A little parsley.
Add Himalayan salt and pepper to taste

Directions:
1. Do not peel any of these special soup vegetables
2. Wash them off
3. Cut them coarsely
4. Simmer them slowly for 2 hours
5. Vary the amount of water used for cooking according to taste and desired consistency.
6. Keep well covered in refrigerator no longer than 2 days
7. Warm up as much as needed each time

Once this soup is made, be sure to warm the soup up on a stove and not in the microwave. Radiating food in the microwave kills the nutrients.

Other possible combinations of juices to have during the day:

1.   Cucumber/1 Apple (in equal amounts)
2.   Carrot/Romaine Lettuce/Apple
3.   Celery/Cucumber/Apple
4.   Celery/Apple
5.   Cucumber/Green Pepper/Apple
6.   One Beet/Beet Leaves/Apple

Raw celery juice has an amazing ability to completely reboot the digestive system and is a juice that is great for healing and detoxifying. The mineral salts in celery help to replenish the body's natural levels of hydrochloric acid. Most people are deficient in this resulting in constipation, low energy, diarrhea, acid reflux, gas and bloating. Celery juice is quite miraculous for balancing out digestion very quickly.

It is suggested that you start this cleanse on a Thursday morning. The reason for this is that days 3-6 of the detoxification can be tough for many people. When the body is getting rid of toxins and you are not getting certain foods that you normally eat, you may get a headache, have lower energy for a few days, and get hunger pains. Usually these symptoms pass away after a few days. It is not the vegetables and fruits causing this, but just your body getting used to these changes. It is much like working out for the first time in 6 months and your body being sore for a few days after the first workout. It doesn't mean you stop working out altogether if you feel sore, but keep going because you know exercise is good for you.

Should I exercise during the detoxification?

It is not advised to do heavy exercising during this detoxification. Brisk walking for a ½ hour 3-5 times per week is all that is needed. If you exercise harder, you may feel a little lightheaded or weak. Be sure to listen to your body. You can also drink as much pure filtered water (Berkey water filters are amazing) as you desire throughout the day. Try to drink water either ½ hour before or after drinking a juice, so as to not dilute juice.

I won't be getting any protein, is that a problem?

Vegetables and fruits do have protein (amino acids). There are 21 amino acids, and all 21 make a complete protein. Vegetables and fruits have amino acids (partial protein), but not all of them. By eating a variety of vegetables and fruits, you will get enough amino acids to make complete proteins. Even if you are not getting enough complete protein, you will be fine for 10 days. Your body may begin to use fat as a source of energy (ketones), which is a good thing, because most of us carry around fat that we would like to burn off.

What should I avoid?

- Avoid all animal products including meats, dairy, and eggs.
- Avoid all diet drinks or anything other than water or fresh made juices.
- Consume no alcohol (it is very hard on the liver).
- Consume no coffee or caffeinated herbal tea. If you normally have more than 1 cup per day, titrate off the coffee slowly in the days/weeks leading up to the detoxification.
- Consume no grains (rice, wheat, bread, pasta, cereals, etc...).
- Consume no soda or sparkling/carbonated water.
- Stay away from trying to sweeten things, even with stevia. Your taste buds will actually change during this time.
- Do not consume any oils, nuts or seeds. They are heavy in fat. Fat is the very hardest thing for your body to digest and we want to give your liver a complete break from fat for 10 days.
- No salad dressings or vinegar either.
- Do not eat avocado or coconut even though they are plant food, they are very high in fat. We want to give the liver a break for 10 days.

What if I don't eat many vegetables or fruits to begin with?

It would be highly suggested that you start juicing at least 2-3 times per day for at least a week or more leading up to the detoxification. You can do this in addition to eating your regular food. If this is not done, you may feel even more of a headache or low energy at the onset and we want this to be as pleasant as possible.

Should I continue taking my medication?

Yes, of course. Unless you are a type 1 diabetic, doing an all vegetable and fruit detoxification is generally very safe. After all, they are the healthiest things you can consume. If you take blood thinning medication, you have to be very careful as well. You can still do the detoxification, but if you consume more green things, you may need to adjust your medication. Again, confer with your doctor before starting the detoxification to ensure your safety.

Here are a few other things to be aware of during a detoxification:

1. If you choose to juice in the morning (HIGHLY suggested), make other juices at the same time (celery, carrot/apple), put them in 16 ounces mason jars and keep chilled. You can then sip on these juices at work throughout the day. You can then juice again when you get home in the evening. Preparation is key!

2. It is so important to be prepared during this time, especially when you go to work. If you don't plan, you will be more susceptible to cheating and giving into cravings. Cut up organic celery, sweet peppers, carrots or other vegetables into plastic containers so that whenever you are hungry you can eat. You can graze and eat all day long, as long as you consume just vegetables or fruits.

3. It is super important to get cruciferous vegetables every day during this detoxification. They are critical in assisting with phase 2 liver detoxification. Cruciferous vegetables include cauliflower, cabbage, Brussels sprouts, bok choy, kale, collard greens, arugula, watercress, turnips and radish. You can include the leafy greens in a vegetable/fruit smoothie or lightly steam in a steamer basket and consume. You can get a metal steamer basket at your local supermarket for less than $10.

4. Take fruits with you to work during the day. Some great ones are organic apples, kiwis, dried black mission figs, papaya, dates, frozen wild blueberries, raisins, grapes, bananas, apricots, or anything else that is fresh or dried organic. If you are already thin, eating more fruits is suggested so that you can have enough calories throughout the course of the day. You will still detoxify just fine. Costco has a wonderful variety of organic produce. In their frozen section, you can find many organic frozen fruits. Wild blueberries are wonderful for detoxifying the liver and are different from regular blueberries. You can get wild blueberries in the frozen section at local supermarkets. Check your local store for such items.

5. Remember, you are eating to detoxify, not necessarily eating for pleasure. It is just 10 days. Challenge yourself, stay with it and you will be glad you did.

6. If you absolutely need to eat outside of the home during this 10 day period of time, many restaurants will be happy to lightly sauté vegetables for you, just tell them to do it with no oil. Use the time to tell others about the 10 day detoxification you are doing rather than feeling left out or like you are missing out on something. It can be something great to talk about.

7. Get your family and friends to do it with you. No better way exists to follow through on something when you have the support of other people that are doing the same things as you are.

8. If you are at least 40 pounds overweight, you can safely do this detoxification for longer than 10 days, even up to 30 days. One gentleman, Joe Cross, was 100 pounds overweight and decided to juice 5 green vegetables juices per day for 60 days. He lost 82 pounds and his chronic autoimmune skin condition (urticaria) completely disappeared. You can watch his documentary called Fat, Sick and Nearly Dead for inspiration. Pay attention to and honor your own body in the process. If you feel like you do need some more protein, add in an organic plant based protein powder to give your body what it needs. We use SP Complete here in the clinic for that purpose. Add in 10-40 grams of protein per day and continue consuming just vegetables and fruits.

9. When coming out of a detoxification, consume things that are more hearty, but don't just jump right into a big steak (lots of fat and protein). Ease into things

with oatmeal, rice, millet, lentils, black beans, a few nuts and seeds and then steadily work up to reintroducing animal meats.

10. You will most likely feel hunger pains during this detoxification. Use a tool such as *The Sedona Method* or *Tapping* to be with and let go of uncomfortable feelings or sensations that may come up for you during this time. Cravings are nothing more than just emotional programs that are coming up. These cravings are just feelings that can be surrendered and let go of.

I have personally seen this 10 day vegetable and fruit detoxification change so many people's lives in a short period of time. I would highly encourage you to try it and see the transformation for yourself.

Start juicing every day

If you do not want to jump into the detoxification and would like to ease into things, I highly suggest making at least 2 – 16 ounce vegetable juices per day. This will only take about 5-10 minutes each day and is one of the most powerful things I have seen that reduces inflammation and helps people to heal very quickly. I would suggest making 16 ounces of celery and 16 ounces of cucumber or 16 ounces of celery and 16 ounces carrot/apple juice every day. A total of 32 ounces of vegetable juice per day can make a wonderful impact on your health.

No more microwaving food

No sensible human being would ever put their body into a human size microwave and turn on the power. Most people are aware of the dangers of radiation, which is why your vital organs are protected while you get x-rays at the dentist office. The radiation of food destroys it. It is better to either warm the food on the stove or in a toaster oven.

3. Eat more raw plant based food.

Nuts/Seeds

Nuts and seeds of all kinds contain protein, fat and many other micro and macro nutrients that support great health. Consider replacing one meal per day where animal products are consumed with a meal that is entirely plant based.

Sprouts

Sprouts of all kinds are a wonderful dietary addition. Many different legumes and beans can be sprouted and consumed. They are very nutrient dense.

Legumes

The most common legumes are kidney beans, black beans, mung beans, lima beans, lentils, and chickpeas. They need to be appropriately soaked in water overnight in order to remove phytic acid. If this is not done, phytic acid can contribute to digestive issues such as gas and bloating.

4. <u>Consume adequate amounts of filtered water each day.</u>

Buy a <u>Berkey water filter</u>

This is the best independently tested water filtration system that is relatively inexpensive, especially if you don't have the resources to install a whole house filtration system. This is better than buying bottled water from the store. Bottled water that has been filtered is fine for consumption, but the sheer amount of plastic that people go through today is staggering. Buy this filter and a 40 ounce stainless steel water bottle and use this to refill throughout the course of the day.

Buy a shower filter or even better a whole house filter

The water that comes from our cities, municipalities and wells has many toxins and chemicals that are toxic to our health. A shower filter can help to protect your skin while your pores are open from toxins in the water.

Avoid pools and hot tubs

Pools and hot tubs have high concentrations of chlorine and bromine, both of which are toxic to our endocrine (hormonal) system.

Alkaline water

I do not recommend buying alkaline water or using a machine to make your water alkaline. I suggest squeezing ½ of a lime or lemon into every 16 ounces of water that is consumed. Lemons and limes are very high on the pH scale and instantly make water alkaline. They are also full of many life-giving nutrients.

5. <u>Body Metal and Chemical Detoxification</u>

The lists below are not exhaustive by any means. Start by questioning all of the things that you ingest, put on your body and smell. Your liver has to process, defend and protect you from all of the toxic things that your body is exposed to. The more you reduce exposure of your body to toxic things, the better you are going to feel.

Personal care products and cosmetics

Remove all personal care cosmetics that are toxic and replace with all organic and/or natural products:

- Shower soap – I personally love Dr. Bronner's products. They have peppermint, baby unscented, almond, lavender, rose, tea tree and citrus body soap. I also use this as a shampoo and shaving cream. It lathers very well.
- Shampoo and Conditioner – Natural Mint with pure essential oils.
- Deodorant – Sky Organics for women and men. You may have to reapply during the course of the day.
- Toothpaste – I personally enjoy Kiss My Face sensitive, others like Dr. Bronners, Periopaste, or Himalaya.
- Mouthwash – Periowash.
- Men's Cologne – Herban Cowboy Dusk (men), Love (women), Sweet Essentials.
- Body Lotion – Dr. Bronners, Ancient Greek Remedy.
- Lip Balm – Sky Organics, Dr. Bronners.
- Hair gel – Herbal Choice Mari Organic.
- Makeup – 100% Pure products – eye cream, mascara, blush, foundation.
- Laundry Detergent – Greenshield Organic. You can also get this at Costco.
- All purpose household cleaner – Natural All Purpose. Or use a combination of hydrogen peroxide and apple cider vinegar.
- Nail Polish – Bontime.

Environmental toxins

Reduce exposure to common household cleaning products, dry cleaning agents, mold, household synthetically scented items, gasoline, car oil, antifreeze, pesticides, herbicides, Febreze, and incense.

If you want to have a house that smells like a million bucks, instead of using those super toxic plugins like Glade, use an essential oil diffuser. Essential oils have been used for thousands of years to help people with all kinds of health problems and ailments. They also smell magnificent. Pick a good diffuser and some essential oils to get you started. Just add water to the diffuser, a few drops of each oil you want and turn the machine on.

Work toxins

Beware of the chemicals, smells and other things that you could come in contact with in your work environment that could contribute to being toxic. Some things to consider are bleaches, ammonia, 409 and other cleaning agents, window cleaner, varnish, degreasers, etc.

6. <u>Supplementation</u>

To alleviate depression, some supplements are critical for healing. I have listed the ones on the top of the list that I find to be the most important and have had the most impact clinically. However, you may find that something else resonates with you better. Follow your own intuition from this list and pick 3-5 supplements to start with.

Omega 3's

I advocate getting these fatty acids from plants rather than through animal products. Oil that comes from flax seeds is very fragile, and many of the flaxseed oil brands on the market are rancid, even though they appear not to be. If you buy oil at the store, consider buying it from the refrigerated section. An even better practice would be to grind 2-3 tablespoons of <u>organic golden flax seeds</u> in a <u>coffee grinder</u> and consume them fresh. <u>Vimergy EPA</u> is another great brand to use. Add them to oatmeal in the morning or to smoothies. Chia seeds, hemp seeds, and walnuts are also fantastic sources of omega 3's. Clinically we also use Hemp Oil Complex from Standard Process (which also contains CBD).

Vitamin D

Vitamin D is a fat soluble vitamin, which the body stores. Anywhere from 5,000IU-10,000IU per day seems to get levels to where they need to be within 1-3 months if people are deficient. A lab test will indicate you are in range between 30 and 100 ng/ml. However, the optimal level I have found for people is 95 ng/ml. <u>Pure Encapsulations</u> is another good brand to use. Even better is trying to be in the sun regularly, especially if you live in a more northern area.

Vitamin C

Vitamin C is one of the safest nutritional supplements to consume. It is needed for iron absorption, all growth and repair of connective tissue/collagen and is useful in high amounts for any bacterial or viral infection. The only side effect if too much is consumed is gas or loose bowels, but most people never reach this level. For those with depression, helpful amounts are between 5,000-10,000mg (5-10 grams) per day.

Since vitamin C is an acid, a buffered form is usually tolerated better from a digestive standpoint. Ester-C is a good buffered brand and so is NOW Calcium Ascorbate Powder. If you want a completely natural source of vitamin C, I would suggest Camu Camu Powder from Terrasoul. It is organic and is a great natural source of this vitamin.

Vitamin B12

One natural substance that is high in B12 and is great for vegetarians and vegans is Hawaiian spirulina. Clinically, we use Cataplex B12, which is a whole food supplement deriving B12 from natural sources. This synergistic product contains intrinsic factors that support the full absorption of B12. Another great form of B-12 is a supplement called Vegansafe B12, which contains two different kinds of B12, making it more useful and absorbable.

Vitamin B3

Niacin can be a very useful vitamin to help someone heal from depression. Clinically we use Niacinamide-B6 from Standard Process, which has worked wonders for some people.

Multivitamin

Clinically we use an organic wholefood multivitamin called Catalyn GF from Standard Process. Other good whole food multivitamins exist on the market as well.

B Complex

Cataplex B GF from Standard Process is a whole food B vitamin supplement that supplies one with a full range of B vitamins. This is not a synthetic vitamin and will not contain thousands of percent of anything. It comes directly from food sources. Pure Encapsulations B Complex Plus is a synthetic version that works well.

SAM-e

A standard dose of SAM-e is 400-800 milligrams per day. Pure Encapsulations offers a good product.

Other Powerful Anti-Inflammatory Supplements

Good State Liquid Zinc Sulfate - wonderfully strengthens the immune system
Pure Encapsulations Calcium/Magnesium - a natural calmative for the central nervous system

7. <u>Start exercising at least 3-5 times per week.</u>

As we discussed earlier in the book, from a Chinese medicine, most depression is a form of stagnation. Stagnation very simply means that something has slowed down and is not moving. The answer is clear – start moving! Exercise is critical for healing from depression. Get out and move and literally shake off the stagnation. Find some kind of movement you love and do it regularly.

8. <u>Get regular acupuncture, chiropractic and massage treatments.</u>

When you are around acupuncturists, chiropractors and massage therapists, you are exposed to the world of natural healing through these practitioners. They can give you access to a world of wonderful information, practices and encouragement to support your healing. Find a practitioner you love and get regular treatments.

9. <u>Try CBD products.</u>

So many people in our world today are seeing such positive effects from the use of this highly medicinal plant. I highly encourage people to try it and see if it makes a difference for you.

CBD oil. In the clinic, we use Hempure Products, which are organically grown and Non-GMO. BEWARE: **Amazon prohibits the sale of CBD on its site.** Even though things may come up in the search results, Amazon does not allow sales of CBD. Only hemp seed oil with no CBD is sold on Amazon, so don't spend your money there if you want to get a CBD product. Hemp seeds/hearts do not contain CBD.

Gummies. These usually taste good, but may contain added sugar and colorings.

Cream and/or Lotion. These are often used externally for muscle soreness or pain.

CBD for pets. It is safe and natural to give to your furry loved ones.

10. <u>Try kratom.</u>

If you are in more pain than anything else, consider using the red strains of kratom. If you want more euphoric and mood lifting effects, consider the white strains. If you want a blend of both, you may consider some of the green strains.

11. <u>Try ayahuasca.</u>

Places around the United States offer weekend retreats where you can consume this substance legally. You can also go to resorts and locations out of the country in such places as Peru, Costa Rica, and Mexico. Be sure to go to a location that has a good reputation and takes good care of the people that attend.

12. <u>Start a regular meditation practice.</u>

I highly recommend the guided meditations of Dr. Jon Kabat Zinn - <u>Series 1</u>, <u>Series 2</u> and <u>Series 3</u>. He also co-authored a book called <u>*The Mindful Way Through Depression*</u>, which also includes guided meditations. Meditation is something that must be consistently done every single day for at least 2 months to experience life transforming effects. Many people have healed from depression after starting a consistent meditation practice.

13. <u>Make your memory list.</u>

Take the time to do this. Set aside 1-3 hours and really be present with the experiences that you have had in your life that have troubled you in the past.

14. <u>Start working through your memory list</u>.

Go through your list memory by memory, especially the memories and emotions that happened when you started getting depressed for the first time. Identify the emotions present in each memory. Tap through each emotion as many times as needed until you feel alleviation of the emotion. Identify any objects, people, sounds, body sensations, or mental pictures that have an emotional charge to them. Take as much time as you need to be with and set free any charge that you sense associated with any of these things.

15. <u>Use tapping everyday as a form of meditative practice.</u>

Each and every day we experience a plethora of negative emotions. Take 15 minutes every day to tap through things that happened to you during that day. You will begin to get insights, awareness and many other things through this practice. Over time with continual daily tapping you will continue to notice more and more positive results.

16. <u>Work with a practitioner.</u>

The wisdom and experience of a competent practitioner can make processing through the past much easier. This person can "hold loving space" by being supportive and encouraging during healing. They can guide you and keep you accountable for making these changes in your life and coaching you through how to work through things emotionally. I highly suggest that you work with someone you trust. I offer appointments over the phone, so even if you are not in the Orlando, Florida area we can still connect and begin to work on your emotional freedom. We can also assess your diet, the supplements you will need to support your healing and so much more. I would be honored to work with you. Please call 407-255-0314 or visit http://www.drscottgraves.com to set up your appointment.

16. <u>General dietary guidelines</u>

In addition to the above items, it is my opinion that our diet can truly help us heal. One book I love on the subject, which is filled with hundreds of healthy recipes, is *Rainbow Green Live Food Cuisine* by Dr. Gabriel Cousens, MD. This book was made specifically for those with diabetes but is still worth its weight in gold with all of the wonderful recipes it contains. Thousands of people have reversed chronic health problems and feel amazing by instituting this type of diet in their lives.

If people are not willing to go full on raw vegan, the paleo diet is seen as another great option that I recommend to people. If we ate one or two meals of the day that were all raw plants, this would make a big difference. But for those that aren't willing to do this, the paleo diet may be right for you. Even though you may not have an autoimmune condition, I recommend *The Autoimmune Paleo Cookbook* by Mickey Trescott and Kyle Johnson. The paleo diet consists of eating moderate amounts of organic animal protein, lots of fresh vegetables and moderate to minimal amounts of fruits, some complex carbohydrates, and fat.

These are the practices that will help you fully heal from depression. All of this requires effort, transformation and personal responsibility. You can heal. I believe in you.

Summary

In my 11 years of torture from depression, I searched endlessly to find a solution to what I felt. I read hundreds of books, changed my diet, spent thousands on counseling and therapy, took antidepressants and thyroid medication and tried many different supplements. I also tried massage, chiropractic, and acupuncture. None of these things helped me that much. I still felt angry, hopeless, apathetic and afraid.

Everyone has a different path to healing and what has been described in the book is just one pathway to healing. I have known people that have healed from depression doing just one or combinations of all of the above things. Additionally, many other things exist not mentioned here that people have done that have helped them heal as well. The above things just seem to be the most common.

People have changed their diets and healed powerfully. They have taken supplements and have balanced their biochemistry and have felt much better. Depression medication has been life-saving for so many people in the midst of their despair. I have put acupuncture needles in people and seen radical changes in people's outlook on life and how they feel. My philosophy is to try anything and everything to help people heal that is safe, makes sense and is affordable.

I have become utterly convinced that letting go of and surrendering emotion is the most powerful form of healing from depression. Surrender addresses the root cause of depression beyond the physical body. Emotions are feelings and feelings are felt in the physical body. They are the signposts expressed through the physical body that point us inward to our rich and deep emotional makeup. We all experience the same emotions. Some of us experience certain emotions more deeply but each person's story is unique and must be uniquely surrendered. We are human beings and within the realm of our being are the states of being that we all experience. Our states of being are our emotions and we were all given the choice to be what we wish to be, to feel the way we wish to feel.

The approach to depression in this book is one that I had searched endlessly to find. In the world of healing from depression, it is by far the road less traveled. I used the understanding of surrender and applied it to my situation specifically.

Surrender can help with any emotion you experience because the process of surrender is the same for any and all emotions. It works for everyone regardless of your previous experiences.

When you are depressed, you take on such an apathetic view of the world, thinking that nothing you do or try is going to change anything. Hopefully this book has brought a spark of hope for you to heal and to feel alive, to know that depression isn't your fault and that you are not to blame, to realize that you can overcome the internal emotional obstacles that have taken over your life, to know that you are not a victim of what you feel and that you can use these tools to surrender and let go of what you feel at any time, and to know that if you muster the courage to face the shadow and darkness that is inside of you, that the light of love, joy, and divinity can radically change you.

Everyone in this world just wants to feel good. We are programmed to avoid pain and pursue pleasure. Most people don't walk straight into their darkness, shadow, pain and negative emotions because they believe it would just simply make them feel worse. Many patients have said to me that they are so afraid that if they allowed themselves to feel what they have buried inside it would totally consume them. It would be like falling back into a pit and never being able to escape. And for many, this is their truth. However, this doesn't have to be true for you.

Healing from depression appears to be very counterintuitive. The irony is that walking straight into and allowing yourself to fully feel what has caused you pain, combined *with* the intention of surrendering and letting go of the feelings and emotions you have, is the very pathway to freedom, feeling good and to love itself. I have observed that the majority of people just simply feel their pain, not knowing that surrender and that love can be fully experienced on the other side of surrender.

Do you want to experience the fullness of the love that you already are? Do you want to truly experience joy and peace? All you have to do is let go of and surrender any feeling and experience that is not love. And when you surrender anything that is not love, love is the only thing that will remain and shine forth as the reality of all of life. God is everything, and therefore love is everything. Love is what you already are. It is your birthright to claim it as your reality.

Truth and freedom are simple. The only thing that makes it hard is our own conditioned mind. The mind likes to make everything so difficult and complicated. Surrender is the pathway. The process of identifying, feeling and surrendering may be the most arduous thing you venture into. It may require every ounce of courage that you can muster. If you are truly ready to surrender, then God will meet you there and will accompany you through all the pain. He wants you to heal. He wants you to have an abundant life.

Dealing with the emotions I held onto from the past was undoubtedly the hardest thing I have ever done. I wouldn't wish that kind of pain on anyone. This pain does exist in all of us, whether we are aware of it or not. Freedom is always waiting for us, just over the mountain of our pain. Walk the pathway, surrender and step into the fullness of who and what you are. In the meantime, all you may have to go on is faith and trust. That is all I had when I began this journey, and I'm sure glad I followed faith and trust into surrender.

After I processed through the memories of being stung at the age of 4 and abandoned by God at age 21, I no longer felt depressed. The depression was gone, and it hasn't returned. Every experience, person, object is an opportunity to see our inner reflection. They are the mechanism which God has built into the fabric of the world so that we can see our reflection or shadow, let go of negative emotions, grow, evolve and be more like Him: full of love, joy, and peace.

May you be free from the depression that has plagued you for so long. May you find what you are looking for that restores balance to your life. May faith and trust guide you into wholeness and healing. May you step into your darkness to allow the Truth of love to set you free. May you become the love and joy that you already are.

1 https://jamanetwork.com/journals/jamainternalmedicine/fullarticle/2592697

2 R. Mojtabai and M. Olfson, "Proportion of Antidepressants Prescribed without a Psychiatric Diagnosis Is Growing," Health Affairs (Millwood) 30, no. 8 (August 2011): 1434-42. Doi: 10.137/hlthaff.2010.1024

3 American Psychiatric Association. (2013). Diagnostic and statistical manual of mental disorders (5th ed.). Washington, DC: Author.

4 https://www.webmd.com/depression/guide/causes-depression#1

5 https://www.mayoclinic.org/diseases-conditions/depression/symptoms-causes/syc-20356007

6 https://www.nimh.nih.gov/health/publications/depression/index.shtml#pub4

7 Hawkins, D. (2012). Letting Go: The Pathway of Surrender. Carlsbad, CA: Hay House, Inc.

8 https://www.merriam-webster.com/dictionary/mindfulness

9 E.Castren, "Is Mood Chemistry?" Nat Rev Neurosci 6, no. 3 (March 2005): 241-46.

10 "Fluoxetine Hydrochloride". The American Society of Health-System Pharmacists. Archived from the original on 8 December 2015. Retrieved 2 December 2015.

11 Volpi-Abadie, J.; Kaye, A. M.; Kaye, A. D. (2013). "Serotonin syndrome". The Ochsner journal. 13 (4): 533–40. PMC 3865832. PMID 24358002.

12 FDA. May 2, 2007. Antidepressant Use in Children, Adolescents, and Adults. Archived 6 January 2016 at the Wayback Machine.

13 Brogan, K. A Mind of Your Own. New York, NY: Harper Wave. 2016.

14 https://www.ncbi.nlm.nih.gov/pmc/articles/PMC4172306/

15 G. Chouinard and V. A. Chouinard, "New Classification of Selective Reuptake Inhibitor Withdrawal," Psychother Psychosom 84, no. 2 (February 21, 2015): 63-71

16 Williams, R. Nutrition Against Disease (New York: Pitman, 1971), 11.

17 Lipton, B. The Wisdom of Your Cells: How Your Beliefs Control Your Biology. Louisville, CO: Sounds True. 2006.

18 https://www.cdc.gov/heartdisease/facts.htm

19 Campbell, T. Colin. The China Study. Dallas, TX: BenBella Books Inc. 2016.

20 https://www.ncbi.nlm.nih.gov/pubmed/9860369

21 Esselstyn, C. Prevent and Reverse Heart Disease. New York, NY: Penguin Group, Inc. 2007.

22 Cousens, G. There is a Cure for Diabetes. Berkeley, CA: North Atlantic Books. 2013.

23 Bestrashniy, J., Winters KC. Variability in medical marijuana laws in the United States. Psychol Addict Behav. 2015;29:639–642

[24] https://www.ncbi.nlm.nih.gov/pmc/articles/PMC3079847/

[25] https://www.ncbi.nlm.nih.gov/pmc/articles/PMC2823358/

[26] https://www.cdc.gov/drugoverdose/data/statedeaths.html

[27] https://www.fda.gov/drugs/drug-interactions-labeling/preventable-adverse-drug-reactions-focus-drug-interactions

[28] https://www.ncbi.nlm.nih.gov/pubmed/21918508

[29] https://www.ncbi.nlm.nih.gov/pmc/articles/PMC3846682/

[30] https://www.ncbi.nlm.nih.gov/pubmed/19188531

[31] https://www.ncbi.nlm.nih.gov/pmc/articles/PMC3903110/

[32] https://www.ncbi.nlm.nih.gov/pubmed/23639523

[33] Agency for Toxic Substances and Disease Registry (August 2007). "ToxFAQs™ for Lead". Center for Disease Control.

[34] www.safecosmetics.org

[35] https://www.huffingtonpost.com/2012/03/12/lead-emissions-children-aviation-fuel_n_1338131.html

[36] https://www.nytimes.com/2008/10/07/business/media/07adco.html

[37] Lear, Linda (1 April 2009). Rachel Carson: Witness for Nature. Mariner Books. ISBN 978-0-547-23823-4.)

[38] Bellon, Tina. "Jury orders J&J to pay $4.7 billion in Missouri asbestos cancer case". U.S. Retrieved 2018-07-13.

[39] http://www.cnn.com/2010/HEALTH/10/26/senate.toxic.america.hearing/index.html

[40] https://ehp.niehs.nih.gov/doi/10.1289/ehp.1307455

[41] https://www.theledger.com/news/20171021/cancer-more-deadly-to-firefighters-than-flames-heart-attacks

[42] https://www.ncbi.nlm.nih.gov/pmc/articles/PMC3238331/?tool=pubmed

[43] https://medlineplus.gov/magazine/issues/summer11/articles/summer11pg6-8.html/

[44] http://www.healthandenvironment.org/partnership_calls/18271

[45] http://pmep.cce.cornell.edu/profiles/extoxnet/metiram-propoxur/parathion-ext.html

[46] "Final report on the safety assessment of sodium laureth sulfate and ammonium laureth sulfate". Journal of the American College of Toxicology. 2 (5): 1–34. 1983.

[47] https://www.ncbi.nlm.nih.gov/pmc/articles/PMC4651417/

[48] https://www.ncbi.nlm.nih.gov/pubmed/18627690

[49] EPA (U.S. Environmental Protection Agency). 2008. Integrated Risk Information System (IRIS). Evidence for human carcinogenicity based on 1986-2005 guidelines.

[50] https://pubchem.ncbi.nlm.nih.gov/compound/311#section=GHS-Classification

[51] J Elberling, P. S. Skov, H. Mosbech, H. Holst, A. Dirksen & J. D. Johansen. 2007. Increased release of histamine in patients with respiratory symptoms related to perfume. Clinical and experimental allergy. Journal of the British Society for Allergy and Clinical Immunology 37(11), 1676-80.)

[52] https://pubchem.ncbi.nlm.nih.gov/compound/6049#section=GHS-Classification

[53] https://pubchem.ncbi.nlm.nih.gov/compound/benzyl_salicylate#section=GHS-Classification

[54] https://pubchem.ncbi.nlm.nih.gov/compound/Lilial#section=Safety-and-Hazards

[55] https://pubchem.ncbi.nlm.nih.gov/compound/5372174#section=Safety-and-Hazards

[56] Chang MW, Nakrani R. 2014. Six children with allergic contact dermatitis to methylisothiazolinone in wet wipes (baby wipes). Pediatrics. 133(2):e434-8.

[57] Burnett CL, Bergfeld WF, et al. 2010. Final report of the safety assessment of methylisothiazolinone. Int J Toxicol. 29(4 Suppl):187S-213S.

[58] https://www.ncbi.nlm.nih.gov/pmc/articles/PMC3238331/?tool=pubmed

[59] https://www.npr.org/2018/08/10/637722786/jury-awards-terminally-ill-man-289-million-in-lawsuit-against-monsanto

[60] https://www.nature.com/news/widely-used-herbicide-linked-to-cancer-1

[61] https://www.ers.usda.gov/data-products/adoption-of-genetically-engineered-crops-in-the-us/recent-trends-in-ge-adoption.aspx

[62] https://www.thelancet.com/journals/lancet/article/PIIS0140-6736(09)60254-3/fulltext

[63] https://enveurope.springeropen.com/articles/10.1186/2190-4715-23-10

[64] https://en.wikipedia.org/wiki/Flour_bleaching_agent

[65] https://onlinelibrary.wiley.com/doi/full/10.1111/apt.12730

[66] Ross, J. The Mood Cure. New York, NY: Penguin Group, Inc. 2002. P. 126

[67] Morrison, J. Cleanse Your Body, Clear Your Mind. New York, NY: Penguin Group, Inc. 2011.

[68] https://www.stopogm.net/sites/stopogm.net/files/EvidenceBenbrook.pdf

[69] Elmore, RW, FW Roeth, LA Nelson, CA Shapiro, RN Klein, SZ Knezevic, A Martin. "Glyphosate-resistant soybean cultivar yields compared with sister lines." Agronomy Journal 93.2 (2001): 408-412. Web. 5 Jan. 2019.

[70] https://www.reuters.com/article/monsanto-investigation-idUSN2515475920100625

[71] https://www.bloomberg.com/news/articles/2014-07-03/gmo-factory-monsantos-high-tech-plans-to-feed-the-world

[72] https://www.nytimes.com/2016/10/30/business/gmo-promise-falls-short.html

[73] Appleton, N. Suicide by Sugar. Garden City Park, NY: Square One Publishers.

2009.

[74] https://link.springer.com/referenceworkentry/10.1007%2F978-1-4419-9863-7_703

[75] https://www.ncbi.nlm.nih.gov/pubmed/28109280

[76] https://www.ncbi.nlm.nih.gov/pmc/articles/PMC4856550/

[77] https://www.ncbi.nlm.nih.gov/pubmed/17921406

[78] https://www.ncbi.nlm.nih.gov/pubmed/24743309

[79] https://www.ncbi.nlm.nih.gov/pubmed/28751637/

[80] https://www.ncbi.nlm.nih.gov/pubmed/26109579

[81] https://www.ncbi.nlm.nih.gov/pmc/articles/PMC4551584/

[82] https://www.ncbi.nlm.nih.gov/pubmed/23633524

[83] https://www.ncbi.nlm.nih.gov/pubmed/18800291

[84] https://www.ncbi.nlm.nih.gov/pmc/articles/PMC2892765/

[85] https://www.ncbi.nlm.nih.gov/pubmed/23364017

[86] https://www.ncbi.nlm.nih.gov/pmc/articles/PMC3497928/

[87] https://www.ncbi.nlm.nih.gov/pubmed/7936222

[88] https://www.ncbi.nlm.nih.gov/pubmed/7614911

[89] http://journals.sfu.ca/africanem/index.php/ajtcam/article/view/4861

[90] https://www.ncbi.nlm.nih.gov/pubmed/24443063

[91] Hill, D.J., et al., "A study of 100 infants and young children with cow's milk allergy," 2 Clinical Reviews in Allergy (1984):125

[92] https://www.ncbi.nlm.nih.gov/pmc/articles/PMC3166669/

[93] Ireland, Corydon, "Hormones in milk can be dangerous," Harvard University Gazette, De. 8, 2006.

[94] USDA, Animal and Plant Health Inspection Service, National Animal Health Monitoring System, Aug. 2004; Dairy 2002, Animal Disease Exclusion Practices on US Dairy Operations, 2002

[95] https://www.newsweek.com/end-antibiotics-185984

[96] https://jamanetwork.com/journals/jamapediatrics/fullarticle/1149502

[97] https://www.webmd.com/ovarian-cancer/news/20000505/milk-ovarian-cancer-risk#1

[98] https://link.springer.com/article/10.1023/A:1008823601897

[99] https://www.ncbi.nlm.nih.gov/pmc/articles/PMC1615057/

[100] https://www.smh.com.au/lifestyle/health-and-wellness/food-with-bad-fats-linked-to-depression-study-finds-20110127-1a6vy.html

[101] https://www.nytimes.com/2007/03/07/dining/07tran.html

[102] https://foodandnutritionresearch.net/index.php/fnr/article/view/413

[103] https://www.ncbi.nlm.nih.gov/pmc/articles/PMC3777290/

[104] http://www.coffeehabitat.com/2006/12/pesticides_used_2/

[105] https://www.ncbi.nlm.nih.gov/pubmed/24761264

[106] https://health.gov/dietaryguidelines/2015/guidelines/appendix-3/

[107] https://www.cdc.gov/mmwr/volumes/66/wr/mm6645a1.htm

[108] https://www.ncbi.nlm.nih.gov/pubmed/11162324

[109] https://www.ncbi.nlm.nih.gov/pmc/articles/PMC3093095/

[110] https://www.ncbi.nlm.nih.gov/pubmed/19880930

[111] https://www.ncbi.nlm.nih.gov/pubmed/16988131

[112] https://www.cdc.gov/nchs/data/databriefs/db61.pdf

[113] Jaret, P., 1998. Are nutraceuticals any good? Hippocrates, 62:63-67

[114] https://www.ncbi.nlm.nih.gov/pubmed/17209208

[115] https://www.ncbi.nlm.nih.gov/pubmed/12936943

[116] https://www.ncbi.nlm.nih.gov/pubmed/18208598

[117] https://lpi.oregonstate.edu/mic/vitamins/vitamin-C

[118] https://www.ncbi.nlm.nih.gov/books/NBK121338/

[119] Chatterjee, I. B., A. K. Majumder, B. K. Nandi, and N. Subramanian. "Synthesis And Some Major Functions Of Vitamin C In Animals." Annals of the New York Academy of Sciences 258.1 Second Confer (1975): 24-47.

[120] Sullivan SS, Rosen CJ, Halteman WA, Chen TC, Holick MF: Adolescent girls in Maine at risk for vitamin D insufficiency. J Am Diet Assoc. 2005, 105: 971-974. 10.1016/j.jada.2005.03.002.

[121] https://www.ncbi.nlm.nih.gov/pubmed/17344510

[122] https://www.ncbi.nlm.nih.gov/pmc/articles/PMC2629072/

[123] https://www.bones.nih.gov/health-info/bone/osteoporosis/overview

[124] https://www.fabresearch.org/viewItem.php?id=8012

[125] https://www.cambridge.org/core/journals/nutrition-research-reviews/article/impact-of-longchain-n3-polyunsaturated-fatty-acids-on-human-health/6C6A8548DD8FCAC300854623CB9C21A2

[126] https://www.ncbi.nlm.nih.gov/pmc/articles/PMC3257695/

[127] https://www.webmd.com/food-recipes/news/20040908/omega-3-fatty-acids-get-new-health-claim#1

[128] Alardi, Stephen. The Depression Cure. Cambrige, MA: Da Capo Press. 2009. P.76.

[129] https://www.sciencedirect.com/science/article/pii/S0163834308000741?via%3Dihub

[130] https://neuro.psychiatryonline.org/doi/abs/10.1176/appi.neuropsych.11020052

[131] https://www.ncbi.nlm.nih.gov/pubmed/25644193

[132] https://academic.oup.com/ajcn/article/71/2/514/4729184

[133] https://www.ncbi.nlm.nih.gov/pubmed/10967371/

[134] https://www.ncbi.nlm.nih.gov/pubmed/16938502

[135] https://www.ncbi.nlm.nih.gov/pmc/articles/PMC2738337/

[136] https://archive.ahrq.gov/clinic/tp/sametp.htm

[137] Benjamin J., et al. Psychopharmacol Bull 31(1): 167-75, 1995.

[138] https://www.ncbi.nlm.nih.gov/pubmed/20561558

[139] https://www.ncbi.nlm.nih.gov/pmc/articles/PMC2738337/

[140] http://www.bourre.fr/pdf/publications_scientifiques/259.pdf

[141] https://www.ncbi.nlm.nih.gov/pmc/articles/PMC3757551/

[142] https://www.ncbi.nlm.nih.gov/pmc/articles/PMC2895281/

[143] https://jamanetwork.com/journals/jama/article-abstract/1881295

[144] https://www.cbsnews.com/news/cdc-80-percent-of-american-adults-dont-get-recommended-exercise/

[145] https://www.ncbi.nlm.nih.gov/pubmed/11836274

[146] http://fluoridation.com/atomicbomb.htm

[147] https://media.utoronto.ca/media-releases/moderate-exercise-not-only-treats-but-prevents-depression/

[148] https://www.sciencedirect.com/science/article/pii/S0749379713004510

[149] Van der Kolk, B. The Body Keeps the Score: Brain, Mind and Body in the Healing of Trauma. New York, NY: Penguin Group, Inc. 2014.

[150] Frankl, V. Man's Search for Meaning. Boston, MA: Beacon Press. 1959.

[151] http://www.klinghardtacademy.com/5-Levels-of-Healing/

[152] Maciocia, G. The Practice of Chinese Medicine. Philadelphia, PA: Elsevier. 1994.

[153] Segal, I. The Secret Language of Your Body. New York, NY: Simon & Shuster, Inc. 2010.

[154] Segal, I. The Secret Language of Your Body. New York, NY: Simon & Shuster, Inc. 2010.

[155] Van der Kolk, B. The Body Keeps the Score: Brain, Mind and Body in the Healing of Trauma. New York, NY: Penguin Group, Inc. 2014.

[156] Kendall, D. The Dao of Chinese Medicine. Oxford, NY: Oxford University Press. 2002.

[157] Keown, D. The Spark in the Machine. London, UK: Singing Dragon. 2014.

[158] Maciocia, G. The Practice of Chinese Medicine. Philadelphia, PA: Elsevier. 1994.

[159] The Holy Bible – New International Version. Psalm 46:10.

[160] Unschild, P., Tessenow, H. Huang Di Nei Jin Su Wen. Los Angeles, CA: University of California Press. 2011.

[161] Roth, Harold. Original Dao: Inward Training. New York, NY: Columbia University Press. 1999.

[162] Huang-Fu, M. The Systematic Classic of Acupuncture and Moxibustion. Boulder, CO: Blue Poppy Press. 1993

[163] William, A. Thyroid Healing. Carlsbad, CA: Hay House Inc. 2017.

[164] Wentz, I. Hashimoto's Thyroiditis. Wentz LLC. 2013.

[165] Maciocia, G. The Practice of Chinese Medicine. Philadelphia, PA: Elsevier. 1994. P. 336.

[166] Zinn, J. Full Catastrophe Living. New York, NY: Random House. 1990.

[167] https://www.brainsync.com/

168   Pahnke WN. (1966). "Drugs and mysticism". International Journal of Parapsychology. 8 (2): 295–315.

169   Smith H. (2000). Cleansing the Doors of Perception: The Religious Significance of Entheogenic Plants and Chemicals. New York, New York: Jeremy P. Tarcher/Putnam. p. 101.

170   Doblin R. (1991). "Pahnke's "Good Friday Experiment": a long-term follow-up and methodological critique." Journal of Transpersonal Psychology. 23 (1): 1–25.

171   https://www.ncbi.nlm.nih.gov/pmc/articles/PMC3412011/

172   Griffiths RR, Richards WA, McCann U, Jesse R (2006). "Psilocybin can occasion mystical-type experiences having substantial and sustained personal meaning and spiritual significance" (PDF). Psychopharmacology. 187 (3): 268–83.

173   https://hub.jhu.edu/2016/12/01/hallucinogen-treats-cancer-depression-anxiety/

174   https://journals.sagepub.com/doi/full/10.1177/0269881116675512

175   https://www.ncbi.nlm.nih.gov/pubmed/25575620?dopt=Abstract&holding=npg

176   Fadiman, J. The Psychedelic Explorers Guidebook. Rochester, VT: Park Street Press.

177

https://www.sciencedirect.com/science/article/pii/S0376871617305586?via%3Dihub

178   https://www.forbes.com/sites/daviddisalvo/2016/09/13/what-the-deas-plan-to-schedule-1-kratom-will-mean-for-millions

179   Thie, J. Touch For Health. Los Angeles, CA: Devorss Press. 2012. P.21.

180   Thie, J. Touch For Health. Los Angeles, CA: Devorss Press. 2012. P.21.

181   Hawkins, D. Reality, Spirituality and Modern Man. Sedona, AZ: Veritas Press. 2008. P. 168.

182   Hawkins, D. I: Reality and Subjectivity. Sedona, AZ: Veritas Press. 2001. P. 43.

183   Diamond, J. Your Body Doesn't Lie. New York, NY: Warner Books, Inc. 1989.

184   Holub, A., Budd-Micheals, E. Psychokinesiology. Carson City, NV: Bridger House Publishers, Inc. 1999. P. 106.

185   Veltheim, J. The Science and Philosophy of Body Talk. 2013.

186   Eden, D. Energy Medicine. New York, NY: Penguin Group, Inc. 1998. p. 51

187   Yuen, K. Instant Pain Elimination. CEM Publishers. 2003.

188   Thie, J. Touch For Health. Los Angeles, CA: Devorss Press. 2012. P.23

189   Nelson, B. The Emotion Code. Mesquite, NV. Wellness Unmasked Publishing. 2007

190   Clarke, A. Profiles of the Future. New York, NY: Henry Holt & Co. 1984.

191   Hawkins, D. Power Vs. Force. Carlsbad, CA: Hay House. P. 305.

192   https://en.wikipedia.org/wiki/Bell%27s_theorem

[193] Callahan, R. Tapping the Healer Within. New York, NY: McGraw-Hill. 2001.

[194] Hay, L. You Can Heal Your Life. Carlsbad, CA: Hay House Inc. 1984.

[195] Hawkins, D. Healing and Recovery. Sedona, AZ: Veritas Press. 2012.

[196] Lipton, B. The Wisdom of Your Cells: How Your Beliefs Control Your Biology. Louisville, CO: Sounds True. 2006.

[197] Goleman, D. Emotional Intelligence. New York, NY. Random House. 2005

[198] Ortner, Nicolas. The Tapping Solution. Carlsbad, CA: Hay House, Inc. 2013.

[199] Dwoskin, Hale. The Sedona Method. Sedona, AZ. Sedona Press. 2007.

[200] Hawkins, D. Letting Go: The Pathway of Surrender. Carlsbad, CA: Hay House, Inc. 2012. P. 30.

[201] Van der Kolk, B. The Body Keeps the Score: Brain, Mind and Body in the Healing of Trauma. New York, NY: Penguin Group, Inc. 2014.

[202] Napier, A., Whitaker, C. The Family Crucible. New Youk, NY: Harper and Row. 2017.

[203] Kubler-Ross, E. On Grief & Grieving. New York, NY: Scribner. 2005.

[204] The Holy Bible – New International Version. Hebrews 13:5.

[205] Hawkins, D. Healing and Recovery. Sedona, AZ: Veritas Press. 2012

[206] Hawkins, D. Transcending The Levels of Consciousness. Sedona, AZ: Veritas Press. 2006. P.138.

[207] Van der Kolk, B. The Body Keeps the Score: Brain, Mind and Body in the Healing of Trauma. New York, NY: Penguin Group, Inc. 2014.

[208] Dwoskin, Hale. The Sedona Method. Sedona, AZ. Sedona Press. 2007.

[209] Hawkins, D. Letting Go: The Pathway of Surrender. Carlsbad, CA: Hay House, Inc. 2012.

[210] The Holy Bible – New International Version. James 1:5.

[211] Lynch, M. Tapping Into Wealth. New York, NY: Penguin Group, Inc. 2013.

[212] The Holy Bible – New International Version. Psalm 46:10.

[213] Segal, I. The Secret Language of Your Body. New York, NY: Simon & Shuster, Inc. 2010.

[214] Boorstein, S. Happiness in an Inside Job. New York, NY: Ballantine Books. 2008.

[215] The Holy Bible – New International Version. Romans 8:28.

[216] https://en.wikipedia.org/wiki/Pareto_principle